Looking Inside the Disordered Brain

Looking Inside
the Disordered Brain

An Introduction to the Functional
Neuroanatomy of Psychopathology

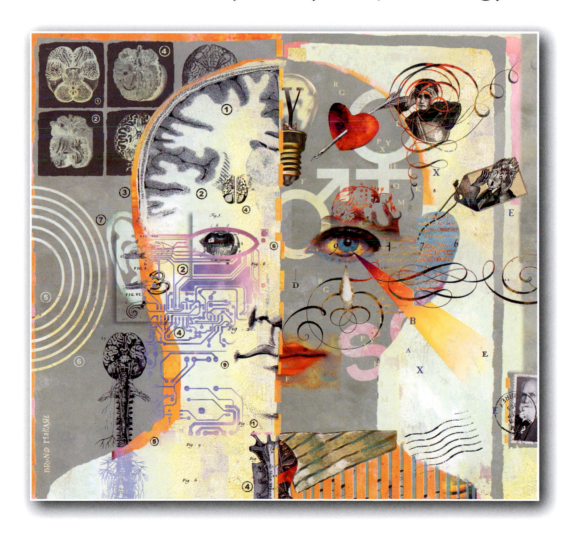

Ahmad R. Hariri

Duke University

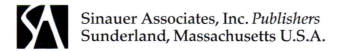

Sinauer Associates, Inc. *Publishers*
Sunderland, Massachusetts U.S.A.

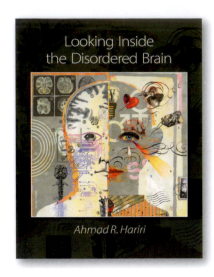

About the Cover Artist

"Head with Symbols" is an original work by **Bruno Mallart**, a talented European artist whose work has appeared in many of the world's premier publications, including *The New York Times*, *The Wall Street Journal*, and *New Scientist*. A freelance illustrator since 1986, Mallart first worked for several children's book publishers and advertising agencies using a classic, realistic watercolor and ink style. Later he began working in a more imaginative way, inventing a unique mix of drawing, painting, and collage. Attracted to all things mechanical, Mallart's work frequently incorporates machine parts such as gears and wheels that suggest movement, action, and functional networks.

Despite the recurring use of the brain in his art, Mallart's background is not scientific (although both his parents were neuroscientists). He uses the brain as a symbol for abstract concepts such as intelligence, thoughts, feelings, and ideas. To see more of Bruno Mallart's art, please visit his website: www.brunomallart.com.

Looking Inside the Disordered Brain: An Introduction to the Functional Neuroanatomy of Psychopathology

Sinauer Associates, Inc.
P.O. Box 407
Sunderland, MA. 01375 U.S.A.

www.sinauer.com
Fax: 413-549-1118
orders@sinauer.com
publish@sinauer.com

Library of Congress Cataloging-in-Publication Data

Hariri, Ahmad R., 1972, author.
 Looking inside the disordered brain : an introduction to the functional neuroanatomy of psychopathology / Ahmad R. Hariri.
      p. ; cm.
 Includes bibliographical references and index.
 ISBN 978-0-87893-979-4
 I. Title.
 [DNLM: 1. Brain--anatomy & histology. 2. Brain--pathology. 3. Mental Disorders--pathology. 4. Neural Pathways. 5. Neuroanatomy--methods. 6. Neurons. WL 300]
 QP376
 612.8'2--dc23   2014038465

Printed in China
5 4 3 2 1

For AB and The Js, Love A

Brief Contents

Contents

UNIT I The Corticolimbic Circuit for Recognition and Reaction

4

The Corticolimbic Circuit

Disorder   55

UNIT II The Corticostriatal Circuit for Motivation and Action

5 *The Corticostriatal Circuit*
Anatomy   93

UNIT III
The Corticohippocampal Circuit for Memory and Executive Control

8 *The Corticohippocampal Circuit*
Anatomy   151

Media and Supplements to accompany
Looking Inside the Disordered Brain

eBook

Looking Inside the Disordered Brain is available as an eBook, in several different formats, including VitalSource CourseSmart, Yuzu, and BryteWave. The eBook can be purchased as either a 180-day rental or as a permanent (non-expiring) subscription. All major mobile devices are supported. For details on the eBook platforms offered, please visit www.sinauer.com/ebooks.

Instructor's Resource Library

(Available to qualified adopters)
The Instructor's Resource Library includes a collection of visual resources from the textbook for use in preparing lectures and other course materials. All textbook figures and tables are included in both JPEG (both high- and low-resolution) and PowerPoint formats. Figures have all been sized and formatted for optimal legibility when projected.

Read Me First!

This textbook has its origins in an advanced undergraduate course on the functional neuroanatomy of psychopathology I have taught annually since 2011 at Duke University. In addition to its place in the undergraduate curriculum, my course also functions to fulfill the biological basis of behavior requirement for our doctoral program in clinical psychology. In my experience, the undergraduate and graduate students who thrive in my course are those who have already successfully completed coursework in *both* abnormal psychology and the biological basis of behavior. However, the textbook, like my course, is designed to allow students from either background to navigate the material. Those lacking a foundation in abnormal psychology will find brief introductions to major psychopathological conditions, while those lacking a background in neuroscience will find descriptions of basic principles of neuroanatomy and neurophysiology.

It is important to note, however, that this book's coverage of these foundational topics is not intended to supplant that provided by rigorous coursework. For maximum benefit students are strongly encouraged to have completed formal coursework in both abnormal psychology and the biological basis of behavior prior to tackling the material presented here.

Style

I adopt a narrative style that is unusual in textbooks. I do so because it provides the freedom to link and build upward—from brain to behavior to psychopathology. The narrative style also allows me to use my experience and knowledge to reconcile a rapidly changing and often conflicting landscape of basic research findings. Using a functional circuit approach, I hope to provide students with an introduction to dominant themes in the study of brain, behavior, and mental illness. These themes, of course, are based on a wealth of primary research, and the text and illustrations have attempted to present this research in an accessible form that focuses not on the experimental details but on the crucially important concepts that are emerging. Thus, the text should be viewed as a jumping-off point for advanced study. It provides a selective focus on key behavioral processes supported by each of three foundational circuits, but is not meant to serve as a comprehensive summary of all the behaviors with which each circuit has been associated.

Spotlighting Research

Similarly, the textbook does not provide a comprehensive overview of neuroscience research in psychopathology. Rather, it focuses on topics for which there is a critical mass of data linking psychopathology with disorder in circuit function. Thus, instructors and students alike are encouraged, even urged, to continually augment the material presented in the textbook with the rapidly developing evidence base provided by empirical reports. To this end, a list of select references and additional readings, largely comprised of primary research papers and empirical studies, is provided at the conclusion of each chapter. Moreover, a handful of particularly important and novel research that has illuminated our understanding of neural circuit anatomy, function, and dysfunction will be considered in detail throughout the textbook using the *Research Spotlight*, which provides details regarding the investigators, key methods, and findings of particularly noteworthy studies.

Acknowledgments

Literally hundreds of colleagues, trainees, and students have contributed in some way to my own study of the brain and behavior. I am uniquely indebted, however, to three individuals who not only launched my career in neuroscience, but also inspired me to share my knowledge through this book.

Professor Susan Bookheimer at the University of California Los Angeles supervised my doctoral training and introduced me to the unique value of fMRI for studying both normal and abnormal behavior. She also taught me the importance of nurturing the independent interests of young scholars and always enjoying the work.

Professor Arnold Scheibel, now retired from the University of California Los Angeles, was the first to take me inside the human brain and impress upon me its endless wonders and beauty. His graduate neuroanatomy course and accompanying textbook, *The Human Brain Coloring Book*, showed me how much fun it can be to learn about the brain, and how this knowledge illuminates what makes each of us unique and individual.

Professor Daniel Weinberger at the Leiber Institute for Brain Development was my postdoctoral mentor at the National Institute of Mental Health. His pioneering research illustrates how the synthesis of otherwise far-flung disciplines can produce transformative discoveries into the nature of mental illness.

To these three scholars, mentors, and friends I owe more than I can fairly describe, and I hope they will find evidence of their lasting impact within the pages of this textbook.

1 Getting Inside and Getting Around

This book adopts a circuit-based approach to understanding how the brain creates ordered perceptions of our world and translates these perceptions into ordered behaviors that allow us to overcome challenges, maximize opportunities, and adapt to change in our environment. We will also discuss how disorder within circuits emerges as abnormalities in these same processes of perception and behavior—what we call psychopathology. Although such a circuit-based approach to brain, behavior, and psychopathology may be relatively novel in an introductory textbook, it is emerging as the dominant research model in neuroscience, psychology, and psychiatry.

Foundational Circuits

A **neural circuit** represents widely distributed yet highly interconnected brain regions or nodes that function in concert to support the orderly processing of information. The structured processing or flow of information within a circuit ultimately generates specific forms of behavioral and physiological responses that help us overcome challenges, maximize opportunities, and adapt to changing circumstances. Likewise, disorder within a neural circuit emerges as specific forms of dysfunctional behavioral and physiological responses that render a person incapable of successfully overcoming challenges, maximizing opportunities, and adapting to change.

Three aspects of three circuits

Using this circuit-based approach, the textbook is divided into three units representing three foundational neural circuits: the corticolimbic, corticostriatal, and corticohippocampal. The presentation incorporates three aspects for each circuit: anatomy (the brain), ordered information processing (behavior), and abnormal or disordered information processing (psychopathology).

- *Anatomy:* Within each unit, the first chapter describes the anatomy of interconnected **circuit nodes** centered on a **hub** structure. We emphasize hub structures—the amygdala, ventral striatum, and dorsolateral prefrontal cortex, respectively—because they coordinate information processing in each of the three circuits.
- *Order:* The second chapter of each unit describes how that circuit supports adaptive behaviors necessary for our successful functioning in the face of a demanding and dynamic world. We describe how the

neural circuit Interconnected brain structures or nodes that together function to process information to generate a discrete set of behavioral and physiological responses necessary for survival.

circuit node Distinct brain structure responsible for a specific aspect of processing information or generating responses within a functional circuit.

hub Circuit node with unique connections that allow it to coordinate the processing or flow of information throughout the rest of a functional circuit.

bilateral symmetry Existence of the same general shape, size, and connections for structures found in both the right and left hemispheres.

ipsilateral Connections between circuit nodes within the same hemisphere (i.e., same side).

contralateral Circuit node connections between the left and right hemispheres (i.e., opposite sides).

upstream As used here, circuit nodes that send information to a circuit hub.

downstream As used here, circuit nodes that receive information from a circuit hub.

corticolimbic circuit supports *recognition* and *reaction*, the corticostriatal circuit supports *motivation* and *action*, and the corticohippocampal circuit supports *memory* and *executive control*.

- *Disorder:* The final chapter of each unit describes how disorder within each circuit emerges as abnormal behaviors and specific symptoms of psychopathology. For the corticolimbic circuit we consider maladaptive or abnormal recognition and reaction to threat and stress; for the corticostriatal circuit, abnormal motivation and maladaptive actions in search of reward; and for the corticohippocampal circuit, the disintegration of memory, thought, and executive control.

Circuit hubs as well as most other circuit nodes are generally **bilaterally symmetrical** structures with predominantly **ipsilateral** connections. There is, however, extensive interhemispheric, or **contralateral**, communication between circuit nodes through major axon pathways ("white matter") linking the right and left hemispheres of the brain (**Figure 1.1**).

We refer to circuit nodes that send information *to* the hub as **upstream**, while nodes that receive information *from* the hub are referred to as **downstream**. We will consider how upstream and downstream information processing through each of these circuits generates order in our perceptions, reactions, actions, and higher cognitive functions, and the disorders that can result when the circuits don't function as expected.

This textbook's nearly exclusive focus on functional neural circuits is intended to provide a foundation for understanding both normal and abnormal behavior at the level most closely associated with its emergence—namely, the processing of information through interconnected brain regions capable of translating a multitude of inputs into an equally diverse set of outputs. Of course, these circuit-level processes can be successively reduced to processes occurring at the cellular, molecular, and genetic levels. Each of these supporting levels of analysis can easily represent the context of not one but many textbooks, and each plays an important role in understanding behavior and psychopathology. However, I believe that the true value of these finer levels of analysis emerges only after first establishing a solid foundation in the functional circuits they support. Thus, our focus on functional neural circuits provides a platform from which the interested scholar can translate otherwise abstract information about cellular, molecular, and genetic processes into the development, maintenance, and regulation of behavior. A foundation in circuit dysfunction and the emergence of disordered behavior likewise helps prepare for an informed examination of strategies for treating

Anterior (rostral)

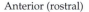

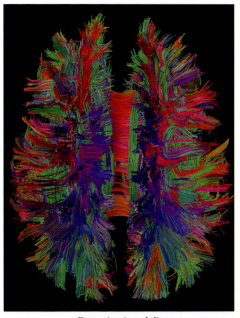

Left hemisphere

Right hemisphere

Posterior (caudal)

Figure 1.1 (A) Diffusion tensor imaging, or DTI, is a technique that allows the axons ("white matter") that carry information between neurons and circuit nodes to be visualized in different colors. This image looks down into the brain from above. Contralateral axon pathways are visualized in red; ipsilateral pathways are green and blue. (From Hagmann et al., 2010.)

and even preventing psychopathology by targeting specific cellular, molecular, and genetic processes.

Core symptoms: A dimensional approach

As with our neural circuit-based approach to the brain, we will deviate from the standard with regard to understanding the neural basis of psychopathology. Prior textbooks have generally adopted the organizational structure of the *Diagnostic and Statistical Manual of Mental Disorders* (*DSM*) by providing a summary of reported abnormalities in brain function and associated behaviors for each of several categorical disorders (e.g., major depressive disorder). These textbooks, in effect, work backward from a *DSM*-based categorical disorder to observed alterations in the brain, which may or may not represent critical foundations for normal behavior. In contrast, we will adopt a forward approach that considers which core symptoms—specific abnormalities in behavior—emerge when there is disorder within our functional neural circuits.

For example, we will consider how disorder of the corticolimbic circuit can emerge as a spectrum of abnormalities in recognizing and reacting to threat and stress, which represent core dimensional symptoms that cut across many categorical disorders, including major depressive disorder, generalized anxiety disorder, specific phobia, posttraumatic stress disorder, and substance use disorder. In fact, we will repeatedly consider many categorical disorders in all three units because some of their core symptoms emerge as a function of disorder within each of the three targeted circuits.

In contrast, other disorders are represented within one specific circuit even though they are associated with symptoms common to disorder of the other circuits. For example, schizophrenia is associated with a broad range of symptoms encompassing dysfunctional emotional and social interactions, abnormal motivations and actions, and grossly disorganized patterns of thinking. Consistent with these broad symptoms, schizophrenia has been linked with disorder in all three functional neural circuits. However, we adopt the perspective that schizophrenia is principally a disorder of the corticohippocampal circuit, emerging as the core symptom of disorganized thought. We consider how the other symptoms—and, in fact, disorder in the other circuits—follow this core breakdown in corticohippocampal circuit function and resulting dysregulation of emotional and motivational processes. Here and elsewhere, the textbook both recognizes the critical importance of targeting the core dimensional features or symptoms of disorders in understanding their fundamental neural basis and also anticipates the forthcoming shift toward dimensional, and away from categorical, diagnoses in the treatment and prevention of mental illness.

Getting Inside: BOLDly Go

Because of the unique ability of functional magnetic resonance imaging, more commonly referred to simply as fMRI, to reveal the activity of distributed neural circuits while humans perform a multitude of simple and complex tasks, we will rely almost exclusively on research that uses it to study our three foundational circuits. Functional MRI is the preferred research tool for studying the structure, function, and connections of the human brain, because it is does not require the use of radioactivity or other administered agents (i.e., it is noninvasive). It also offers the best available balance between capturing fairly detailed anatomy of neural structures and measuring their activity in near real time (**Figure 1.2A**). This optimal combination of spatial and temporal resolution without the need

core symptoms The abnormal behaviors and responses that are typically observed in a disorder.

dimensional symptoms Scores derived from a variety of self-report and observational measures that reflect the severity of core symptoms in an individual.

fMRI (functional magnetic resonance imaging) Widely used noninvasive technique for measuring neural circuit function.

Figure 1.2 (A) Compared with other widely used techniques, including electroencephalography (EEG), magnetoencephalography (MEG), and positron emission tomography (PET), fMRI represents the best balance between visualizing anatomical detail (spatial resolution) and speed of recording signals associated with changes in brain activity (temporal resolution). (B) The use of fMRI in neuroscience and psychology has skyrocketed since the technique emerged. The graph plots the number of indexed studies with the terms "fMRI" or "functional MRI" in their titles or abstracts for each year since the first fMRI studies were published in 1992.

(A)

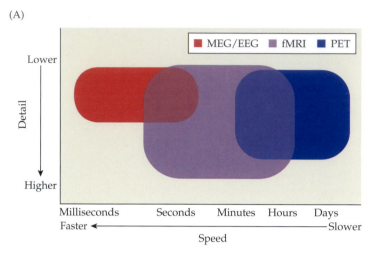

(B)

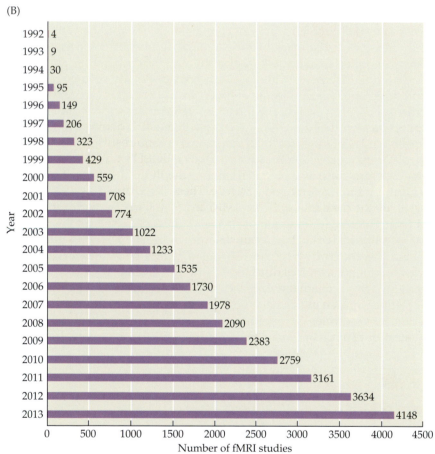

for invasive procedures has driven the nearly exponential expansion of fMRI as the tool of choice for studying human brain function (**Figure 1.2B**).

The fundamental basis of fMRI is the detection of the **BOLD**, or **blood oxygen level-dependent** signal. As activity in ensembles of neurons increases during the processing of information, there is a significant increase in blood flow to the area where these neurons are located. This change in blood flow brings a

BOLD (blood oxygen level-dependent) Signal correlated with neuronal activity and detected using fMRI.

Control or baseline condition

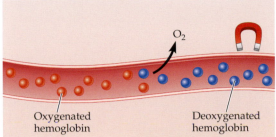

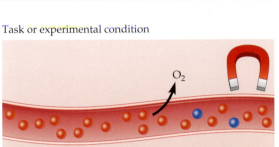

Task or experimental condition

Figure 1.3 When groups of neurons function to process information or complete a task, there is an associated increase in blood flow to the general brain region where these neurons exist. This increase in blood flow is accompanied by an increase in the ratio of oxygenated to deoxygenated hemoglobin, which results in a stronger magnetic signal from the brain region where the increase in blood flow has occurred. By showing differences in the magnitude of this blood oxygen level-dependent, or BOLD, signal between a control, or baseline, condition and a task, or experimental, condition, fMRI can generate an indirect measure of neural activity associated with a specific mental process.

concurrent increase in the local ratio of oxygenated to deoxygenated hemoglobin (**Figure 1.3**). This increase in oxygenated blood results in a stronger local magnetic signature, which is detected as the BOLD signal by fMRI scanners. Most modern fMRI scanners can resolve the BOLD signal in brain areas as small cubes some 2–3 mm on each side. These three-dimensional cubes, called **voxels**, are the basic unit of BOLD fMRI and localize activity within a standard anatomical space (**Figure 1.4**).

Typically, fMRI studies conduct voxelwise statistical comparisons of the change in the magnitude of the BOLD signal between two conditions—that is, they identify BOLD signal during the performance of an experimental task that is greater than the signal during the performance of a control task or while at rest. This is written as "task > control" or "task > rest." This relative change in BOLD signal between two conditions, or **contrast image**, is interpreted as reflecting activity of a brain region that is important in the processes under study.

voxel Three-dimensional unit of brain volume (usually a cube about 2–3 mm on a side) for reporting neural activity using BOLD fMRI.

contrast image A statistical image or map of differences in neural activity between two conditions such as an experimental task and a baseline or control state for an individual.

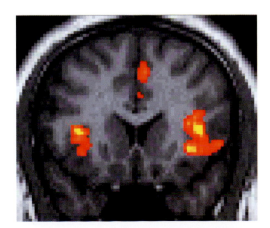

Figure 1.4 Data from fMRI scans emerge as a statistical map of voxels, small three-dimensional "blocks" within the brain. Voxels in which BOLD signal changes between a task and control condition exceed a designated threshold value can then be depicted along a color gradient, with "hotter" colors representing stronger activity. This statistical map is then superimposed on a structural MRI image. (From Huettel et al, 2014.)

RESEARCH SPOTLIGHT

Although first introduced as a tool for studying human brain function more than two decades ago and almost instantly adopted by neuroscientists, psychologists, and psychiatrists for studying human behavior and psychopathology, the fundamental neural basis of the BOLD signal was not clear until only a few years ago. In 2001, Nikos Logothetis and colleagues at the Max Planck Institute for Biological Cybernetics in Germany conducted a seminal study revealing that the BOLD signal measured with fMRI is, in fact, highly correlated with the activity of neuronal ensembles. To establish this correlation, Logothetis and colleagues engineered a unique recording rig (**Figure 1.5A**) that allowed the simultaneous measurement of neuronal activity and BOLD signal in the visual cortex of rhesus macaques when they were looking at a rotating checkerboard pattern (a commonly used stimulus in vision studies).

As expected, there was significant neuronal activity in the visual cortex during stimulation. More importantly, there was a highly correlated increase in BOLD signal beginning approximately 2 seconds after the onset of neuronal activity and reaching a plateau approximately 10 seconds after onset (**Figure 1.5B**). This temporal delay between the BOLD signal and neuronal activity reflects the time required for blood flow (and associated changes in the ratio of oxygenated to deoxygenated hemoglobin) to increase subsequent to activation of a neuronal ensemble in response to stimulation. This was a subtle yet important observation that highlights the indirect relationship between neuronal activity and BOLD signal. Thus, the work of Logothetis and colleagues established that the BOLD signal represents a faithful albeit indirect measure of neuronal activity during the processing of information. With the publication of this seminal finding, neuroscientists, psychologists, and psychiatrists breathed a collective sigh of relief as their long-standing use of fMRI to measure human brain function was validated.

Figure 1.5 (A) Custom designed equipment allowing for the simultaneous recording of electrical activity of neurons and BOLD fMRI from the visual cortex of rhesus macaques. (B) Using this equipment, Logothetis and colleagues were able to provide the first demonstration that the BOLD signal and actual activity of neurons in the monkey visual cortex (the area outlined in green in the photograph) in response to a visual stimulus are highly correlated. (From Logothetis et al., 2001.)

(A)

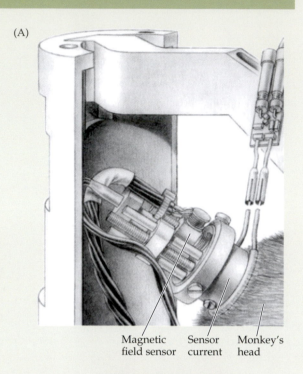

Magnetic field sensor   Sensor current   Monkey's head

(B)

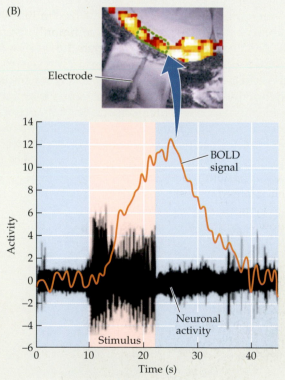

Electrode

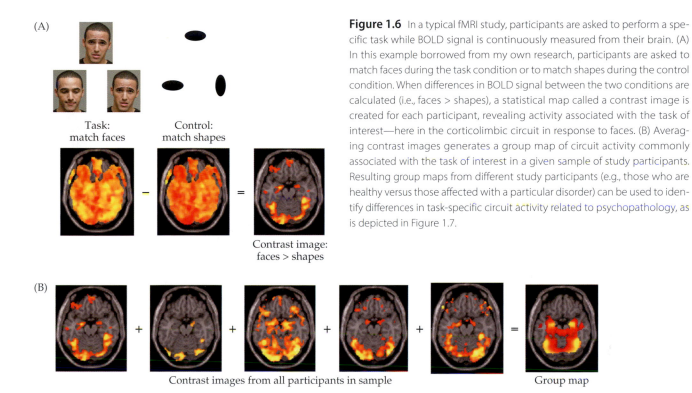

Figure 1.6 In a typical fMRI study, participants are asked to perform a specific task while BOLD signal is continuously measured from their brain. (A) In this example borrowed from my own research, participants are asked to match faces during the task condition or to match shapes during the control condition. When differences in BOLD signal between the two conditions are calculated (i.e., faces > shapes), a statistical map called a contrast image is created for each participant, revealing activity associated with the task of interest—here in the corticolimbic circuit in response to faces. (B) Averaging contrast images generates a group map of circuit activity commonly associated with the task of interest in a given sample of study participants. Resulting group maps from different study participants (e.g., those who are healthy versus those affected with a particular disorder) can be used to identify differences in task-specific circuit activity related to psychopathology, as is depicted in Figure 1.7.

Averaging contrast images from many individuals allows investigators to identify activity in brain regions commonly supporting a specific task or form of information processing (**Figure 1.6**). The group map created by such averaging techniques are critical for understanding how activity in neural circuits can be mapped onto specific functions and how circuit activity helps establish order. By comparing the average neural activity seen in a group map from healthy volunteers with that seen in a group map from affected individuals, investigators can identify patterns of either greater or lesser activity associated with a specific disorder. Using such a difference map is one common strategy for identifying how disorder within a specific neural circuit is associated with psychopathology. This approach parallels that of the *DSM*, which creates diagnostic categories of individuals who share some constellation of symptoms not typically present in healthy volunteers, and provides a window into general patterns of circuit dysfunction in a disorder (**Figure 1.7**).

group maps A 3-D rendering of where in the brain there is activity across a group of individuals when performing the same task; created from averaging contrast images.

difference maps A 3-D rendering of where in the brain activity between two groups of individuals (e.g., healthy study participants compared with affected individuals) is significantly different for a given task. Derived from statistical comparisons of group maps.

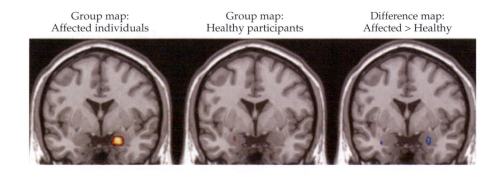

Figure 1.7 A common approach to mapping disorder is to identify the average differences in activity between a group of affected individuals and a group of healthy participants by statistically comparing their group maps of activity associated with a specific task thereby generating a difference map.

Figure 1.8 A second approach to mapping disorder involves extracting activity levels in a specific brain region for affected individuals and then correlating these activity levels to differences in the severity or experience of symptoms. In this example, symptom severity (*x*-axis) is graphed on an arbitrary scale, while brain activity (*y*-axis) is graphed as the percent change in BOLD signal between a task and control condition, with 0 representing the mean value across all individuals. Another common approach to reporting BOLD fMRI data is through arbitrary units representing standardized values across individuals.

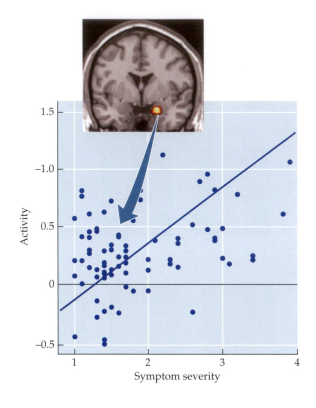

individual differences Patterns of correlation between the magnitude of brain activity in an individual and their behaviors, including the severity of symptoms in individuals with a disorder.

A complementary approach involves mapping a single individual's magnitude of activity in a given brain region—identified from group maps—onto self-reported or observational measures of behavior, physiological changes in response to a challenge, or symptom severity (**Figure 1.8**). Resulting maps of these **individual differences** allow investigators to implicate activity in a specific circuit node in the emergence of a specific behavior or the severity of symptoms, which may be present in multiple categorical disorders. This second approach to mapping disorder aligns with the dimensional approach to psychopathology described above and emphasized throughout this textbook.

Regardless of the specific mapping approach adopted, BOLD fMRI research can only establish that there is a correlation between regional brain activity and a behavior, at either the group or individual level. BOLD fMRI does not provide causal data that demonstrate that activity in a brain region is necessary for a behavior. Such causal links are rare in human research but occasionally can be established through studies of individuals with specific brain lesions; the direct electrical stimulation of brain regions during intraoperative procedures; or the indirect, transient disruption of regional function by use of techniques such as transcranial magnetic stimulation. When possible and appropriate, we will highlight such data throughout the textbook, as they augment the primary fMRI research.

Getting Around: Brain Planes

The human body plan is generally symmetrical, with left and right halves that are largely mirror images of each other. The brain is representative of this general plan, with symmetrical structures occurring within the left and right hemispheres, as described at the start of this chapter. Structures of the brain or body that fall nearer either the left or right side are referred to as being lateral; structures nearer the center are medial.

Beyond lateral and medial, directional designations for the human brain differ somewhat from those used for the rest of the body. This is because the vertical axis of the body bends forward when it reaches the brain (**Figure 1.9**). Thus, toward the top of the body (i.e., the head) is anterior, while the "tail end" is posterior; in the brain, however, anterior indicates the front of the head, properly referred to as rostral, "toward the beak" (i.e., the nose), and posterior indicates the back of the head, properly referred to as caudal, "toward the tail." The dorsal (back) and ventral (belly) axes of the body shift in the brain such that dorsal refers to the perspective from the top of the brain looking down, while ventral refers to the view from the bottom looking up (**Figure 1.10**).

The outer layers of the left and right hemispheres are made up of neurons (i.e., gray matter) referred to as the cerebral cortex. Beneath the cortex lie the subcortical structures of the brain, often made up of clusters of anatomically distinct neurons referred to as nuclei. Our study in this textbook centers on information pathways between neurons in different regions of the cortex and neurons in subcortical structures (e.g., the

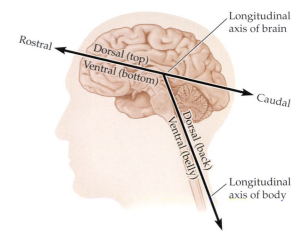

Figure 1.9 As upright posture evolved in humans, the long axis of the central nervous system flexed, leading to an angle between the axis of the body and that of the forebrain. The terms *rostral* and *caudal* refer specifically to the axis of the brain.

lateral Refers to the sides.

medial Refers to the middle or center.

rostral Refers to the front (anterior) of the brain (noseward).

caudal Refers to the back (posterior) of the brain (tailward).

dorsal Refers to the top of the brain (or the back of the body).

ventral Refers to bottom of the brain (or the belly of the body).

cortex/cortical Refers to gray matter (the cell bodies of neurons) on the surface of the brain.

subcortex/subcortical Refers to gray matter of the brain below the cortex.

nuclei Anatomically discrete and identifiable clusters of neurons within the central nervous system.

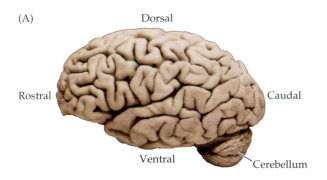

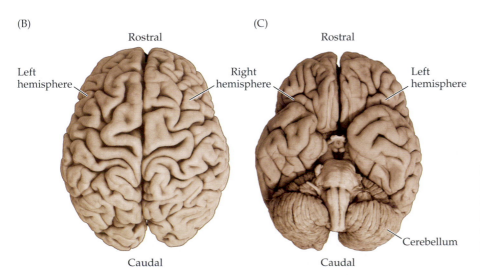

Figure 1.10 Surface views of the human brain. (A) Lateral surface of the left cerebral hemisphere. (B) The dorsal surface is seen looking at the brain from above. (C) The ventral surface views the brain from below looking up.

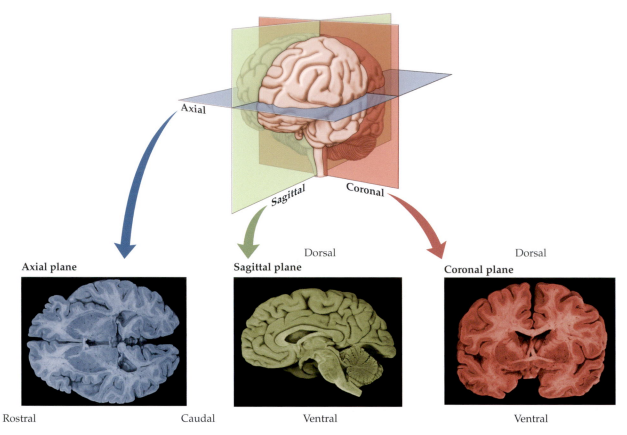

Axial
Sagittal   Coronal

Axial plane   Dorsal   Dorsal
                       Sagittal plane   Coronal plane

Rostral   Caudal   Ventral   Ventral

Figure 1.11 The internal anatomy of the brain in postmortem sections (below) corresponding to the axial, sagittal, and coronal sections depicted above. (Photographs courtesy of S. Mark Williams and Dale Purves, Duke University Medical Center.)

top-down As used here, information processing initiated and orchestrated by cortical structures.

bottom-up As used here, information processing initiated by subcortical structures, especially the amygdala and ventral striatum.

axial A horizontal plane dividing the brain into dorsal and ventral sections.

coronal A vertical plane dividing the brain into rostral and caudal sections.

sagittal A vertical plane dividing the brain into left and right sections.

midsagittal The vertical plane that divides the brain into equal left and right sections (i.e., hemispheres).

amygdala, ventral striatum, and hippocampus). When information is sent from the cortex to subcortical structures, it is referred to as top-down information processing; bottom-up information processing is initiated by subcortical structures sending signals to the cortex.

The beauty of magnetic resonance imaging is that it provides a window through which we can, without harm and with minimal inconvenience to the individual undergoing the procedure, view the interior of the intact and living brain. In the past, this internal anatomy could be studied closely only by dissecting, or sectioning, the brain postmortem, which remains a valuable source of information. In fact, in fMRI studies we still refer to the planes of these sections by their historical postmortem designations: axial, coronal, and sagittal (**Figure 1.11**). The axial section divides the brain horizontally into dorsal and ventral sections. The coronal section divides the brain vertically into rostral and caudal sections. The sagittal section also divides the brain vertically, but into left and right sections. A sagittal section through the center of the brain divides the left and right hemispheres; this commonly seen section is referred to, understandably, as the midsagittal plane. You will see examples of fMRI research depicting circuit activity in all of these planes throughout this text, starting with Chapter 2 as we begin our examination of the corticolimbic circuit.

Literature Cited & Further Reading

Angell, M. (2011). The epidemic of mental illness: Why? *The New York Review of Books*, June 23.

Angell, M. (2011). The illusions of psychiatry. *The New York Review of Books*, July 14.

Cressey. D. (2011). Psychopharmacology in crisis. *Nature*, doi:10.1038/news.2011.367.

Hagmann, P., & 9 others. (2010). MR connectomics: Principles and challenges. *Journal of Neuroscience Methods*, 194: 34–45.

Huettel, S. A., Song, A. W., & McCarthy, G. (2014) *Functional magnetic resonance imaging, 3rd ed.* Sunderland, MA: Sinauer Associates, Inc.

Insel, T. R. (2014). The NIMH Research Domain Criteria (RDoC) Project: Precision medicine for psychiatry. *American Journal of Psychiatry*, 171: 395–397.

Kendler, K. S. (2009). An historical framework for psychiatric nosology. *Psychological Medicine*, 39: 1935–1941.

Logothetis, N. K., Pauls, J., Augath, M., Trinath, T., & Oeltermann, A. (2001). Neurophysiological investigation of the basis of the fMRI signal. *Nature*, 412: 150–157.

Weinberger, D. R., & Goldberg, T. E. (2014). RDoCs redux. *World Psychiatry*, 13: 36–38.

UNIT I

The Corticolimbic Circuit for Recognition and Reaction

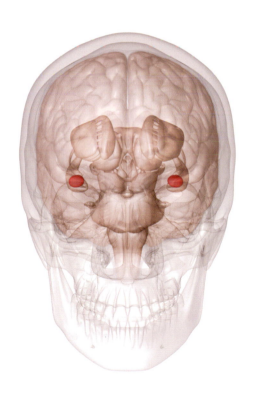

2 Anatomy

The corticolimbic circuit supports many life-sustaining functions and behaviors that can be broadly categorized as *recognition* and *reaction*. In this chapter, we will review the general anatomy of the corticolimbic circuit and identify how key nodes of this circuitry interact to first make us aware of our continually changing world (i.e., facilitate recognition) and then coordinate adaptive responses to the challenges at hand (i.e., generate an appropriate reaction). Over time, the corticolimbic circuit supports learning. Learning through the corticolimbic circuit—a process we will review in Chapter 3—represents the neuroanatomical foundation for anticipating and adaptively responding to events that emerge in our everyday lives, especially threat. As we will see in Chapter 4, disorder within the corticolimbic circuit leads to dysfunction in this form of learning and to the emergence of inappropriate recognition of and reaction to threatening stimuli, which can eventually result in pathological behaviors such as depression and posttraumatic stress disorder.

The corticolimbic circuit (**Figure 2.1**) is comprised of the following interconnected structures:

1. Amygdala
2. Thalamus and sensory cortices
3. Hypothalamus
4. Brainstem
5. Substantia innominata
6. Insula
7. Hippocampal formation
8. Prefrontal cortex

A review of these key anatomical nodes is necessary for a comprehensive understanding of how information is processed within the corticolimbic circuit to ultimately mediate recognition and reaction, which we will consider in detail in Chapter 3. As we turn to examine how disorder within the circuit manifests as abnormal behavior and specific symptoms of psychopathology in Chapter 4, we will focus on dysfunction in select nodes that are critical for regulating this information flow, with a particular emphasis on the circuit's hub.

Figure 2.1 The key nodes of the cortico-limbic circuit and their basic connections. The amygdala is the hub of the circuit, through which sensory inputs from the thalamus and sensory cortices ("upstream" structures) are translated into appropriate changes in behavior and physiology via outputs mediated by the hypothalamus, brainstem, substantia innominata, insula, hippocampal formation, and prefrontal cortex ("downstream" structures). Feedback from neurons in the prefrontal cortex eventually can lead to new changes in behavior via the inhibition of specific neurons in the amygdala.

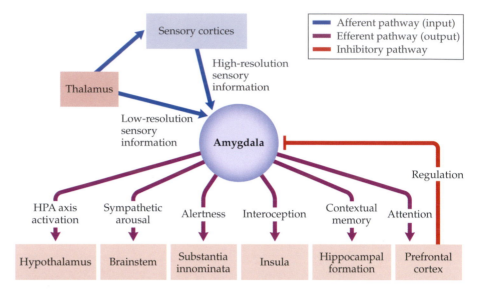

basolateral complex of the amygdala (BLA) Single term referring to the lateral, basal, and accessory basal nuclei of the amygdala. The principal input structure of the amygdala, serving to process and relay multiple inputs (e.g., sensory, contextual, regulatory) from cortical and subcortical structures on to the central nucleus of the amygdala.

central nucleus of the amygdala (CeA) The principal output structure of the amygdala, serving to process and relay input from the BLA on to multiple downstream targets that control behavioral and physiological changes.

The Amygdala

The hub of the corticolimbic circuit is the amygdala, a bilaterally symmetrical subcortical structure located deep within in the anterior medial temporal lobe (**Figure 2.2**). The amygdala was named for its anatomical appearance: the word *amygdala* is Latin for "almond," which is a fair description of its general shape and size. The amygdala is a quintessential circuit hub, with its extensive patterns of afferent (input) and efferent (output) connections that help us first recognize and then react to the challenges that arise and confront us in our environment.

Although the amygdala is often referred to as a single, homogeneous structure, it is in fact both structurally and functionally heterogeneous, consisting of 13 distinct nuclei. We will focus on the following five nuclei, which play a critical role in the basic corticolimbic circuit functions of recognition and reaction:

1. Lateral nucleus
2. Basal nucleus
3. Accessory basal nucleus
4. Central nucleus
5. Intercalated cell masses

The lateral, basal, and accessory basal nuclei are often lumped together as the **basolateral complex of the amygdala**, or **BLA** (see Figure 2.2D). Although each of these individual nuclei has some unique connections, all three generally function as afferent relay structures. The lateral nucleus receives afferent input from auditory, visual, gustatory, and somatosensory cortices, as well as from the sensory nuclei of the thalamus, hippocampal formation, and prefrontal cortex. The majority of these lateral nucleus neurons relay this input on to the basal and accessory basal nuclei, which then feed the input forward to the **central nucleus of the amygdala**, or **CeA**. In turn, the CeA provides a major source of efferent projections to multiple downstream targets, including the brainstem, hypothalamus, and substantia innominata. Thus, the BLA is the

CeA   central nucleus of the amygdala
BLA   basolateral complex of the amygdala

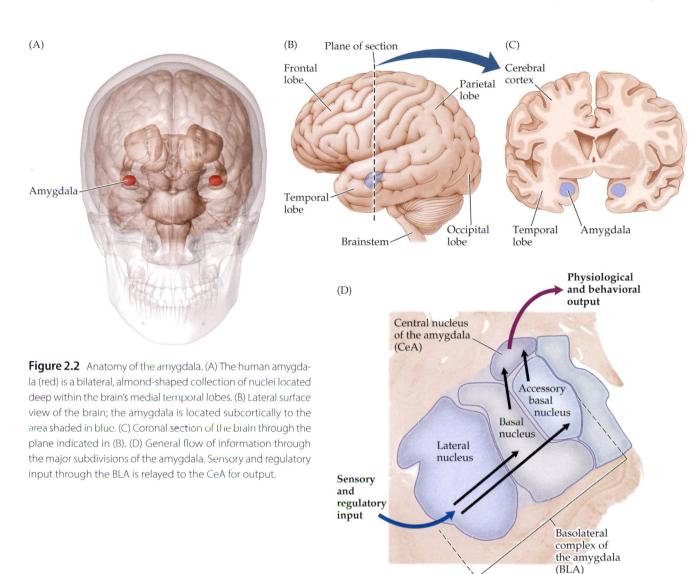

Figure 2.2 Anatomy of the amygdala. (A) The human amygdala (red) is a bilateral, almond-shaped collection of nuclei located deep within the brain's medial temporal lobes. (B) Lateral surface view of the brain; the amygdala is located subcortically to the area shaded in blue. (C) Coronal section of the brain through the plane indicated in (B). (D) General flow of information through the major subdivisions of the amygdala. Sensory and regulatory input through the BLA is relayed to the CeA for output.

principal input structure of the amygdala, while the CeA functions as the principal output structure.

Finally, the **intercalated cell masses**, or **ICMs**, are small pockets or islands of inhibitory neurons strategically positioned to regulate communication between the BLA and CeA (**Figure 2.3**). A distinct subpopulation of neurons in the BLA (different from those neurons projecting to the CeA) drives the activity of the ICMs. The ICMs project to the CeA and inhibit its output. As we will learn later, neurons in the prefrontal cortex also inhibit activity of the CeA through the ICMs. It is thus useful to think of ICMs as representing "inhibitory moats," or gates, that regulate amygdala output through inhibition of the CeA.

In summary, the amygdala functions as the hub of the corticolimbic circuit by routing sensory and regulatory input through the BLA to the CeA, which then drives output through multiple downstream targets. Broadly, these amygdala connections are critical for the process of establishing associations between one

intercalated cell masses (ICMs)
"Islands" of inhibitory neurons that regulate communication between the amygdala's basolateral complex (BLA) and central nucleus (CeA).

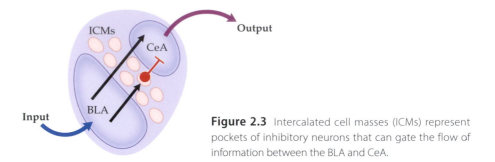

Figure 2.3 Intercalated cell masses (ICMs) represent pockets of inhibitory neurons that can gate the flow of information between the BLA and CeA.

stimulus and another (such as the buzzing of a bee followed by a painful sting) that predict threat or safety. In many ways, this broad role of the amygdala is best represented by fear learning, which we will review in detail in Chapter 3. For now, let us return to neuroanatomy and consider the interactions of the amygdala with upstream structures that provide sensory input as well as with downstream structures that mediate specific behavioral and physiological output.

RESEARCH SPOTLIGHT

In the central nucleus of the amygdala, we encounter a further structural and functional subdivision of the amygdala. Specifically, the CeA is subdivided into medial and lateral divisions. The medial division (CeA-M) mediates activation of downstream targets (i.e., output). In contrast, the lateral division (CeA-L) is positioned to terminate amygdala output to downstream targets by inhibiting the CeA-M. Interestingly, recent work by Huber and colleagues has demonstrated that the distribution of receptors for two different neuropeptides across the CeA-L and CeA-M is consistent with their effects on our social behavior. Receptors for the hormone vasopressin, which generally decreases social behavior, are found in the CeA-M. Receptors for oxytocin, which generally increases social behavior, are located in the CeA-L. Thus, oxytocin may have its prosocial effects by activating the CeA-L, which in turn inhibits the CeA-M and amygdala output. Vasopressin, in contrast, may have antisocial effects through direct activation of the CeA-M, triggering amygdala output such as fear.

The Thalamus and Sensory Cortices

Within the context of the corticolimbic circuit, the thalamic nuclei relay multimodal sensory information to the BLA. Of particular relevance, the medial geniculate nucleus relays auditory information, the pulvinar relays visual information, and the ventral posterior nucleus relays somatosensory (e.g., touch, pain) as well as gustatory (taste) information (**Figure 2.4**). Olfactory information (smells), in contrast, lacks a thalamic relay and reaches the amygdala directly, through projections to the BLA via the olfactory tract. This direct link to the amygdala is believed to contribute to the strong emotional meanings often attached to specific aromas (e.g., the perfume of a sweetheart, or Mom's apple pie). These thalamic relays allow stimuli to be rapidly processed by the BLA and, in turn, quick (even reflexive) responses to be orchestrated through the CeA even before we may be fully conscious or aware of the stimuli.

BLA   basolateral complex of the amygdala
CeA   central nucleus of the amygdala
ICMs   intercalated cell masses

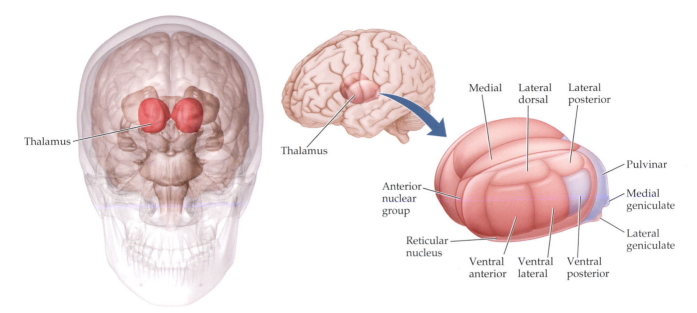

Figure 2.4 Thalamic nuclei relay sensory information to the BLA. Of particular importance for the core corticolimbic circuit functions of recognition and reaction are the medial geniculate nucleus (which relays auditory information), the pulvinar (visual information), and the ventral posterior nucleus (somatosensory information, including pain).

The information relayed by the thalamus is relatively crude and lacks the details necessary to let us know exactly what we are encountering. These details are filled in by sensory regions of the cortex, to which the thalamic relays convey modality-specific information (e.g., auditory information to the primary auditory cortex via the medial geniculate nucleus) parallel to that forwarded directly to the BLA. These sensory cortices also project to the BLA, providing a second, higher-resolution input that can further drive amygdala output. Because this second input is indirect (i.e., it passes from the thalamus to the amygdala through the sensory cortices), the high-resolution details are slower to arrive at the BLA.

The neuroscientist Joseph LeDoux at New York University describes the subcortical pathway from the thalamus to the amygdala as the **"low road"** and the cortical pathway through sensory cortices as the **"high road."** The classic example used by LeDoux to describe the low and high roads in action involves a young man hiking along a narrow trail. After moving quickly along the trail for an hour, he suddenly encounters a long, thin object on the trail directly in front of him. Transmitted along the low road, this visual information reaches the pulvinar of the thalamus, which directly relays a crude representation of the object (imagine a fuzzy long line) to the BLA, which in turn drives the CeA to activate specific regions of the brainstem that cause the hiker to freeze in his tracks. This is a critical processing circuit because it keeps the hiker from stepping on the object, which could be potentially dangerous (possibly even fatal) if the object is, say, a venomous snake. At the same time, the visual information travels along the high road from pulvinar to visual cortices where the object is identified, in fact, as a diamondback rattlesnake (**Figure 2.5**). The subsequent availability of this detailed object information through the high road leads the hiker to re-route his trek around the snake and safely pick

"low road" Term used by Joseph LeDoux for the subcortical pathway from the thalamus directly to the BLA; allows sensory stimuli to be processed rapidly, but at low resolution.

"high road" LeDoux's term for the cortical pathway from the thalamus through the sensory cortices and then to the BLA; allows sensory stimuli to be processed at higher resolution, but less rapidly.

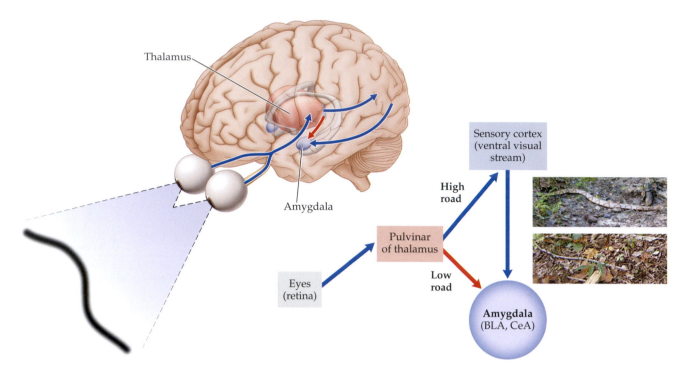

Figure 2.5 The low and high roads to the amygdala. Through the low road, thalamic nuclei (e.g., the pulvinar) relay relatively crude representations of our external world from sensory organs (e.g., retina of the eye) to the BLA. Through the high road, these thalamic nuclei relay the same information to sensory cortices (e.g., the ventral visual stream; see Chapter 8), which provide relatively detailed information to the BLA. (After LeDoux, 1996.)

up the trail on the other side. Thus, the initial freezing response mediated by the low road saves him from a possible strike and allows him the time to avoid the snake. Had the object been a dead branch fallen from a nearby tree, however, the hiker could have simply resumed his trek (after shaking off the embarrassment of having frozen in his tracks for a branch).

Why should our initial (i.e., low road) response assume the object is potentially dangerous? LeDoux comments that it is better to mistake a fallen branch for a snake than the other way around. That is, we're better off freezing unnecessarily for a branch than stepping carelessly on a snake and receiving a nasty bite. As exemplified by the hiker on the trail, the evolutionary process of natural selection has shaped a corticolimbic circuit that errs on the side of caution, opting to help keep us safe rather than sorry. Later in this unit we will review evidence from fMRI studies demonstrating the sensitivity of these parallel low road and high road pathways to the amygdala in response to a variety of stimuli as the corticolimbic circuit functions to keep us safe from harm.

The Hypothalamus

The hypothalamus is made up of multiple interconnected nuclei that regulate a host of the basic physiological functions that maintain homeostasis (internal stability), including thirst, hunger, and body temperature. The amygdala, particularly the CeA, can drive activity in many of these hypothalamic nuclei. Of specific importance within the corticolimbic circuit for recognition

BLA   basolateral complex of the amygdala
CeA   central nucleus of the amygdala

(A)

(B)

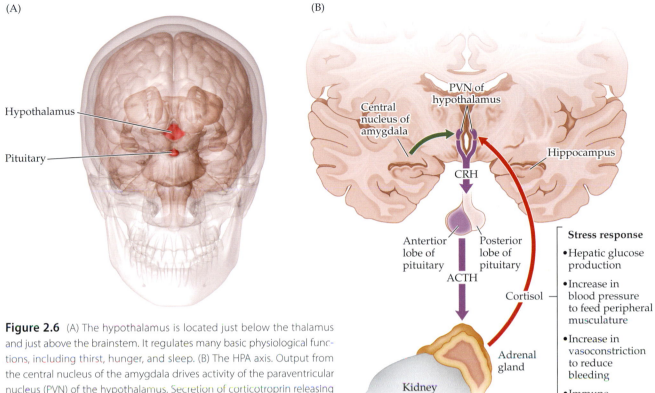

Hypothalamus

Pituitary

PVN of hypothalamus

Central nucleus of amygdala

Hippocampus

CRH

Antertior lobe of pituitary

Posterior lobe of pituitary

ACTH

Cortisol

Adrenal gland

Kidney

Stress response

• Hepatic glucose production

• Increase in blood pressure to feed peripheral musculature

• Increase in vasoconstriction to reduce bleeding

• Immune suppression

Figure 2.6 (A) The hypothalamus is located just below the thalamus and just above the brainstem. It regulates many basic physiological functions, including thirst, hunger, and sleep. (B) The HPA axis. Output from the central nucleus of the amygdala drives activity of the paraventricular nucleus (PVN) of the hypothalamus. Secretion of corticotroprin releasing hormone (CRH) from the PVN stimulates the anterior pituitary to release adrenocorticotropic hormone (ACTH) into the bloodstream. ACTH reaches the adrenal glands, stimulating the adrenals to release cortisol, which drive's the body's stress response. Cortisol also functions to provide negative feedback inhibition of the HPA, in part, by driving activity in the hippocampus, which functions to inhibit the PVN. Thus, the activation of the body's stress response is self-limited.

and reaction, the paraventricular nucleus (PVN) controls the activation of the major hormonal systems in the body. One of these hormonal systems is the **hypothalamic-pituitary-adrenal (HPA) axis** (**Figure 2.6**). When the PVN is activated by CeA inputs, it releases corticotropin-releasing hormone into the anterior pituitary gland. The anterior pituitary gland then releases adrenocorticotropic hormone (ACTH) into the bloodstream. When ACTH reaches the cortex of the adrenal glands, it stimulates the release of the steroidal hormone cortisol into the circulatory system. Multiple physiological processes are influenced by cortisol, including the production of glucose in the liver for energy, an increase in blood pressure to move blood into the peripheral musculature for rapid movement, an increase in vasoconstriction to reduce bleeding, and a suppression of the immune response. In total, cortisol functions to mobilize available resources and energy in response to an immediate challenge from the environment.

A major component of our physiological response to threat and stress is initiated through this activation of the PVN. Critically, there are intrinsic negative feedback loops (including one within the corticolimbic circuit that will be covered later in this chapter) that limit the effects of cortisol once the stressor or threat has been eliminated through appropriate responses. Failure

hypothalamic-pituitary-adrenal (HPA) axis A series of complex connections between the hypothalamus, pituitary gland, and adrenal gland that result in the release and regulation of cortisol in response to stress. Input from the amygdala to the paraventricular nucleus of the hypothalamus can activate this major hormonal system.

to inhibit the HPA axis response contributes to a host of problems, both medical (e.g., weight loss, bone loss, muscle wasting, insulin resistance, decreased immunity) and psychological (e.g., anxiety, depression, memory impairment).

In addition to its critical role in regulating the release of cortisol via the HPA axis, the PVN releases a number of neuropeptides that are involved in modulating the function of the corticolimbic circuit and, in turn, the expression of arousal and reaction. These include oxytocin, vasopressin, and neuropeptide Y. Importantly, many neurons within the corticolimbic circuit, and particularly within the amygdala, express receptors for these modulatory neuropeptides (see the Research Spotlight on p. 20).

The Brainstem

Broadly, the brainstem is the most ancient and highly conserved structure of vertebrate brains. The brainstem lies between the cerebrum and spinal cord, and all major afferent and efferent fibers of the central nervous system pass through this structure (**Figure 2.7**). Within the three major anatomical divisions of the brainstem—the medulla oblongata, pons, and midbrain—there are numerous nuclei that control many basic life-sustaining functions, including breathing, heart rate, sleeping, and eating.

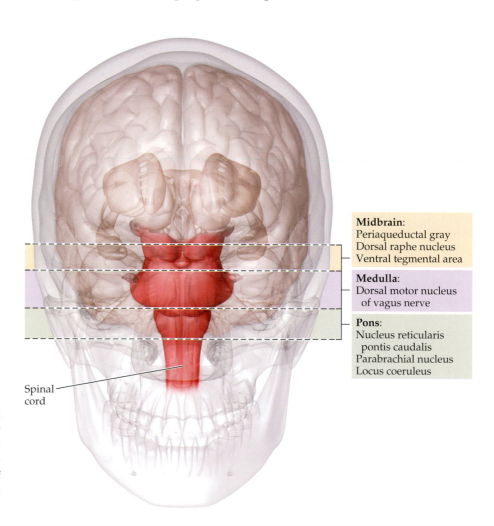

Midbrain:
Periaqueductal gray
Dorsal raphe nucleus
Ventral tegmental area

Medulla:
Dorsal motor nucleus
  of vagus nerve

Pons:
Nucleus reticularis
  pontis caudalis
Parabrachial nucleus
Locus coeruleus

Spinal cord

Figure 2.7 The three major anatomical divisions of the brainstem contain many nuclei that sustain critical autonomic functions such as heartbeat and breathing. The figure highlights the locations of several nuclei important to the corticolimbic circuit.

HPA   hypothalamic-pituitary-adrenal
PVN   paraventricular nucleus

TABLE 2.1 Brainstem nuclei in the corticolimbic circuit	
Brainstem nucleus	**Effect of efferent input from CeA**
Nucleus reticularis pontis caudalis	Exaggerates the startle response
Periaqueductal gray	Triggers the "freeze" response
Dorsal motor nucleus of vagus nerve	Triggers increased heart rate
Ventral tegmental area	Triggers release of dopamine
Dorsal raphe nucleus	Triggers release of serotonin
Locus coeruleus	Triggers release of norepinephrine
Parabrachial nucleus*	Triggers increased breathing rate

*The parabrachial nucleus also has afferent projections that transmit nociceptive (painful) stimuli to the amygdala.

Within the corticolimbic circuit, the effects of the CeA on recognition and reaction are further mediated through direct projections to multiple brainstem nuclei (**Table 2.1**). Through its projections to the nucleus reticularis pontis caudalis (or caudal pontine nucleus of the reticular formation), the CeA can exaggerate our startle response under threatening conditions (e.g., we will jump faster and higher when we hear a loud banging sound if we are walking down a dark, abandoned alley than if we are in a supermarket aisle). Through the periaqueductal gray, the CeA can trigger our freezing response, particularly when a threat (e.g., a snake) is relatively far away and we can escape detection or avoid the threat simply by not moving. Projections to the parabrachial nucleus allow the CeA to trigger an increase in respiration, while those to the dorsal motor nucleus of the vagus nerve trigger an increase in heart rate. Interestingly, efferents from the parabrachial nucleus provide direct nociceptive input (i.e., sensations of pain) to the amygdala. This pathway allows the amygdala to monitor incoming painful and other noxious stimuli and to immediately generate adaptive responses. As we will see in Chapter 3, this is a key component of fear learning.

The CeA can also have more general effects through its projections to the brainstem. Specifically, CeA projections to the ventral tegmental area, dorsal raphe nucleus, and locus coeruleus of the brainstem can trigger the release of dopamine, serotonin, and norepinephrine, respectively. These neuromodulators can have widespread effects on the relative responsiveness of many nodes of the corticolimbic circuit. Thus, through direct projections to targets in the brainstem, the CeA is able to trigger specific patterns of reaction such as freezing and startle, as well as general arousal through changes in circuit responsiveness (e.g., the release of neuromodulators).

The Substantia Innominata

The substantia innominata (Latin for "unnamed substance") is a region that is largely contiguous with the dorsal and anterior boundaries of the CeA (**Figure 2.8**). The name of this region reflects its functional and structural heterogeneity, which makes it difficult to identify clear anatomical boundaries. However, two distinct groups of neurons within the substantia innominata are closely connected with the amygdala and significantly contribute to the effects of the corticolimbic circuit on recognition and reaction. The first of these is the nucleus basalis of Meynert (NBM), a dense region of cholinergic neurons

neuromodulators Broad class of molecules, released by a nucleus or small group of neurons, that modulate the responsiveness of other neurons. Examples include dopamine, serotonin, norepinephrine, and acetylcholine.

CeA   central nucleus of the amygdala
NBM   nucleus basalis of Meynert

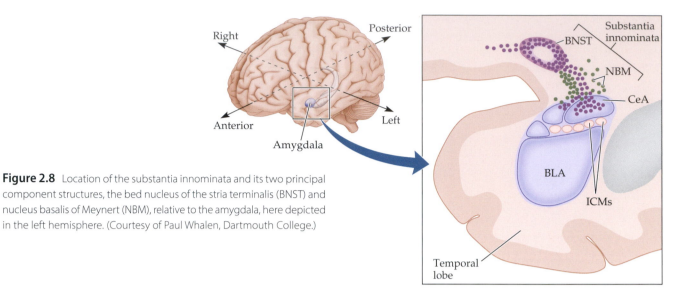

Figure 2.8 Location of the substantia innominata and its two principal component structures, the bed nucleus of the stria terminalis (BNST) and nucleus basalis of Meynert (NBM), relative to the amygdala, here depicted in the left hemisphere. (Courtesy of Paul Whalen, Dartmouth College.)

potentiation Increasing the responsiveness of a neuron to input (e.g., the effects of the neuromodulator acetylcholine, referred to as *cholinergic potentiation*).

whose efferents are distributed widely throughout the cortex. Projections of the CeA driving the NBM result in the release of acetylcholine, a neuromodulator that functions to increase the responsiveness of neurons to converging input. Such cholinergic **potentiation** of neurons in the prefrontal cortex helps us process more information about our environments (i.e., broaden our attention) so that we can develop a better picture of what is happening around us. Cholinergic potentiation of neurons in sensory cortices allows for more accurate identification of objects in our environment (e.g., recognizing that it is a snake on the trail). One specific sensory cortical target of cholinergic neurons from the NBM is the posterior fusiform gyrus, which is important for recognizing faces. As we will see in Chapter 3, faces (and facial expressions) are powerful provocateurs of the amygdala and the interconnected corticolimbic circuit.

Thus, by increasing the responsiveness of multiple downstream targets, particularly the prefrontal and sensory cortices, the NBM is positioned to translate activity of the CeA into general increases in arousal, attention, and recognition of the stimuli we encounter in our lives (**Figure 2.9**).

The second relevant region of the substantia innominata, located dorsal to the NBM, is the bed nucleus of the stria terminalis (BNST; see Figure 2.8). The name of this structure reflects the position of its neurons adjacent to the stria terminalis, the major efferent pathway of the amygdala. In addition to

Figure 2.9 Key direct and indirect output pathways from the central nucleus of the amygdala. The indirect pathway includes the nucleus basalis of Meynert, a group of neurons in the substantia innominata whose release of acetylcholine functions to increase the responsiveness of multiple downstream targets in the corticolimbic circuit. This cholinergic potentiation results in increases in arousal, attention, and recognition of stimuli.

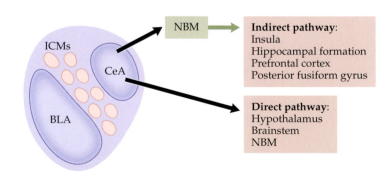

| BNST | bed nucleus of the stria terminalis | CeA | central nucleus of the amygdala |
| NBM | nucleus basalis of Meynert | BLA | basolateral complex of the amygdala |

having direct connections with the amygdala, neurons of the BNST project to many of the same downstream regions as the CeA, including all of the previously mentioned targets in the brainstem and hypothalamus. Thus, the BNST is positioned to initiate many of the same changes in physiology and behavior as the amygdala. As we will learn in Chapters 3 and 4, divergence in the responsiveness of the amygdala and BNST to specific types of stimuli, as well as the relative presence or absence of the ICMs, may be critically important in anxiety disorders.

RESEARCH SPOTLIGHT

Studies in rats using chemicals to trace connections between neurons reveal the presence of direct connections not only between neurons in the BLA and CeA, but also between the BLA and neurons in the BNST (see Davis et al., 2010). Injection of an anterograde tracer (i.e., a chemical marker that labels the efferent connections of neurons) into the BLA, results in dense labeling of neurons in both the CeA and the BNST (**Figure 2.10**). This suggests that the BLA can drive activity not only of the CeA but also of the BNST.

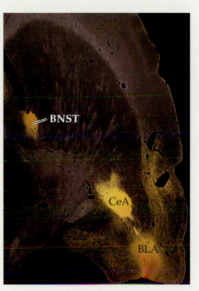

Figure 2.10 Tracing studies reveal that neurons in both the CeA and BNST have direct connections with the BLA. (From Davis et al., 2010; micrograph prepared by Chungjun Shi.)

The Insula

As we have learned above, the extensive connections between the CeA and downstream targets in the hypothalamus, brainstem, and substantia innominata provide a system through which the amygdala can transduce the constant stream of sensory information from our changing environments into moment-by-moment adjustments in our levels of general arousal as well as our specific reactions to the challenges we face. Our awareness of these adjustments, particularly those in our physiological states, begins in the insula.

The insula (or insular cortex) is located deep within the Sylvian fissure in both hemispheres. In terms of gross anatomy, the insula is obscured from sight by the frontal, temporal, and parietal opercula (Latin for "lids") and is only visible when the opercula are retracted (**Figure 2.11**). The insula is generally divided into anterior and posterior regions, and it is the anterior insula that receives dense projections from the amygdala, primarily from the BLA. This pathway allows the BLA to drive activity in the anterior insula much as it does in the CeA. In addition, the general responsiveness of the insula is potentiated indirectly through the drive of the CeA on the NBM. This potentiation

ICMs   intercalated cell masses

Figure 2.11 The insula (or insular cortex; black outline) is buried deep within the Sylvian fissure (highlighted in white) and is revealed when the the frontal and temporal opercula ("lids") are retracted.

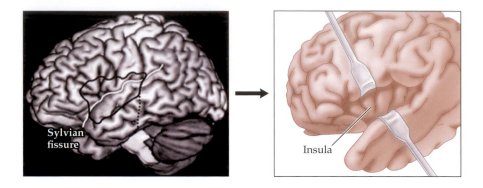

interoception The conscious awareness of internal bodily states (e.g., gastrointestinal activity).

of activity in the anterior insula is critical for generating awareness of the other changes instantiated by the CeA, because the anterior insula represents a convergence of somatosensory (externally originating signals, such as heat or touch) and interoceptive (internally originating signals, such as heart rate) projections from the body. This convergence allows for a representation of our bodily states, including heart rate, respiration, gastrointestinal activity, perspiration, and muscle tension.

In the broader context of the corticolimbic circuit, the direct and indirect drive from the amygdala onto the anterior insula promotes **interoception**: our awareness of how our bodily states are changing in response to any number of stimuli, including threat. Most of us experience this phenomenon, for example when we get "butterflies" before an important presentation, or when we feel our heart race and muscles tighten when confronted by someone we have made angry. In these situations, interoceptive awareness helps us understand what we are experiencing and how we can mount a successful response to the situation. However, as we will see in Chapter 4, disorder in the response of the anterior insula can contribute to the emergence of anxiety disorders.

The Hippocampal Formation

While our subjective awareness of the physiological changes mediated by the amygdala is shaped through the insula, our memory for where and when these changes occurred is dependent on the hippocampal formation (**Figure 2.12**). The hippocampal formation (HF) refers broadly to highly interconnected adjacent regions of the medial temporal lobes, including the parahippocampal cortex, entorhinal cortex, perirhinal cortex, and hippocampus located immediately posterior to the amygdala. The discrete role of the HF in mnemonic processes, particularly declarative memory, will be covered in detail in Unit III. Within the context of the corticolimbic circuit we will focus on two parallel functions of the HF.

The first entails the role of the HF for encoding the specific environmental circumstances or context in which the amygdala triggers changes in our physiology and behavior. Through excitatory projections—largely from the BLA—the amygdala can directly potentiate the activity of the HF. The amygdala can also indirectly potentiate activity of the HF through increasing cholinergic tone via projections of the CeA to the NBM. These direct and indirect pathways for potentiating HF activity function to increase our capacity to encode (i.e., form new memories) and subsequently recall (i.e., remember

CeA   central nucleus of the amygdala
NBM   nucleus basalis of Meynert
HF   hippocampal formation

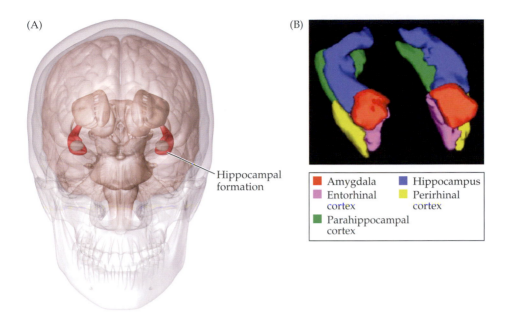

Figure 2.12 (A) The hippocampal formation begins just behind the amygdala and follows a curved path within the medial temporal lobe of each hemisphere. (B) Based on MRI data, this three-dimensional depiction shows the general shape, arrangement, and position of the hippocampal formation relative to the amygdala within the left and right medial temporal lobes. (B adapted from Dolcos et al., 2004.)

the memories) the context in which we have experienced or encountered a specific stimulus that triggered an amygdala response. This phenomenon is often referred to colloquially as a "flashbulb" memory because the details of such memories are often very vivid and encompass multiple sensory modalities, including sight, sound, and smell.

Returning to our example of the hiker, it is the potentiation of activity in the HF by the amygdala concurrent with its stimulation of other downstream targets (e.g., the brainstem and hypothalamus) that allows him to know on which specific trail in the park he almost stepped on a snake. This memory is critical because it allows for a finely tuned expression of amygdala output *only in the appropriate context* (e.g., the hillside trail but not the lakeside trail). We will revisit the importance of the HF for the contextually appropriate expression of amygdala output when we examine fear learning in Chapter 3.

The second function of the HF within the corticolimbic circuit is to mediate negative feedback inhibition of the HPA axis response triggered by the amygdala through the PVN (see Figure 2.6). Specifically, cortisol released as the final product of the HPA axis binds to mineralocorticoid receptors in the hippocampus to potentiate activity. This increase in activity in turn inhibits the activity of the PVN. Thus, the HF is positioned to mediate negative inhibition of the HPA axis at its source in the hypothalamus. In this way, the HF serves as the brake to the amygdala's accelerator of the stress response. This braking function of the HF is essential to limiting the duration of the stress response and preventing the development of the chronic stress phenotypes noted above (weight loss, muscle wasting, memory impairment, etc.) and commonly observed in mood and anxiety disorders. Interestingly, amygdala activity not only accelerates the stress response, but also actually enables

BLA   basolateral complex of the amygdala
HPA   hypothalamic-pituitary-adrenal
PVN   paraventricular nucleus

this braking function through increasing the responsiveness of the HF via cholinergic potentiation. In many ways, this interplay between the amygdala and HF is characteristic of the nuanced dynamics occurring throughout the corticolimbic circuit in the service of generating adaptive responses to the challenges we face.

The Prefrontal Cortex

Of all the corticolimbic circuit nodes with which the amygdala interacts to generate recognition and reaction, the most critical is the prefrontal cortex, particularly its medial surface. The functional dynamics between the amygdala and medial prefrontal cortex are paramount for the expression of adaptive responses to the challenges we face. These functional dynamics are mediated through extensive reciprocal connections between the amygdala and mPFC. As we will see in Chapter 4, disorder between these two nodes of the corticolimbic circuit underlies much of the psychopathology associated with mood and anxiety disorders.

Generally, the mPFC is positioned to provide a two-stage response to amygdala activity and the resulting changes in physiology and behavior. First, the mPFC functions to evaluate and integrate these changes to appropriately update our ongoing responses. Once this occurs, the mPFC then functions to inhibit further amygdala signaling and subsequently terminate its output, allowing us to return to our baseline, or pre-provoked, state. The mPFC is often divided into ventral and dorsal sections along an imaginary boundary extending rostrally from the genu (anterior end) of the corpus callosum (**Figure 2.13A**).

The ventromedial PFC is responsible for the initial integration and evaluation of changes in physiology and behavior driven by amygdala output. There is further anatomical and functional subdivision of the vmPFC into the orbitofrontal cortex and, in some work, the ventral anterior cingulate cortex. With regard to the general circuit anatomy, however, we will refer more broadly to the vmPFC. Direct efferents from the BLA allow the amygdala to drive activity in local neuronal circuits within the vmPFC. These connections with the vmPFC are particularly important for assigning valence to the stimuli detected by the amygdala, because these prefrontal regions also receive projections from primary sensory cortices, the hippocampal formation, and the insula, as well as subcortical regions concerned with hedonic tone (perceived degree of pleasantness or unpleasantness), which will be reviewed in detail as components of the corticostriatal circuit in Unit II. Projections from the BLA increase sensitivity of vmPFC neurons to input from the above regions. Indirectly, the responsiveness of neurons in the vmPFC is further heightened through increased cholinergic tone mediated by the pathway from the CeA to the NBM. Thus, direct and indirect input from the amygdala increases the processing of salient sensory, mnemonic (memory), interoceptive (internal physiology), and hedonic information through the vmPFC. It is this convergence of information within the vmPFC that produces conscious awareness of our experiences and colors them as being subjectively pleasant or unpleasant (i.e., of positive or negative valence). It is important to note that the amygdala does not directly determine these subjective feelings, but rather drives associated changes in physiology and behavior. It is the evaluation of this drive by the vmPFC that generates the emotional charge of each experience.

HF	hippocampal formation	**BLA**	basolateral complex of the amygdala
mPFC	medial prefrontal cortex	**CeA**	central nucleus of the amygdala
vmPFC	ventromedial prefrontal cortex	**NBM**	nucleus basalis of Meynert

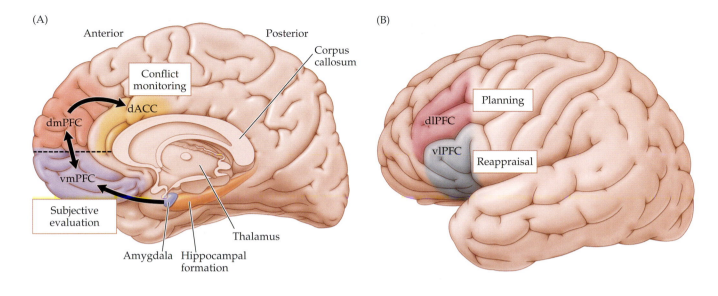

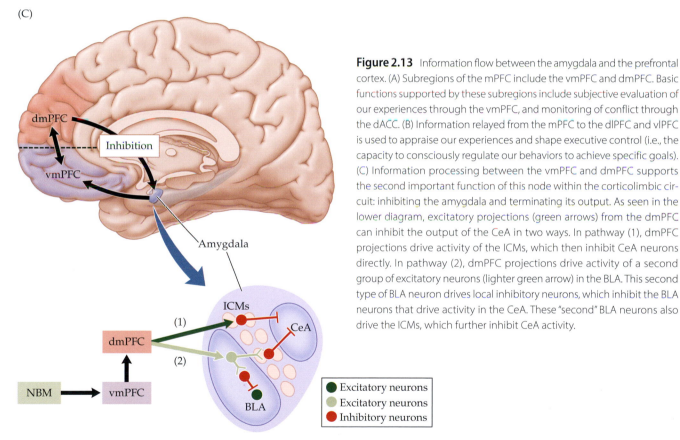

Figure 2.13 Information flow between the amygdala and the prefrontal cortex. (A) Subregions of the mPFC include the vmPFC and dmPFC. Basic functions supported by these subregions include subjective evaluation of our experiences through the vmPFC, and monitoring of conflict through the dACC. (B) Information relayed from the mPFC to the dlPFC and vlPFC is used to appraise our experiences and shape executive control (i.e., the capacity to consciously regulate our behaviors to achieve specific goals). (C) Information processing between the vmPFC and dmPFC supports the second important function of this node within the corticolimbic circuit: inhibiting the amygdala and terminating its output. As seen in the lower diagram, excitatory projections (green arrows) from the dmPFC can inhibit the output of the CeA in two ways. In pathway (1), dmPFC projections drive activity of the ICMs, which then inhibit CeA neurons directly. In pathway (2), dmPFC projections drive activity of a second group of excitatory neurons (lighter green arrow) in the BLA. This second type of BLA neuron drives local inhibitory neurons, which inhibit the BLA neurons that drive activity in the CeA. These "second" BLA neurons also drive the ICMs, which further inhibit CeA activity.

Returning to our hiker example, this processing stream between the amygdala and vmPFC would emerge as follows: Having already frozen in his tracks through the low-road processing of stimuli via pathways between the amygdala (thalamus to BLA to CeA) and brainstem (the periaqueductal gray), the hiker becomes consciously aware of his circumstance as the amygdala

dACC dorsal anterior cingulate cortex	**dmPFC** dorsomedial prefrontal cortex
dlPFC dorsolateral prefrontal cortex	**ICMs** intercalated cell masses
vlPFC ventrolateral prefrontal cortex	

drives activity in the vmPFC. Almost simultaneously, information about the visual nature (snake or branch?) of the stimulus arrives in the vmPFC via his ventral visual stream; about his location (lakeside trail or hillside trail?) via the hippocampus; and about autonomic changes in his physiology (racing heart, sweaty palms) via the insula. The vmPFC then translates all this information into his subjective feeling that the experience he is having is unpleasant and frightening.

From this stage of early conscious awareness, the vmPFC signals other regions of the prefrontal cortex, including the dmPFC, dACC, dlPFC, and vlPFC. Activity in these prefrontal regions supports more explicit levels of information processing, culminating in executive control, which is the capacity to consciously regulate our behaviors to achieve specific goals (**Figure 2.13B**). We will consider the importance of executive control through these prefrontal regions, particularly the dlPFC, in the regulation of bottom-up drives and emotional responses when we describe the corticohippocampal circuit in Unit III. For now, we turn to a parallel pathway between the vmPFC and dmPFC supporting the second important function of the medial PFC within the corticolimbic circuit: inhibiting the amygdala and terminating output. Populations of neurons in the vmPFC that have been made more responsive through the direct and indirect bottom-up effects of the amygdala now provide excitatory drive to neurons in the adjacent dmPFC. These dmPFC neurons, in turn, project onto two specific populations of neurons in the amygdala that function ultimately to inhibit the CeA and terminate amygdala output (**Figure 2.13C**).

The first of these neuronal populations consists of the ICMs. By driving activity of the ICMs, which synapse directly onto output neurons of the CeA, the dmPFC inhibits amygdala output. Thus, the excitatory drive from the dmPFC activates the "inhibitory moat" function of the ICMs, effectively terminating output of the CeA.

The second target population of the dmPFC is comprised of excitatory neurons within the BLA. These specific BLA neurons synapse onto local inhibitory neurons, which project onto the population of excitatory BLA neurons that drive activity of the CeA. Through this local amygdala circuitry, the excitatory drive from the dmPFC indirectly inhibits CeA output by driving the inhibition of excitatory BLA input.

Such multistage patterns of local inhibition and disinhibition represent one of the more subtle yet more important processes through which the brain shapes and controls our behavior. One of my mentors, the psychiatrist and neuroanatomist Arnold Scheibel at the University of California Los Angeles, elegantly describes this characteristic of the brain as "sculpting in negativity." The critical role of this top-down inhibitory pathway will be highlighted in the next chapter as we review fear learning, and specifically fear extinction.

In addition to this implicit inhibition of the amygdala, the direct projections from the dmPFC to the amygdala likely mediate more explicit forms of emotion regulation, which we will consider in Unit III, initiated by other regions of prefrontal cortex, most notably the dlPFC. However, as there are no direct anatomical connections between these prefrontal regions and the amygdala; their functional interaction is mediated through the dmPFC, which is structurally connected to these regions as well as to the amygdala.

vmPFC	ventromedial prefrontal cortex	**dlPFC**	dorsolateral prefrontal cortex	**BLA**	basolateral complex of the amygdala
dmPFC	dorsomedial prefrontal cortex	**vlPFC**	ventrolateral prefrontal cortex		
dACC	dorsal anterior cingulate cortex			**CeA**	central nucleus of the amygdala

Summary

Through a network of connections between subcortical, cortical, and brainstem structures, the corticolimbic circuit mediates momentary changes in recognition and reaction that help us meet and overcome the challenges we face in our lives. The amygdala functions as the hub of this circuit, integrating incoming information about external triggers and internal states into adaptive changes in our physiology, behavior, and general awareness of our surroundings. The multidimensional changes triggered through the amygdala are integrated into complex behavioral responses encompassing planning and decision making through the medial prefrontal cortex, particularly its ventral division. This bottom-up processing stream culminates in the regulation of the amygdala through top-down inhibitory signals from the dorsal division of the medial prefrontal cortex. Thus, the corticolimbic circuit is engaged by external stimuli, and its very response to these stimuli results in its disengagement and return to a baseline state, where it can monitor the environment for the next trigger.

Literature Cited & Further Reading

Davis, M., Walker, D. L., Miles, L., & Grillon, C. (2010). Phasic versus sustained fear in rats and humans: Role of the extended amygdala in fear versus anxiety. *Neuropsychopharmacology,* 35: 105–135.

de Kloet, E. R., Vreugdenhil, E., Oitzl, M. S., & Joël., M. (1998). Brain corticosteroid receptor balance in health and disease. *Endocrine Reviews,* 19: 269–301

Dolcos, F., LeBar, K. S., & Cabeza, R. 2004. Interaction between the amygdala and the medial temporal lobe memory system predicts better memory for emotional events. *Neuron,* 42: 855–863.

Huber, D., Veinante, P., & Stoop, R. (2005). Vasopressin and oxytocin excite distinct neuronal populations in the central amygdala. *Science,* 308: 245–248.

Kurth, F., Zilles, K., Fox, P. T., Laird, A. R., & Eickhoff, S. B. (2010). A link between the systems: Functional differentiation and integration within the human insula revealed by meta-analysis. *Brain Structure & Function,* 214: 519–534

LeDoux, J. E. (1996). *The emotional brain: The mysterious underpinnings of emotional life.* London: Simon & Schuster.

3

Order

In this chapter, we will initially approach the dynamic functions of the corticolimbic circuit from the perspective of fear learning, as this phenomenon allows for a dissection of the circuit nodes critical for *recognition* and *reaction* discussed in Chapter 2. We then cast our net wider and consider different types of stimuli processed by the corticolimbic circuit (i.e., triggers) and how circuit function helps create order in the way we recognize and react to such stimuli in our environments. In Chapter 4, we will consider how disorder within the corticolimbic circuit emerges as specific symptoms of psychopathology.

Fear Learning

A great deal of our current knowledge of the corticolimbic circuit derives from studies of how animals learn to predict and avoid stimuli that are threatening and/or can cause bodily harm. In controlled laboratory experiments, this phenomenon is best captured through fear learning (**Figure 3.1**) whereby an animal learns that a previously neutral stimulus (e.g., an auditory tone) predicts an aversive stimulus (e.g., an electric shock). After repeated pairings of the two stimuli, the animal expresses a fear response (e.g., freezing in place) to the previously neutral stimulus even in the absence of the aversive stimulus. This initial stage of fear learning is known as **fear conditioning** because the animal learns to fear the previously neutral stimulus (the **conditioned stimulus**, or CS, in this case a tone) through the systematic pairing of that stimulus with an intrinsically aversive stimulus (the **unconditioned stimulus**, or US, here an electric shock).

Quite often, but not necessarily, there is a second stage of fear learning during which the animal gradually learns through repeated presentation of the CS in the absence of the US that the CS no longer predicts the US. This stage of learning is known as **fear extinction** because the conditioned fear response is eliminated or extinguished. In animal studies, fear extinction is generally conducted in a different context from the preceding fear conditioning (e.g., different enclosures with unique features or distinguishing markings easily noticed by the animal). This is done to test the ability of the animal to selectively express a conditioned fear response in a threatening environment and not to express this fear response in a safe or nonthreatening environment. After all, in nature it is adaptive to express fear only in specific threatening

fear conditioning A form of associative learning wherein a previously neutral stimulus (e.g., tone) is repeatedly paired with an aversive stimulus (e.g., electric shock) until the previously neutral stimulus alone elicits a fear response.

conditioned stimulus (CS) A neutral stimulus such as a tone that through fear conditioning comes to elicit a learned fear response.

unconditioned stimulus (US) An aversive stimulus such as an electric shock that is capable of directly causing bodily harm and elicits a reflexive or automatic fear response.

fear extinction A second form of associative learning, independent of fear conditioning, where in a conditioned stimulus is repeatedly presented in a new context and in the absence of an unconditioned stimulus. Leads to the extinction of fear responses to the conditioned stimulus in the new context.

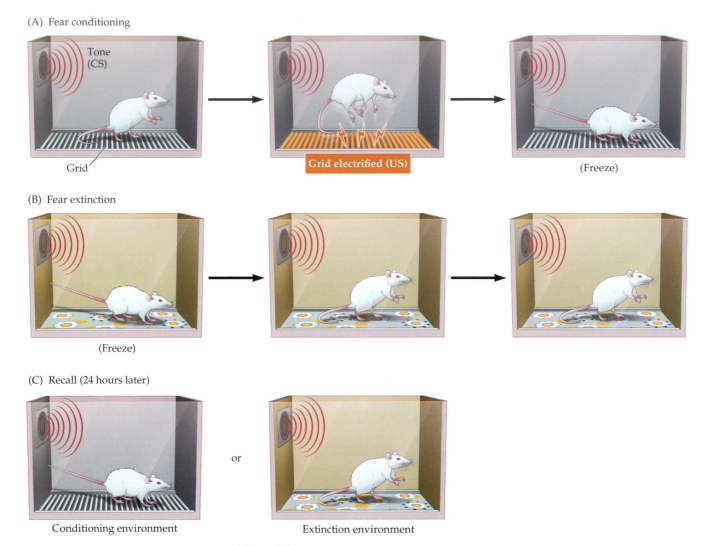

(A) Fear conditioning

Tone (CS)

Grid

Grid electrified (US)

(Freeze)

(B) Fear extinction

(Freeze)

(C) Recall (24 hours later)

or

Conditioning environment

Extinction environment

Figure 3.1 The three common components of fear learning as exemplified by an animal model. (A) In *fear conditioning*, rats are conditioned to fear a previously neutral auditory tone (the conditioned stimulus, or CS) that is repeatedly paired with an electric shock (the unconditioned stimulus, or US). Over time, rats exhibit a fear response (freezing) to the CS alone. (B) In *fear extinction*, the same rats are again repeatedly exposed to the CS, but in a new context and in the absence of the US. The rats learn that there is no cause for fear in this new context and no longer exhibit a fear response to the CS. (C) In the final component, *recall*, rats are placed in either the original context where conditioning occurred or the second context where extinction occurred and, depending on this context, will or will not exhibit fear.

fear recall The context-dependent expression of fear conditioning or fear extinction

contexts (e.g., in a dark abandoned alley) and to suppress fear in nonthreatening contexts (e.g., in the aisle of a supermarket).

Critically, both fear conditioning and fear extinction are learned through key nodes of the corticolimbic circuit described in Chapter 2. Likewise, the ability to express either conditioned fear or extinction after learning, which is often referred to as **fear recall**, is supported by the corticolimbic circuit. In the following sections, we will identify the specific contributions of the amygdala, medial prefrontal cortex, and hippocampal formation to these components of

CS   conditioned stimulus
US   unconditioned stimulus

fear learning. Although we will not explicitly describe the role of all circuit nodes detailed in Chapter 2, it is nevertheless important to consider how they contribute to the overall phenomenon of fear learning by directing information flow through the circuit via input (e.g., from the thalamus) and output (e.g., to the brainstem).

The Amygdala and Fear Conditioning

The amygdala is critical for the first component of fear learning: conditioning. The ability to learn that an aversive stimulus (i.e., the US) is faithfully predicted by a co-occurring signal in the environment (i.e., the CS) depends on the processing of both the US and CS through the amygdala (**Figure 3.2**). The CS inputs typically arrive from the sensory thalamus and sensory cortices (e.g., auditory thalamus and auditory cortex processing an auditory tone). The US inputs typically arrive either directly or indirectly (through the thalamus) from spinal pathways conveying nociceptive information (e.g., free nerve endings responding to an electric shock). Specifically, the CS and US inputs, which occur very close together in time (e.g., only a few milliseconds apart), converge in the BLA. This convergence leads to a stronger activation of neurons in the BLA that project onto those of the CeA. These BLA neurons are sometimes called fear neurons. As the pairing of the CS and US is repeated, the synaptic connections between the BLA fear neurons and CeA are strengthened through the process of long-term potentiation, or LTP. This strengthening of connections between the BLA fear neurons and CeA forms the fundamental basis of fear conditioning.

The end result of this conditioning is that the CS alone activates BLA fear neurons leading to appropriate changes in physiology and behavior through the downstream targets of the CeA (e.g., freezing, through the periaqueductal gray of the brainstem). In this manner, the amygdala learns to recognize stimuli in our environment that predict aversive consequences through converging inputs to the BLA. And, through its output at downstream targets such as the hypothalamus, brainstem, and substantia innominata, the CeA initiates reactions that help us avoid these consequences.

So, how does this fear conditioning mechanism relate to more realistic or natural fears that many of us share and could encounter in the real world? After all, it is not often that we are repeatedly exposed to an electric shock at the same time we hear a loud tone. Thank goodness! To better appreciate this important question, let's return to the example of the hiker encountering a venomous snake on the trail. It is certainly possible that our hiker has encountered snakes before on his treks along the trail and, after several repeated encounters, perhaps even one where he was bitten, has formed a conditioned fear response. If this has occurred, then whenever he encounters a snake (or even a fallen branch), he will freeze to ensure that he will not be bitten. This represents a conditioned, or learned, fear response where the snake represents the CS and the snakebite the US. In all likelihood,

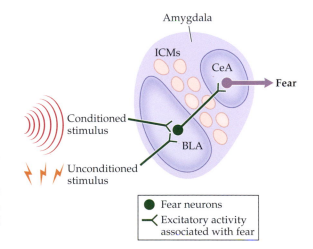

Figure 3.2 During fear conditioning, convergence of inputs representing the CS and US onto "fear" neurons in the basolateral amygdala (BLA) drives activation of neurons in the central nucleus (CeA), which in turn initiate physiological and behavioral responses characteristic of fear. (After Sah & Westbrook, 2008.)

BLA	basolateral complex of the amygdala	LTP	long-term potentiation
CeA	central nucleus of the amygdala	ICMs	intercalated cell masses

one-trial learning A single pairing of a conditioned and an unconditioned stimulus results in a learned association (e.g., fear conditioning) that subsequently elicits a consistent fear response when encountering the CS alone.

indirect fear learning Development of a conditioned fear response after only observing or hearing of the aversive consequences of others' experiences. Also known as observational fear learning.

however, most of us would freeze in this situation, regardless of whether or not we have previously had negative encounters with a snake.

In fact, repeated pairing of a CS and US is not a prerequisite for expressing a fear response; rather, it is only one example of how a conditioned, or learned, fear response can develop. Most of our natural fear responses occur after only a single negative experience (so-called one-trial learning), or even in the absence of any explicit experience altogether. One-trial learning likely reflects both the relative magnitude and the proximity of the association between the CS and US. For example, snakebite is a more serious consequence with greater pain and tissue damage than a mosquito bite. This difference in magnitude of the US results in a stronger and faster learning process in the amygdala (i.e., LTP of connections between BLA and CeA). This learning results in immediate and persistent changes in physiology and behavior whenever a snake is encountered in the future. Many of us would exhibit fear of a snake, but not many of us would be afraid of a mosquito. Moreover, the CS and US are perfectly linked with snakebite—that is, the CS is the very source of the US. This proximity also increases the strength of the learning in the amygdala and the expression of fear. Compare snakebite to the rather distant relationship between an auditory tone and an electric shock, and an appreciation emerges for why you may need only one bad encounter with a snake but many repeated encounters with a tone and shock to learn that fear is an appropriate response. But most of us have never been bitten by a snake or had any negative experiences with them, and still we are fearful. How can this be?

Arguments have been made that certain stimuli are inherently frightening (i.e., we are born with these fears) because of the dire, often fatal consequences associated with them. In fact, studies do suggest that we are faster and better at detecting certain natural threats like snakes and spiders in our environment. This may reflect some intrinsic properties of these stimuli that result in faster processing through neural circuits (e.g., the low road) that have been shaped over time by natural selection. However, there is little empirical evidence to support that these same stimuli are inherently fear-provoking. That is, even though we may detect these stimuli faster, we are not necessarily fearful of them.

What is more likely is that we can form conditioned fear responses not only through a negative experience such as being bitten by a snake, but also through observation or even description of such an experience happening to another person. In other words, we can learn to fear snakes by observing the consequences of someone else being bitten or by hearing how painful and deadly snakebites can be through stories of others' experiences or from nature documentaries on television. Strengthening of the connections between the BLA and CeA supports this indirect form of fear conditioning as well, and it is likely dependent on concurrent activation of CS and US input pathways, albeit in the absence of their direct stimulation. Such indirect fear learning gives us a great advantage in surviving the dangers of our worlds by allowing us to learn important associations without having to suffer the direct consequences. (It's also likely why we actually feel afraid when watching a scary movie, even though the action is confined to the screen.) We will discuss the importance of learning about threat in our environments through the experiences of others later in the chapter, when we review the research on human faces and facial expressions as triggers of the amygdala and corticolimbic circuit.

CS	conditioned stimulus	BLA	basolateral complex of the amygdala
US	unconditioned stimulus	CeA	central nucleus of the amygdala
LTP	long-term potentiation		

RESEARCH SPOTLIGHT

Indirect, or observational, fear learning may not be unique to humans. As reported by Jeon and colleagues (2010), mice who merely observe other mice receiving an electric shock will exhibit freezing behavior even though they have never been shocked directly (**Figure 3.3**). The observers continue to display this fear response when placed in the original surroundings 24 hours after the experiment. Such observational fear learning in mice appears to depend on the functioning of the corticolimbic circuit, particularly of the amygdala and the mouse equivalent of our medial prefrontal cortex.

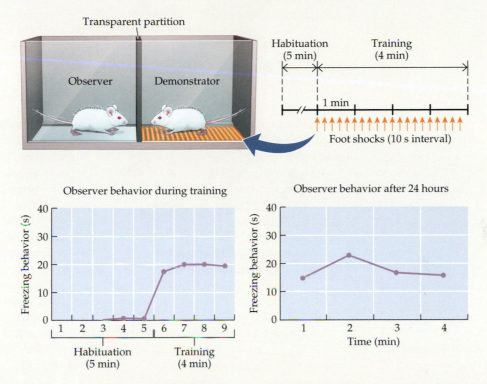

Figure 3.3 When a mouse is allowed to observe another mouse undergoing fear conditioning by receiving electric shocks to the feet, the observer exhibits fear responses (freezing), even though it has never experienced the US. When placed back in the context of having observed the fear conditioning, the observer's conditioned fear response continues to be expressed the next day. (After Jeon et al., 2010.)

The Medial Prefrontal Cortex and Fear Extinction

The medial prefrontal cortex is critical for the second component of fear learning: extinction. Before reviewing the changes in corticolimbic circuit function supporting extinction, it is important to note that fear extinction is an active process, requiring a form of learning that is independent of that supporting fear conditioning. In other words, fear extinction represents a second pathway of learning that operates in parallel to the learning that supports fear conditioning (**Figure 3.4**). Fear extinction is not simply forgetting or eliminating the learning of fear conditioning, as might be inferred from the experimental paradigm of extinction wherein the CS is presented in the absence of the US.

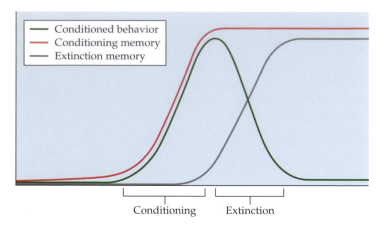

Figure 3.4 Fear conditioning and fear extinction represent two parallel but independent forms of learning that function to control the expression and extinction of conditioned fear. (After Quirk et al., 2006.)

During extinction, the absence of the US input to the BLA reduces the activation of the pathway between the BLA and CeA that drives fear conditioning. The CS input to the BLA is still present during extinction but, without the converging US input, the CS does not drive BLA activity as strongly. What is critical for extinction is *concurrent processing* of the CS input through sensory cortices by the mPFC. Recall that as a component of the general flow of information through the corticolimbic circuit, the bottom-up signal from the amygdala drives the vmPFC, which in turn drives activity of the dmPFC. Thus, the processing of the CS input as well as the top-down inhibitory activity of the dmPFC is enhanced. We will now consider how this top-down inhibitory activity is accomplished.

The dmPFC actively prevents the expression of conditioned fear responses, and it promotes the expression of fear extinction through the inhibition of the CeA (**Figure 3.5**). This is accomplished through two primary pathways

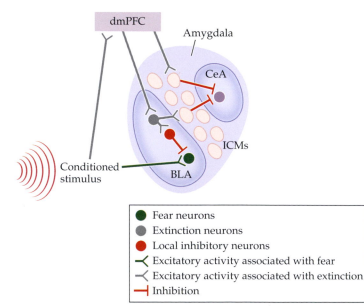

Figure 3.5 During fear extinction, inputs from the dorsomedial prefrontal cortex activate inhibitory neurons of the intercalated cell masses (ICMs)—either directly or through activation of a distinct subset of extinction neurons in the BLA, which further function to inhibit fear neurons in the BLA. These parallel pathways result in the inhibition of neurons in the CeA and the extinction of fear. (After Sah & Westbrook, 2008.)

● Fear neurons
● Extinction neurons
● Local inhibitory neurons
⊰ Excitatory activity associated with fear
⊰ Excitatory activity associated with extinction
⊣ Inhibition

CS	conditioned stimulus	mPFC	medial prefrontal cortex
US	unconditioned stimulus	dmPFC	dorsomedial prefrontal cortex
BLA	basolateral complex of the amygdala	vmPFC	ventromedial prefrontal cortex
CeA	central nucleus of the amygdala		

described in Chapter 2. In the first, dmPFC neurons drive activity of the ICMs, which inhibit the CeA directly. In the second, dmPFC neurons drive activity of a subpopulation of BLA neurons, sometimes called extinction neurons. These BLA extinction neurons then effect two changes: direct stimulation of the ICMs working to inhibit the CeA; and activation of another subpopulation of BLA neurons, which in turn inhibit those BLA fear neurons driving the CeA. The repeated presentation of the CS drives activity in the dmPFC and strengthens (again through LTP) its connections with the amygdala. These pathways between the dmPFC and amygdala represent the second **learning trace** that mediates extinction of the original trace (e.g., freezing) through top-down inhibition.

Importantly, if the US occurs again in the presence of the CS, the original fear conditioning is quickly reestablished through the amygdala. The fear conditioning pathway generally dominates the two learning traces because information is processed through it more directly (e.g., thalamic sensory and spinal pain signals). We can speculate that this pathway also dominates because it is better to express a conditioned fear response in the absence of a threat than to express an extinction response in the presence of a threat.

Much as with the broader relevance of the pathway between the BLA and CeA for the expression of nonconditioned fear (e.g., observational fear learning), the extinction pathway between the dmPFC and CeA is important for inhibiting all forms of fear, including those learned indirectly. Returning to our hiker example, after freezing to avoid the snake ahead of him on the path, he reroutes around the snake and resumes his trek. Activity of the dmPFC and activation of the inhibitory pathways between the dmPFC and amygdala suppress CeA output driving the periaqueductal gray (PAG) and generating freezing. By inhibiting the CeA, the dmPFC allows the hiker to break his frozen stance and initiate an adaptive response (i.e., going off the trail and around the snake). This top-down inhibitory pathway takes over as part of the normal flow of information through the corticolimbic circuit even if we have not undergone formal extinction learning (i.e., repeated encounters with a snake where we are not bitten). If the dmPFC failed to inhibit CeA output, the fear response would persist and the hiker would remain frozen in his tracks (at least until someone came along to help). This is certainly not an adaptive response. As we will learn in Chapter 4, disorder in this top-down extinction pathway often contributes as much as the bottom-up conditioning pathway to psychopathology, especially anxiety disorders.

The Hippocampal Formation and Fear Recall

Now that we have learned how fear conditioning is mediated through the amygdala and fear extinction through the dmPFC, we will consider how it is that we appropriately express one and not the other form of fear learning. The hippocampal formation helps shape such context-appropriate expression or recall of either conditioning or extinction. This gating function reflects the critical importance of the HF for determining the location and context for specific experiences (e.g., environment A for fear conditioning and environment B for fear extinction; see Figure 3.1).

During fear learning, the HF is encoding information about the environment, which as we saw in Chapter 2, is directly (via the BLA) and indirectly (via the NBM) potentiated by the amygdala. During fear conditioning, this potentiated HF activity helps create a memory for the context in which the

learning trace Increased communication within specific neural pathways supporting associative learning such as fear conditioning and fear extinction.

ICMs	intercalated cell masses	HF	hippocampal formation
LTP	long-term potentiation	NBM	nucleus basalis of Meynert
PAG	periaqueductal gray		

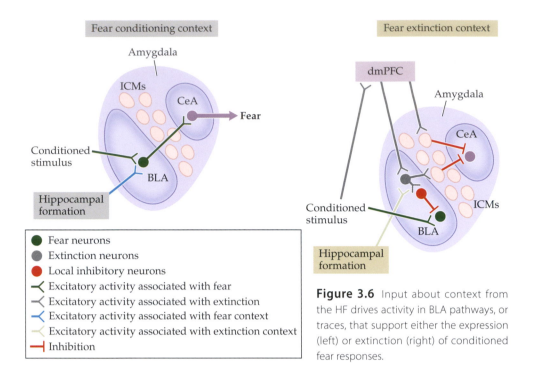

Figure 3.6 Input about context from the HF drives activity in BLA pathways, or traces, that support either the expression (left) or extinction (right) of conditioned fear responses.

CS and US were repeatedly paired together. This is commonly referred to as context conditioning and manifests as a heightened fear response when the animal is placed in the same context in which the CS was paired with the US. In contrast, the amygdala is mediating what is commonly referred to as cue conditioning (i.e., fear of the CS directly).

After fear conditioning and fear extinction have been learned, it is this memory for context created through the HF that helps determine which of the learning traces shown in **Figure 3.6** is expressed. The available evidence suggests that HF activity associated with encoding the context where fear conditioning occurred drives pathways resulting in activation of the CeA and the expression of fear. In contrast, HF activity associated with encoding the safe context, where fear extinction occurred, drives pathways resulting in inhibition of the CeA and suppression of the fear response (i.e., extinction).

Let's now consider how this gating function of the HF operates more generally to control the expression or inhibition of fear, by returning to our hiker. A week has passed since his encounter with the snake, and he bravely returns for another trek along the hillside trail. He begins at the trailhead and, after an hour, approaches the section of the trail where he only narrowly avoided being bitten a week ago. Thanks to the context memory provided by the HF, he recognizes this section of the trail and remembers to be cautious. Activity in the HF associated with this fearful context also functions to drive the fear neurons in the BLA, resulting in activation of the CeA. As we have seen, activity of the CeA mediates a host of changes. Most relevant here is the increase in general arousal (via the NBM) and increased processing of information about our hiker's immediate environment (via the sensory cortices).

CS	conditioned stimulus	ICMs	intercalated cell masses
US	unconditioned stimulus	CeA	central nucleus of the amygdala
HF	hippocampal formation	BLA	basolateral complex of the amygdala
dmPFC	dorsomedial prefrontal cortex	NBM	nucleus basalis of Meynert

This state of heightened vigilance prepares him to react quickly if a threat is recognized. If another snake is detected he will freeze (via the PAG) and again avoid being bitten. In fact, his freezing response will likely be larger than when he first encountered the snake, because of the heightened arousal and general activation of the corticolimbic circuit associated with merely being back on the hillside trail. These exaggerated reactions are described as **fear potentiation**.

If, however, there is no snake and he passes on to other sections of the trail where he hasn't encountered danger—and there is neither CS nor context signals of fear—he can return to a baseline state (calm and relaxed) and enjoy the rest of his hike. Thus, the context memory of where he is hiking (hillside or lakeside trail) as represented by activity in the HF helps determine when fear should, or should not be expressed.

Beyond Fear Learning

Consistent with experiments in animals, imaging studies have revealed similarly important contributions of the corticolimbic circuit to fear learning in humans. For example, the magnitude of amygdala activity in response to a CS predicts the strength of a fear response, whereas the magnitude of activity in the vmPFC and hippocampal formation predict the ability to successfully inhibit fear following extinction (**Figure 3.7**). The selective contributions of specific corticolimbic circuit nodes to discrete components of fear learning have been further documented in studies of patients with specific lesions (**Figure 3.8**). For example, studies of patients with isolated amygdala lesions have demonstrated specific impairments in generating conditioned fear responses while retaining the ability to describe facts about the experiment itself, even including details of the CS-US pairing. In contrast, patients with isolated lesions of the hippocampal formation have shown normal conditioned fear responses but impairments in retaining facts about the experiment. The latter pattern reflects the importance of the HF in forming declarative memories, which will be considered in Unit III.

Much like their animal counterparts, human fear-learning experiments represent a highly specific form of behavior (e.g., tone–shock pairings) that are not representative of our daily lives and common experiences. They are also very difficult to conduct, because of the need for specialized equipment that

fear potentiation Increased quickness and strength of response (typically of reflexive responses like startle) when in a state of fear.

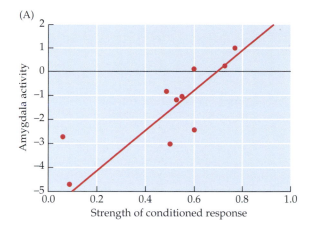

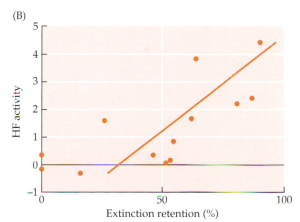

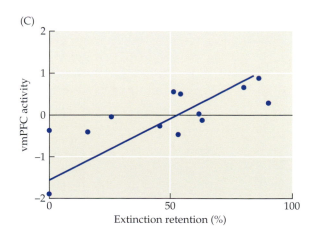

Figure 3.7 (A) The magnitude of amygdala activation in response to a conditioned stimulus after fear conditioning predicts the strength of the conditioned response, measured here as changes in skin conductance or electrodermal activity (sweating). (B,C) In contrast, the magnitude of activity in the vmPFC and hippocampal formation predict the ability to successfully inhibit fear following extinction. Note that 0 represents mean activity in these data. (A after Phelps et al., 2004; B,C after Milad et al., 2007.)

PAG   periaqueductal gray
vmPFC ventromedial prefrontal cortex

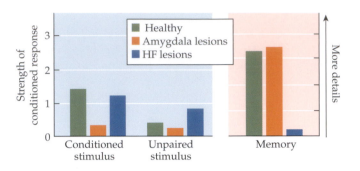

Figure 3.8 Specific lesions to the amygdala impair conditioned fear responses, as indexed by increased sweating in response to conditioned stimuli in comparison with unpaired stimuli (left). However, these amygdala lesions do not affect the ability to consciously remember details of the experiment (right). In contrast, specific lesions to the hippocampal formation impair conscious recollection of the experiment but do not affect conditioned fear responses. (After LaBar & Phelps, 2005.)

is compatible with MRI (e.g., nonmagnetic sensors and stimulators) as well as the requirement to deliver highly unpleasant if not painful electric shocks or similar aversive stimulation. The latter becomes particularly difficult when studying patients with mood and anxiety disorders. Because of these limitations and challenges, the majority of human fMRI studies of corticolimbic circuit function employ pictorial stimuli representing different forms of threat. These stimuli can include pictures of natural threats in our environment, such as snakes, spiders, sharks, and snarling dogs; or threats unique to our modern lives, such as car crashes, shipwrecks, and acts of terror. However, one particular category of stimulus is by far the most common and most effective in triggering the corticolimbic circuit in fMRI studies. What is this ubiquitous stimulus that triggers incredibly strong responses from the corticolimbic circuit, especially the amygdala? You need look no further than a mirror.

About Face!

From the moment of our birth, there may be no more important stimulus in our lives than human faces. The critical importance of these stimuli is readily apparent in the almost instantaneous search for and fixation with human faces displayed by nearly every baby. Arguably, human faces represent the most important source of information about our environment. In fact, we have what at times is a rather amusing tendency to recognize faces in inanimate objects (**Figure 3.9**). This is because we are a highly social species and our survival depends as much on others as ourselves. What we lack in physical tools to conquer challenges in our world (we don't have the jaws of a lion, the girth of a hippo, the speed of an antelope, or a dog's sense of smell) we make up for in our ability to work together, or cooperate.

In the context of cooperation, human faces not only serve as a direct means of establishing identity (this is my wife; this is my child; this a friend; this is a stranger), but also provide critical cues about what's going on around us and what appropriate actions we should take in response. All facial expressions convey important information about our environment, but a few specific expressions—particularly fear and anger—may be the most critical for our survival. As we will see, facial expressions actually get us closer to fear learning than may be obvious at first glance.

Hopefully, the parallels between human faces and facial expressions as important signals from our environment, and the amygdala and the rest of the corticolimbic circuit as a system for recognizing and reacting to such

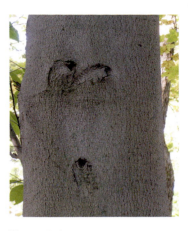 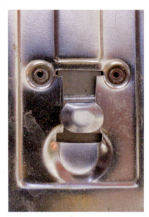 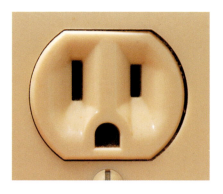

Figure 3.9 Most humans exhibit a strong tendency to recognize faces and even emotional expressions—surprise, happiness, fear—in inanimate objects. (Photographs courtesy of D. McIntyre.)

signals, are now clear. Next we will consider why certain specific emotional expressions act as powerful triggers of the amygdala. Note that we will largely focus on the response of the amygdala to different facial expressions and will not discuss the response of the other nodes of the corticolimbic circuit. This is because, as the hub of the circuit, the amygdala's activity generally carries forward to these other nodes (e.g., the brainstem) in the context of generating appropriate reactions (e.g., freezing) and regulating these reactions in an adaptive fashion (e.g., inhibiting the amygdala after the threat is eliminated via the dmPFC). As we will see in the next chapter, disorder in this flow of information, particularly in the communication between the amygdala and mPFC, contributes to psychopathology of mood and anxiety.

RESEARCH SPOTLIGHT

Among his many contributions to science, Charles Darwin may have been the first to systematically study and describe the critical importance of human faces, particularly human facial expressions, in shaping our behaviors. In his 1872 book *The Expression of the Emotions in Man and Animals*, Darwin astutely noted that rapid changes in our facial expressions are outward signals of basic emotional states such as fear and anger. He further argued that because such emotional facial expressions are difficult if not impossible to display volitionally in the absence of the underlying emotion (i.e., they cannot be faked), they represent "honest indicators" of our intentions or experiences. Thus, we can learn a great deal about each other, as well as our shared environment, by detecting and learning to interpret facial expressions. We will discuss this aspect of facial expressions in detail below. The contemporary psychologist Paul Ekman has extended these observations by Darwin through demonstration that some facial expressions are recognized universally and that even subtle changes in facial features can reveal important information about a person's intentions and state of mind.

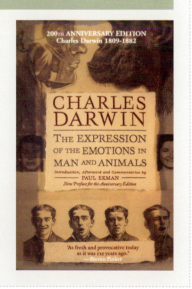

dmPFC   dorsomedial prefrontal cortex
mPFC   medial prefrontal cortex

Specific Expressions

Researchers have identified six basic emotional facial expressions that are recognized across most individuals and cultures. They are anger, fear, disgust, happiness, sadness, and surprise (**Figure 3.10**). When presented during fMRI, all of these facial expressions can trigger amygdala activity, and this is particularly true for fear and anger. In addition, so-called neutral expressions, which display no clear expression, also elicit amygdala activity in certain contexts. In the following sections, we briefly discuss what specific qualities of fearful, angry, surprised, and neutral expressions are associated with amygdala activity. We focus on these expressions because they all convey information about potential threat in our environment and, accordingly, trigger the amygdala and extended corticolimbic circuit to generate appropriate reactions and responses. We will briefly consider amygdala activity in response to happy and sad facial expressions when we describe corticolimbic circuit dysfunction in depression in Chapter 4.

You're in trouble now! (Anger)

Angry facial expressions are the clearest signals of threat or danger in our immediate environment. We learn through experience that when a person displaying an expression of anger confronts us, they intend to inflict bodily harm or some other ill will. An angry facial expression is effectively a CS (like the tone in fear conditioning) that predicts a US (an aversive consequence,

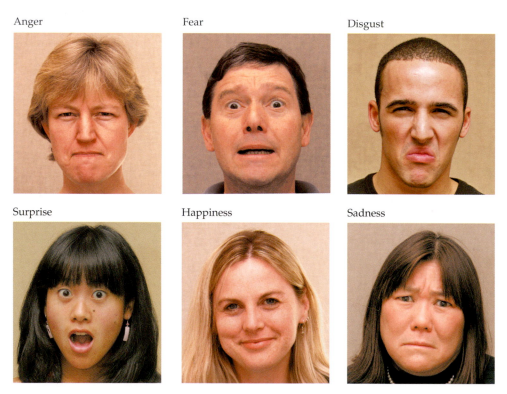

Anger Fear Disgust

Surprise Happiness Sadness

Figure 3.10 The six basic emotional facial expressions that can trigger amygdala activity: anger, fear, disgust, surprise, happiness, and sadness. (Photographs courtesy of D. McIntyre.)

CS conditioned stimulus
US unconditioned stimulus

RESEARCH SPOTLIGHT

Almost all of the facial expression stimuli used in fMRI research involve individuals with what is commonly referred to as direct gaze. That is, the individual posing the expression is looking straight at the viewer. In reality, the direction of eye gaze varies as a function of the situation and conveys important information above and beyond the facial expression. The importance of eye gaze becomes clear when we consider our two canonical CS facial expressions: fear and anger. In virtually every study using fearful and angry facial expressions, the eye gaze for both is directed at the viewer (i.e., the faces are looking straight at you). This makes sense with angry facial expressions, since in real life they are almost always directed toward the target of aggression. With fearful expressions, however, it is far less common that someone experiencing fear would be looking straight at you (unless, perhaps, you were angry and threatening them).

More commonly, someone is fearful of something they have encountered in the environment (e.g., the rattlesnake on the hillside path). As a consequence, a fearful facial expression typically involves eye gaze directed at the source of threat (i.e., averted from you). In a now classic fMRI study, Adams and colleagues manipulated the direction of eye gaze for angry and fearful facial expressions and recorded the differential activity of the amygdala to four possible combinations: anger with directed gaze, anger with averted gaze, fear with directed gaze, and fear with averted gaze (**Figure 3.11A**). What they found was a remarkable pattern of amygdala activity that followed the relative clarity with which each combination signaled threat (**Figure 3.11B**). The strongest amygdala activity was observed to the combinations that least clearly signaled threat: anger with averted gaze and fear with directed gaze. The weakest amygdala activity was observed to combinations that most clearly signaled threat: anger with directed gaze and fear with averted gaze.

Thus, when the source of threat in the environment is clear, less amygdala activity is needed to generate an appropriate reaction (e.g., he is angry with me, or he is afraid of something in front of him on the path). But, when the source of the threat is unclear, more amygdala activity is needed to drive downstream targets that will work to help you determine what the actual threat may be (e.g., With whom is he angry? Why is he afraid of me?). This role of the amygdala to help resolve where (or what) exactly is the source of threat depends on the increased arousal mediated through cholinergic tone via the NBM and increased activity of neuromodulatory centers in the brainstem. This clever experiment sheds light on the importance of the amygdala and extended corticolimbic circuit for helping us learn about our environment by diffusing our attention, particularly when the signals are unclear. This sensitivity to ambiguity is key in the activity of the amygdala to the two other expressions we consider: surprise and neutral.

(A)

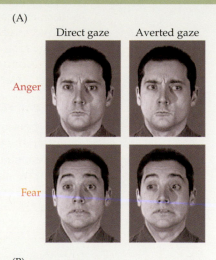

(B)

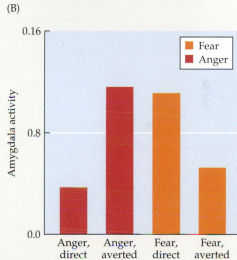

Figure 3.11 The magnitude of amygdala activity in response to fearful and angry facial expressions depends on the direction of eye gaze (A) and the associated ambiguity about where the threat is located in the environment. (B) Greater ambiguity regarding the source of the threat is communicated by anger with averted gaze than by anger with direct gaze. Likewise, fear with direct gaze elicits stronger amygdala activity than the less ambiguous signaling of threat by fear with averted gaze. Note that 0 represents baseline activity in these data. (After Adams et al., 2003.)

NBM   nucleus basalis of Meynert

such as the electric shock in conditioning). In fact, much like a snake, an angry expression is a very powerful CS because it perfectly represents the US, or aversive consequence, with which it is associated. Thus, amygdala activity in response to angry expressions is a reflection of the fear learning that has occurred over time and results in specific defensive behaviors (e.g., freezing if the angry person is far enough away and you can escape detection, or increased muscle tension and blood flow to your extremities if the person is close and ready to attack).

Look out! (Fear)

Similar to angry faces, facial expressions of fear represent a CS. With fear, however, the US is not always clear. The fear expressed by another person could be elicited by any number of stimuli in your shared environment, but a fearful facial expression is a clear signal that something harmful or threatening exists and that you should take appropriate action in much the same way the person making the expression should. Perhaps, for example, you are traveling along the hillside path and meet our hiker moving toward you just as he almost steps on the rattlesnake. The fearful expression on his face triggers activity in your amygdala, which initiates a cascade of responses—most prominently increased arousal leading to a search for the threatening stimulus in your shared local environment (i.e., the snake on the path). Thus, a fear expression is generally a trigger of increased sensory and attentional processing of stimuli in your environment (i.e., scanning for threat) mediated through the amygdala and extended corticolimbic circuit.

What's happening? (Surprise)

It should come as no surprise that the two quintessential expressions associated with threat—fear and anger—are very powerful amygdala triggers. What about facial expressions that are less clearly linked to a negative outcome? The best example of such an ambiguous expression is surprise. The valence of a surprised expression—that is, whether it is associated with a positive or negative emotion—is determined largely by the context in which it is observed. Paul Whalen at Dartmouth College uses the following manipulation to demonstrate this context-dependent nature of surprised expressions. Imagine seeing someone with a surprised expression as it is revealed that they have won the lottery. For most of us, this surprised expression would be subjectively identified as being clearly positive in valence. Now take the same person and the same surprised expression, but change the context to that person having just discovered they are a prime suspect in a double homicide. Most of us would find this example of a surprised expression as clearly negative in valence as we would find the earlier example clearly positive. Thus, the context is critical in determining the potential relevance and meaning of surprised expressions, which are otherwise ambiguous in valence (i.e., neither clearly positive nor clearly negative).

The amygdala activity observed in response to surprised expressions functions to generate arousal broadly (via cholinergic potentiation through the NBM or other neuromodulatory signals supplied by brainstem nuclei) and increased activity specifically in the prefrontal cortex. This bottom-up flow of information works to help us determine what exactly is the nature or context of the surprised expression we are observing (e.g., it's a surprise birthday party, or it's someone just noticing the blue and red lights of a

CS	conditioned stimulus
US	unconditioned stimulus
NBM	nucleus basalis of Meynert

police car behind them on the highway). It's only after such elaboration occurs that we can respond most appropriately (e.g., smile and sing happy birthday, or advise the driver to remain calm and slowly pull off to the side of the highway).

RESEARCH SPOTLIGHT

The eyes are the windows to the soul and to… the amygdala? There are many individual elements or features that comprise a face, and there are unique configurations of these elements that characterize the basic emotional expressions. So what, if any, specific features trigger the amygdala? As evident in the musings of many philosophers, poets, and writers, it appears that the eyes have it when it comes to reaching not only our soul but also our amygdala. While this may be somewhat obvious simply from comparing differences in the shape and position of the eyes across the different facial expressions, a landmark study by Paul Whalen and colleagues at Dartmouth College provides us with concrete evidence for the importance of the eyes, and more specifically the white of the eye, or sclera.

In their fMRI study, healthy participants viewed neutral facial expressions. Unbeknownst to the subjects, each of these facial expressions was very briefly preceded (for 33 milliseconds) by just the eyes from either a happy facial expression or a fearful facial expression. This procedure, in which a different stimulus is

rapidly (i.e., subconsciously) presented immediately before a perceived stimulus, is known as backward masking (**Figure 3.12**, left). In this case, backward masking was used so the eyes were not consciously perceived by the participants. After the experiment, subjects reported having been aware of (i.e., seeing) only the neutral facial expressions. However, differences in activity revealed that the amygdala detected either fearful or happy eyes even when the subjects did not remember seeing them. Specifically, amygdala activity was greater to neutral expressions preceded by fearful eyes, which show more of the sclera, than to those same neutral expressions preceded by happy eyes, which show less of the sclera and more of the pupil and iris (**Figure 3.12**, right). These results indicate that the eyes—and specifically the amount of the sclera displayed—are a key element of emotional facial expressions that trigger amygdala activity. As we will discover in Chapter 4, such sensitivity to the information conveyed by the eyes may contribute to the emergence of disorders such as autism.

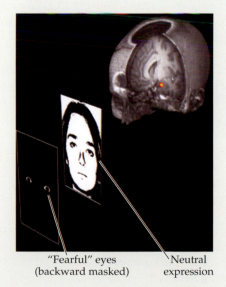

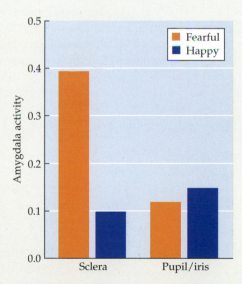

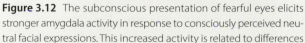
"Fearful" eyes (backward masked)   Neutral expression

Figure 3.12 The subconscious presentation of fearful eyes elicits stronger amygdala activity in response to consciously perceived neutral facial expressions. This increased activity is related to differences in the sclera, which is more visible with fearful expressions compared with other expressions (including happy) than differences in the pupil or iris. (After Whalen et al., 2004.)

Friend or foe? (Neutral)

While we might assume that a face displaying no identifiable facial expression (i.e., a blank stare) carries no useful information, in fact a so-called neutral expression can convey a very important signal about a person and, possibly, our environment. This is evident from the generally strong amygdala activity to neutral expressions observed in fMRI studies. In particular, the amygdala exhibits a strong response to neutral expressions from faces we have never seen before.

In fact, a neutral expression from a familiar face (e.g., a parent or a sibling) doesn't trigger a large amygdala response, presumably because we know these people and can expect or predict their general behavior and whether they are friend or foe. In contrast, an unfamiliar or novel face with a neutral expression is a particularly potent source of uncertainty. This uncertainty lies in the fact that we have no prior history with those people and thus cannot predict their behavior; and because there is no clear expression presented, our ability to determine a momentarily appropriate response is limited.

Because of this dearth of information, in many ways a blank stare from a stranger may be the most disconcerting stimulus we commonly encounter. The results are not dissimilar to the amygdala response observed to the ambiguity conveyed by surprised expressions. However, uncertainty (i.e., I don't have any basis for a response) can be even worse than ambiguity (i.e., it could be good or bad). The amygdala response triggered by the uncertainty of a neutral expression on a newly encountered face functions to help us learn more about the person and the context in which we encounter them and, if necessary, to quickly defend ourselves if the person turns out to be a threat.

The amygdala response to neutral, novel faces, however, does not necessarily imply a threat response. Novel people (or things) can just as easily represent sources of benefit (e.g., a new source of food or help in fighting off predators). Remember that one of the important roles of the amygdala is to generate increased arousal and diffuse attention, particularly through prefrontal circuits, allowing us to learn more about our environment. In the case of novel, neutral expressions, amygdala activity is most likely related to this broader learning phenomenon. That is, the amygdala is generating a change in our arousal and attention that helps us determine who this new person is and what, if any, importance they may have in our own lives.

Just Chill Out: Amygdala Habituation

habituation The gradual decrease in amygdala activity over time when a conditioned stimulus is not followed by an unconditioned stimulus.

While facial expressions signaling important information about our environment consistently trigger amygdala activity and through this activity engage the rest of the corticolimbic circuit, amygdala activity and its downstream effects are normally limited in duration. In fact, repeatedly presenting any of these facial expressions over a short period of time (the 5 to 10 minutes of a typical fMRI scan, for example) results in a significant decrease in amygdala activity (**Figure 3.13**). This decrease over repeated presentations is commonly referred to as **habituation**. Inasmuch as amygdala activity in response to facial expressions is representative of fear conditioning, amygdala habituation to facial expressions is representative of fear extinction. This is particularly true for fearful and angry expressions, but also holds for surprised and neutral expressions.

CS	conditioned stimulus
US	unconditioned stimulus

Investigators have argued that amygdala habituation to the repeated presentation of fearful or angry expressions in fMRI studies effectively represents fear extinction wherein the CS (facial expression) is unpaired from the US (e.g., being attacked in the case of anger, or encountering a rattlesnake in the case of fear). Of course, the original fear conditioning has occurred before the fMRI scan ever begins, representing each person's experiences (direct or indirect) with angry and fearful facial expressions over a lifetime.

When these expressions are first presented during fMRI, there is robust amygdala activity reflecting the fear conditioning that has occurred. As this activity is propagated through the corticolimbic circuit, the broader context (i.e., I am inside a scanner with no one else around) of the expressions' appearance is processed through the hippocampal formation. Having been stimulated by CeA outputs to the NBM and brainstem, the vmPFC functions to integrate all of the information available (i.e., I'm not experiencing any negative consequences when I see these expressions and I'm in a scanner as part of a research study). The successful integration of this information over time results in the top-down inhibition of amygdala activity via the dmPFC as a function of having learned that these expressions in this context no longer predict threat.

Amygdala habituation to surprised and neutral facial expressions reflects a similar flow of information processing; however, this decrease in activity likely reflects the growing familiarity with neutral facial expressions, because with repeated presentations they are no longer novel and, moreover, have not predicted any changes in our environment. The absence of meaningful changes in our environment (either good or bad) is likely why amygdala habituation to surprised expressions occurs. A failure of the vmPFC to integrate bottom-up signaling and initiate top-down inhibition through the dmPFC results in sustained amygdala activity (i.e., no habituation) and, as we will see in the next chapter, may be present in mood and anxiety disorders.

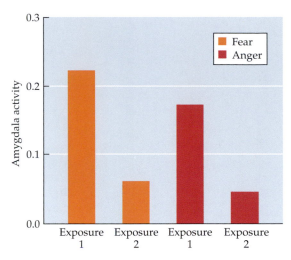

Figure 3.13 Amygdala activity habituates with repeated presentations of threat-related stimuli like angry and fearful facial expressions when they are not paired with aversive or unpleasant stimulation. Note that 0 represents baseline activity in these data. (After Fisher et al., 2009.)

Anxiety

The overall functioning of the corticolimbic circuit described above is usefully captured through dimensional measures of state and trait anxiety. **State anxiety** reflects the experience of unpleasant emotional arousal (i.e., fear) when confronted with a threat or in a dangerous situation. **Trait anxiety**, in contrast, reflects the tendency of an individual to experience state anxiety if confronted with a threat, or in a dangerous situation. Obviously, the experience of state anxiety or fear is necessary for adaptive responding to threat (i.e., you don't want to be oblivious to an actual threat), but high levels of trait anxiety can lead to maladaptive responding (e.g., worrying about being harmed even in the absence of threat). In comparison to someone who is relatively low in trait anxiety, for example, a person who is relatively high would be more apprehensive and nervous about walking home through an otherwise familiar and safe park if it's after dark. Importantly, this apprehension emerges even in the absence of any clear threat or danger, such as a menacing person lurking at the edge of the park or a loud commotion

state anxiety The experience of unpleasant emotional arousal such as fear in response to threat or danger.

trait anxiety The general tendency to experience state anxiety if confronted by threat or danger.

mPFC	medial prefrontal cortex
CeA	central nucleus of the amygdala
NBM	nucleus basalis of Meynert
vmPFC	ventromedial prefrontal cortex
dmPFC	dorsomedial prefrontal cortex

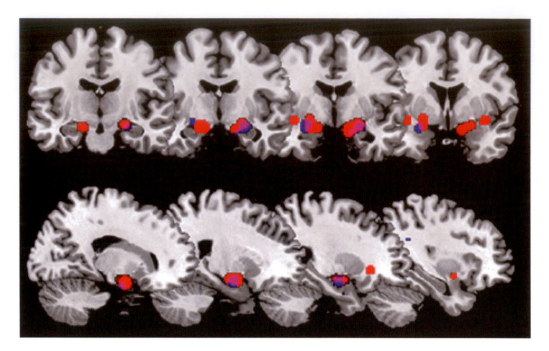

Figure 3.14 Increased amygdala activity to fearful and angry facial expressions is associated with higher levels of trait anxiety (red areas) and state anxiety (blue areas). Areas of overlap are seen as pale purple. (From Calder et al., 2011.)

coming from within the park. These scenarios would lead to appropriate levels of fear. It is the presence or absence of clear and present danger that most differentiates state anxiety or fear from trait anxiety. Although high trait anxiety is not in and of itself a disorder or psychopathology, higher levels are commonly observed in individuals at risk for developing mood and anxiety disorders, and presence of high trait anxiety cuts across many categorical disorders.

As you might imagine, high trait anxiety is associated with relatively increased amygdala activity (and decreased habituation) to threat cues (**Figure 3.14**). This is particularly true for threat cues that are ambiguous in nature, such as fearful and surprised facial expressions, because there is higher intrinsic uncertainty about the potential threat with these cues. High trait anxiety is also associated with increased activity in the insula, which may reflect a greater sensitivity to even subtle changes in physiology such as heart rate or respiration, which may then be misinterpreted as interoceptive signals of threat. More importantly, high trait anxiety is associated with decreased activity of the prefrontal cortex, particularly the vmPFC and dmPFC. There is also evidence of decreased functional connectivity between the amygdala and these prefrontal regions with higher trait anxiety. These alterations result in a diminished capacity to integrate bottom-up signals from the amygdala and insula, and then institute top-down regulation of the amygdala. Such disorder or imbalance between bottom-up and top-down information flow through the corticolimbic circuit is a hallmark of psychopathology reflecting maladaptive recognition of and reaction to threat, as we will see in the next chapter.

vmPFC ventromedial prefrontal cortex
dmPFC dorsomedial prefrontal cortex

Summary

The ultimate expression of the corticolimbic circuit is as changes in our recognition of and reaction to threat in our environment. In many ways, this expression can be portrayed by analogy with the behaviors and interactions of a keen watchdog and his responsible owner. A watchdog will respond by barking whenever he notices a change in his surroundings (e.g., when someone rings the doorbell or walks up the driveway). This initial barking response parallels the functions of the amygdala in recognizing changes in our environment. When we are at home and hear our watchdog bark, we quickly turn our attention to him and determine why he is barking. We may check the front door or look out the window to see who is on our property. This change in our behavior in response to the dog's barking parallels the results of amygdala output, especially engagement of the prefrontal cortex.

If we do see someone on our property, we next determine who it is: a friend dropping by unexpectedly, the postman delivering a package, or a burglar in a ski mask. This determination requires activity not only of our executive decision making skills via the prefrontal cortex, but also of our long-term memory via the hippocampal formation and our visual acuity via the ventral visual stream. Activity in these areas is elevated as a result of amygdala activity, helping us determine exactly who is on our property and if they might pose a threat. Once we determine who the person is, we approach our watchdog and instruct him appropriately—to stop barking and sit beside us if it is the postman, or to keep barking and make himself visible in the front window if it is a burglar. The feedback we give our watchdog to control his barking parallels the feedback provided by the prefrontal cortex to the amygdala.

The above scenario works only when all parts of the circuit, particularly the amygdala and medial prefrontal cortex, are working effectively. As we will see in Chapter 4, a breakdown in corticolimbic circuit function wreaks havoc on our behaviors, just as a watchdog wreaks havoc if his owner does not shape and control his responses. If we are not at home, for example, the watchdog will bark as long as a stranger remains on the property—and sometimes well after the person has left if, much like people who have high levels of anxiety, the dog is unable to recognize that the potential danger is gone.

While this analogy provides a useful way to consider the very broad functioning of the corticolimbic circuit, the process of fear learning as reviewed in detail at the beginning of this chapter is arguably most representative of the critical importance of the circuit for our survival. It will be useful to keep in mind both this analogy and the component processes of fear learning as we discuss how disorder within the corticolimbic circuit is expressed as specific forms of psychopathology.

Literature Cited & Further Reading

Adams, R. B., Jr., Gordon, H. L., Baird, A. A., Ambady, N., & Kleck, R. E. (2003). Effects of gaze on amygdala sensitivity to anger and fear faces. *Science*, 300: 1536.

Bechara, A., Tranel, D., Damasio, H., Adolphe, R., Rockland, C., & Damasio, A. R. (1995). Double dissociation of conditioning and declarative knowledge relative to the amygdala and hippocampus in humans. *Science*, 269: 1115–1118.

Calder, A. J., Ewbank, M., & Passamonti, L. (2011). Personality influences the neural responses to viewing facial expressions of emotion. *Philosophical Transactions of the Royal Society (B)*, 366: 1684–1701.

Darwin, C. (1872). *The Expression of the Emotions in Man and Animals*. 200th anniversary edition with commentary by Paul Ekman (2009). New York: Oxford University Press.

Debiec, J., & Sullivan, R. M. (2014). Intergenerational transmission of emotional trauma through amygdala-dependent mother-to-infant transfer of specific fear. *Proceedings of the National Academy of Sciences USA*, 111: 12222–12227.

Fisher, P. M., & 8 others. (2009). Medial prefrontal cortex 5-HT$_{2A}$ density is correlated with amygdala reactivity, response habituation, and functional coupling. *Cerebral Cortex*, 19: 2499–2507.

LaBar, K. S. & Phelps, E. A. (2005). Reinstatement of conditioned fear in humans is context-dependent and impaired in amnesia. *Behavioral Neuroscience*, 119: 677–686.

Jeon, D., & 8 others. (2010). Observational fear learning involves affective pain system and Ca$_v$1.2 Ca^{2+} channels in ACC. *Nature Neuroscience*, 13: 482–488.

Maren, S., Phan, K. L., & Liberzon, I. (2013). The contextual brain: Implications for fear conditioning, extinction and psychopathology. *Nature Reviews Neuroscience*, 14: 417–428.

Milad, M. R., Quirk, G. J., Pitman, R. K., Orr, S. P., Fischl, B., & Rauch, S. L. (2007). A role for the human dorsal anterior cingulate cortex in fear expression. *Biological Psychiatry*, 62: 1191–1194.

Morris, J. S., Friston, K. R., & Dolan, R. J. (1997). Neural responses to salient visual stimuli. *Proceedings of the Royal Society of London (B)*, 264: 769–775.

Phelps, E. A., Delgado, M. R., Nearing, K. I., & LeDoux, J. E. (2004). Extinction learning in humans: Role of the amygdala and vmPFC. *Neuron*, 43: 897–905.

Sah, P., & Westbrook, R. F. (2008). The circuit of fear. *Nature*, 454: 589–590,

Quirk, G. J., Garcia, R., & González-Lima, F. (2006). Prefrontal mechanisms in extinction of conditioned fear. *Biological Psychiatry*, 60: 337–343.

Whalen, P. J., & 10 others (2004). Human amygdala responsivity to masked fearful eye whites. *Science*, 306: 2061.

4

The Corticolimbic Circuit
Disorder

In Chapter 2 we established the neuroanatomical basis for and functional interactions of key nodes comprising the corticolimbic circuit. In Chapter 3 we saw how the orderly processing of information through this circuit helps us recognize and generate adaptive reactions to the challenges we face in our environments. In this chapter, we consider how disorder within the corticolimbic circuit manifests as abnormal or maladaptive reactions to environmental challenge. Broadly, corticolimbic circuit dysfunction is most closely linked with symptoms common to mood and anxiety disorders (e.g., major depressive disorder, generalized anxiety disorder) as well as disorders of social behavior (e.g., autism spectrum disorders, antisocial personality disorder).

Consistent with the perspective we adopted in the preceding chapters, the amygdala will serve as the entry point for our study of how dysfunction within the corticolimbic circuit emerges as disordered behavior or psychopathology. In part, this amygdala-centric approach reflects the predominant focus on this structure in fMRI studies of mood and anxiety disorders as well as disorders of social behavior. This perspective, however, is not simply one of convenience. Rather, it strongly reflects the critical importance of the amygdala as the hub of the corticolimbic circuit—a hub that functions to detect stimuli in our environment and trigger adaptive reactions by channeling information through the appropriate nodes of the circuit.

As we will discover throughout this chapter, psychopathology associated with disorder of the corticolimbic circuit is quintessentially one of abnormal or maladaptive reactions to challenges, especially threat, in our environment. While the amygdala is the hub of the corticolimbic circuit through which our reactions to the environment are triggered, as well as the focus of understanding related disorders, it is only one component of the circuit. In many cases, the disorder observed in the amygdala may, in fact, reflect dysfunction in other circuit nodes, most notably the ventromedial prefrontal cortex (vmPFC) and dorsomedial prefrontal cortex (dmPFC), and the failure of these nodes to effectively integrate and regulate the bottom-up drive of the amygdala. When possible and appropriate, we will consider dysfunction in other nodes of the corticolimbic circuit as they contribute to specific forms of psychopathology.

Although at this point in time we cannot abandon the existing diagnostic nosology, and even though almost all fMRI studies are conducted in groups of individuals with *DSM*-defined categorical disorders (i.e., disorders defined by the *Diagnostic and Statistical Manual of Mental Disorders*), we will attempt to underscore the emergence of highly conserved and overlapping symptoms related to the changes occurring in the underlying corticolimbic circuit. In other words, we will begin by considering how relative increases or decreases in amygdala activity manifest as specific symptoms of psychopathology; we will then discuss categorical disorders sharing this alteration in amygdala activity and the related changes in their unique and shared symptoms.

Amygdala Hyperactivity

What happens when the activity of the amygdala is increased or exaggerated? As would be predicted based on the critical importance of the circuit in generating reactions to challenges we encounter in our environment, when there is amygdala hyperactivity, we become hypersensitive to these challenges. We may even perceive otherwise harmless or nonthreatening stimuli as representing threat or danger, leading to inappropriate fear and stress responses.

Such exaggerated recognition and reaction to threat and stress—real or imagined—is a hallmark symptom that unifies mood and anxiety disorders. This core symptom likely explains the substantial overlap that exists between different categorical mood and anxiety disorders, which often co-occur within individuals. This phenomenon is commonly referred to as "comorbidity." Further, this unifying symptom is evident in the grouping of mood and anxiety disorders together under the broad label of **internalizing disorders**. The label *internalizing* references the general tendency of those suffering from these disorders to experience disabling levels of internal or inwardly directed distress (e.g., fear, anxiety, sadness, guilt, despair, helplessness) when confronted by threat or stressful situations. In contrast, those suffering from **externalizing disorders** express their distress outwardly in the form of disruptive behaviors such as crime, violence, and drug abuse. We will review some externalizing disorders, including antisocial personality disorder, later in this chapter, although most of these will be reviewed in Unit 2, on the corticostriatal circuit.

Consistent with the exaggerated recognition of and reaction to threat and stress, which manifest as internal states of distress, amygdala hyperactivity has been repeatedly observed in fMRI studies of mood and anxiety disorders. This is wholly expected, given the strong potentiating effects of amygdala activity on our physiological arousal (e.g., increased heart rate, respiration, and HPA axis activity) and our subjective awareness of these effects (e.g., through increased responsiveness of the insula). Typically, these potentiating effects are perfectly normal and, in fact, critical for adaptive responses that help us overcome the challenges we face. As we will review below, the emerging picture in mood and anxiety disorders entails not only amygdala hyperactivity but also dysfunctional activity of the medial prefrontal cortex. It is likely that a failure of the mPFC to integrate and, ultimately, regulate the amygdala further exacerbates its hyperactivity, resulting in the internalizing distress characteristic of mood and anxiety disorders. In many ways, the amygdala appears to be *shouting* in these disorders, and the PFC appears to be *not listening* to the amygdala's call for attention.

Despite the core symptom of internal distress in response to perceived threat and stress, as well as amygdala hyperactivity, shared across mood

internalizing disorders Characterized by inwardly directed distress (e.g., fear, guilt, anxiety) when confronted by threat or stressful situations.

externalizing disorders Characterized by outwardly directed distress in the form of disruptive or destructive behaviors (e.g., violence or substance abuse).

HPA   hypothalamic-pituitary-adrenal axis
mPFC   medial prefrontal cortex

and anxiety disorders, the existing research is most amenable to a review of findings within specific diagnostic categories. The following sections will consider select evidence implicating corticolimbic circuit dysfunction, with a focus on amygdala hyperactivity, within the most prevalent disorders of mood, and anxiety. However, it is important to consider the shared symptoms and circuit-level features across disorders as summarized above. We will also consider evidence for amygdala hyperactivity in disorders of social behavior such as autism spectrum disorders and will highlight similarities at the level of both circuit dysfunction and symptomatology across all these disorders.

Mood Disorders

Mood disorders are characterized by a sustained disturbance in predominant internal emotional experience. As emphasized above, mood disorders involve an exaggerated reaction or hypersensitivity to threat and stress. Mood disorders are the most prevalent form of psychopathology identified in the *DSM*. Here we will consider the evidence for corticolimbic circuit dysfunction in the two most common mood disorders: major depressive disorder and bipolar disorders.

Major depressive disorder

Major depressive disorder (MDD), commonly referred to simply as depression, is characterized by experiencing at least one major depressive episode, or MDE. Typically, individuals experience multiple episodes leading to the diagnosis of recurrent MDD. Critically, individuals with MDD cannot have experienced any periods of manic or hypomanic states, which we will describe later, in the discussion of bipolar disorders.

An MDE must include depressed mood, or markedly diminished interest or pleasure in all (or almost all) activities most of the day, nearly every day, for at least two weeks, as indicated by either subjective report or observation made by others. An MDE must also include four or more additional symptoms, including disturbances in sleep, appetite, or physical activity; feelings of guilt and worthlessness; difficulty concentrating; and suicidal ideation (i.e., preoccupation with the idea of suicide).

More fMRI studies of amygdala activity and corticolimbic circuit function have been conducted in MDD than in any other mood or anxiety disorder. Wayne Drevets and colleagues, then at Washington University in St. Louis, conducted the first study finding abnormal amygdala function in MDD in 1992. Unlike the majority of studies now being conducted, these investigators used positron emission tomography (PET) to measure direct changes in cerebral blood flow rather than fMRI, since the latter was not commonly available at that time.

In their seminal study, Drevets and colleagues found that amygdala activity was elevated in individuals with MDD, in comparison to healthy participants, even when they were resting comfortably during a PET scan and not viewing any triggers (e.g., emotional facial expressions). Interestingly, another group of individuals who had suffered from MDD in the past but were currently in remission (i.e., asymptomatic) also exhibited elevated amygdala activity in comparison to the healthy group. This pattern suggests that amygdala hyperactivity is likely a trait marker for depression, and that

mood disorders Characterized by sustained disturbance in internal emotional experiences and patterns of thinking, whether negative (depression) or positive (mania).

major depressive disorder (MDD) Commonly referred to simply as depression; characterized by typically recurring major depressive episodes, with no occurrence of manic or hypomanic episodes.

major depressive episode (MDE) Persistent depressed mood or anhedonia, typically experienced with disturbances in appetite, sleep, or activity as well as feelings of guilt, difficulty concentrating, or suicidal ideation.

depressed mood Feeling sad, tearful, empty, or irritable; easily upset and overwhelmed by otherwise typical experiences.

MDD   major depressive disorder
MDE   major depressive episode

(A)

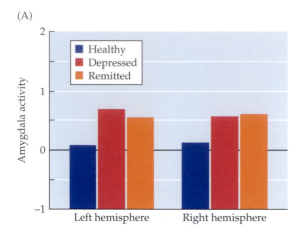

(B)

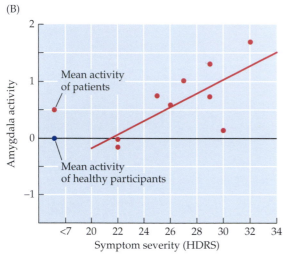

Figure 4.1 (A) In comparison with healthy participants, there is evidence of amygdala hyperactivity both in individuals currently suffering from depression (depressed) and in those who have a history of depression but are not currently experiencing symptoms (remitted). (B) Amygdala hyperactivity not only distinguishes an MDE, it also predicts the severity of symptoms as measured by the Hamilton Depression Rating Scale (HDRS). Note that 0 represents baseline activity in these data. (After Drevets et al., 1992.)

it exists regardless of the presence or absence of symptoms (**Figure 4.1A**). In other words, amygdala hyperactivity appears to represent a risk factor for depression. The magnitude of amygdala hyperactivity in the patients with current MDD, moreover, predicted the severity of their symptoms (**Figure 4.1B**). Thus, even within a group of patients all meeting *DSM* diagnostic criteria for MDD, differences in amygdala hyperactivity predict the depth of depression.

Interestingly, while the increased amygdala activity observed by Drevets and colleagues was not in response to any specific stimulus (e.g., emotional facial expressions), most subsequent fMRI studies have found increased amygdala activity in response to a broad range of negative emotional stimuli, including prototypical facial expressions conveying threat (i.e., expressions of fear, anger, or surprise) or neutral expressions as well as other emotions, notably sadness. This pattern of generally increased amygdala activity is commonly interpreted as consistent with hypersensitivity of individuals with MDD to negative experiences, as well as their tendency to assign or experience events as negative.

Not surprisingly, hyperactivity of the amygdala is not the only disorder of the corticolimbic circuit observed in individuals suffering from depression. Increased activity is also commonly observed in the insula and dorsal anterior cingulate cortex (**Figure 4.2A**). While amygdala hyperactivity is reflected in the hypersensitivity of individuals to stress and threat, their greater subjective awareness of the resulting physiological changes may be reflected in hyperactivity of the insula. The dACC hyperactivity may reflect the experience of emotional conflict in patients who struggle to maintain normal relationships in the face of depressed mood.

Interestingly, in the original study by Drevets and colleagues, individuals with depression also exhibited more activity in the dmPFC than did healthy participants. In contrast to amygdala hyperactivity, which was found in both currently depressed individuals and those in remission, hyperactivity of the dmPFC was unique to those currently depressed. This pattern suggests that, while amygdala hyperactivity is a trait marker in depression, dmPFC hyperactivity may be a state marker of an MDE. That is, amygdala activity may always be higher in those vulnerable for depression, but the actual experience of an MDE follows when the dmPFC attempts but ultimately fails to effectively regulate the amygdala.

There is also evidence for increased activity in the visual thalamus, including the pulvinar, during the processing of emotional facial expressions in MDD (**Figure 4.2B**). This suggests the intriguing possibility that individuals at risk for MDD may have heightened primary sensory processing of threat-related

MDD	major depressive disorder
MDE	major depressive episode
dACC	dorsal anterior cingulate cortex

(A)

(B)

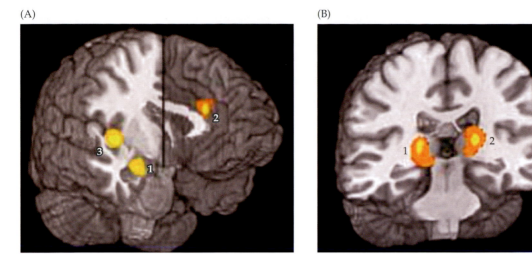

Figure 4.2 (A) Meta-analysis of 38 fMRI studies involving viewing of emotional facial expressions reveals consistent evidence for relative hyperactivity of the amygdala (1); dACC (2); and the anterior insula (3) in MDD in comparison with healthy participants. (B) The analysis also revealed relative hyperactivity of the pulvinar nucleus of the thalamus (1, 2), which relays visual information to the amygdala, in MDD. (From Hamilton et al., 2012.)

cues. Thus, trait-like amygdala hyperactivity could reflect augmented threat processing in MDD, which is likely further exaggerated by dysfunctional top-down regulation of amygdala hyperactivity via the dmPFC.

Dysregulation of communication between the amygdala and dmPFC in MDD is most clearly reflected in studies using functional connectivity, which is a measure of how strongly activity in two regions of the brain is correlated. Functional connectivity can be either positive (i.e., activity in both regions increases together) or negative (i.e., activity in one region increases while activity in the other decreases). Measures of functional connectivity do not readily allow for determination of temporal order (i.e., activity occurs first in region A and subsequently in region B) or directionality (i.e., region A is driving activity in region B). Nevertheless, functional connectivity can be used to estimate how effectively two nodes within a circuit are generally communicating information.

In healthy, nondepressed people, functional connectivity between the amygdala and both vmPFC and dmPFC is positive. This positive functional connectivity is significantly weaker in MDD and can predict the severity of depression symptoms (**Figure 4.3**). This weakened connectivity simultaneously suggests impairments in the capacity to integrate bottom-up arousal and effect top-down inhibition following a triggering event or stimulus.

The above fMRI data reveal that dysfunction of the corticolimbic circuit, particularly amygdala hyperactivity and decreased amygdala-mPFC functional connectivity, is a core component of MDD. Consistent with this model, MDEs often

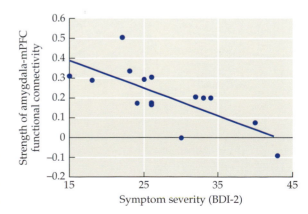

Figure 4.3 Increased severity of current depressive symptoms in MDD, seen here as a higher score on the Beck Depression Inventory-II (BDI-2), is related to weaker functional connectivity between the amygdala and the mPFC. Note that 0 represents mean connectivity in these data. (After Matthews et al., 2008.)

dmPFC dorsomedial prefrontal cortex
vmPFC ventromedial prefrontal cortex
mPFC medial prefrontal cortex

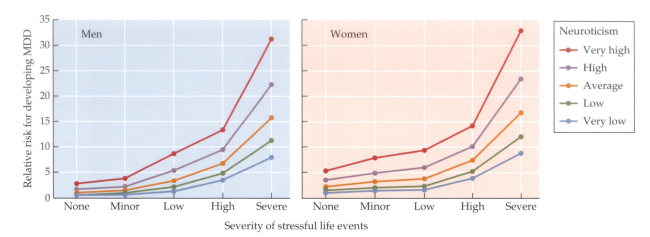

Figure 4.4 In both men and women, the risk of developing MDD in response to stressful experiences is greater in individuals with higher levels of negative affect and anxiety, as indexed here by the personality trait of neuroticism. (After Kendler et al., 2004.)

neuroticism A personality trait or disposition to experience strong negative emotions, including anxiety.

follow stressful life events such as being harshly reprimanded by an angry supervisor at work, getting divorced, or even being in a car accident. Moreover, the development of depression following a stressful life event is more likely for individuals who are high in trait anxiety and dispositional negative affect, sometimes characterized as **neuroticism** (**Figure 4.4**). Such trait measures reflect the tendency to be sensitive and vigilant for threat in the environment and, as prototypical dimensional features of personality, are expressed to some degree in us all. Those individuals at risk for depression, however, have particularly high levels of trait anxiety and negative affect. Taken together, these data suggest that stressful life events and the stimuli in our environments that signal threat (e.g., angry facial expressions) trigger amygdala hyperactivity, thereby unmasking the inability of the mPFC to integrate and regulate this activity, resulting in depression, particularly in those who are more sensitive to threat generally.

A final component of understanding corticolimbic circuit dysfunction in depression arises from the growing number of pre- and posttreatment fMRI studies, which are far more numerous for MDD than for other mood or anxiety disorders. Remarkably, fMRI evidence suggests that successful treatment of MDD acts to restore order in corticolimbic circuit function. For example, selective serotonin reuptake inhibitors, or SSRIs, which are the most commonly prescribed medication in MDD, appear to simultaneously increase the functional connectivity between the amygdala and both vmPFC and dmPFC and decrease amygdala hyperactivity (**Figure 4.5A**). Similarly, cognitive behavioral therapy (CBT) results in decreased amygdala hyperactivity and, possibly, increased amygdala-mPFC functional connectivity (**Figure 4.5B**).

Finally, deep brain stimulation (DBS) has emerged as a treatment option of last resort in depressed individuals who have not responded to any other form of treatment, including SSRIs and CBT. DBS treatment in depression often targets subregions of the mPFC, particularly the subgenual anterior cingulate cortex, directly stimulating activity in this region. It is believed that such direct stimulation restores functional connectivity between the mPFC and other nodes of the corticolimbic circuit, including the amygdala. That three such disparate treatment approaches—targeting, respectively, brain

MDD	major depressive disorder	vmPFC	ventromedial prefrontal cortex
SSRIs	selective serotonin reuptake inhibitors	dmPFC	dorsomedial prefrontal cortex
		mPFC	medial prefrontal cortex

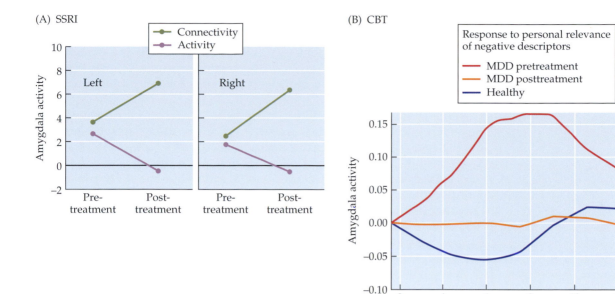

(A) SSRI

Connectivity
Activity

(B) CBT

Response to personal relevance
of negative descriptors

MDD pretreatment
MDD posttreatment
Healthy

Figure 4.5 Two common treatment approaches to alleviate symptoms of MDD are associated with changes in corticolimbic circuit function. (A) Drug therapy. After 6 weeks of treatment with a selective serotonin reuptake inhibitor (SSRI), one study observed an increase in the functional connectivity between the amygdala and mPFC, and a decrease in amygdala hyperactivity in response to negative versus neutral pictures. (B) Cognitive behavioral therapy (CBT). After 14 weeks of CBT, one study observed decreased amygdala hyperactivity in patients with MDD when rating the personal relevance of negative words such as "ugly" and "worthless." This decrease in amygdala hyperactivity following CBT was associated with increased activity of the prefrontal cortex, which we will consider in Unit III. Note that 0 represents baseline activity in these data. (A after Anand et al., 2007; B after DeRubeis et al., 2008.)

chemistry, behavior, and brain electrical activity—all alleviate symptoms of depression by restoring order in the corticolimbic circuit is a strong indication of the circuit's critical importance in the etiology of MDD.

Bipolar disorders

As their name implies, bipolar disorders (BD) are characterized by cycling between extremes of emotional reaction. Individuals with BD experience manic episodes (or in some cases hypomanic states) that can involve a number of abnormal behaviors. These include extreme "high" or euphoric feelings; excessive energy and activity; restlessness, racing thoughts, and rapid talking; denial that anything is wrong; being easily irritated or distracted; decreased need for sleep; unrealistic beliefs in one's ability and powers; uncharacteristically poor judgment; provocative, intrusive, paranoid, or aggressive behaviors; unusual sexual drive; and abuse of drugs, particularly cocaine, alcohol, or sleeping medications. To define a manic episode, these symptoms must be present for 7 days or be severe enough to require hospitalization. Individuals with BD often also suffer from MDEs as seen in MDD. Generally, individuals with BD will alternate between manic episodes, MDEs, and periods of normal mood known as euthymia.

Compared with MDD, fMRI studies of BD are relatively few. However, a consistent picture of corticolimbic circuit dysfunction is emerging from these studies. Of particular note, Lori Altshuler and colleagues at UCLA have been examining corticolimbic circuit dysfunction across the major states of BD:

bipolar disorders (BD) Characterized by typically recurring cycles of manic episodes, euthymia, and major depressive episodes.

manic episodes Persistent feelings of euphoria, increased energy, diminished need for sleep, grandiosity, denial, and generally poor decision making.

euthymia Normal mood and affect.

CBT   cognitive behavioral therapy
BD   bipolar disorders
MDE   major depressive episode

manic, depressed, and euthymic. In the first of their studies published in 2005, Altshuler and colleagues reported amygdala hyperactivity in response to emotional facial expressions in individuals with BD during a manic episode. In many ways, such amygdala hyperactivity is highly consistent with the euphoria, irritability, insomnia, inattention, and distractibility that often define a manic episode.

When individuals with BD are in a depressive episode, however, there is relatively decreased amygdala activity. In addition, there is decreased activity in several prefrontal regions, including the vlPFC and dlPFC. Interestingly, the vlPFC also exhibits a relatively attenuated response in individuals during a manic episode. Moreover, a similar decrease in vlPFC activity has been documented in individuals during a euthymic, or normal, mood state. Notably, amygdala activity appears normal when individuals with BD are in a euthymic state.

When we look across these studies of BD, a striking pattern emerges. First, amygdala activity follows a state-dependent course—increased in manic, decreased in depressed, and normal in euthymic states (**Figure 4.6A**). Second, prefrontal cortex activation exhibits a state-independent, or trait-like, course that is decreased in all three states (**Figure 4.6B**). Critically, the vlPFC region exhibiting trait-like hypoactivation across manic, depressed, and euthymic states plays an important role in the downregulation of amygdala activity. In healthy participants, the vlPFC appears to exert top-down regulatory control over the amygdala (likely through the dmPFC, which has direct amygdala connections), as indexed by negative functional connectivity between the

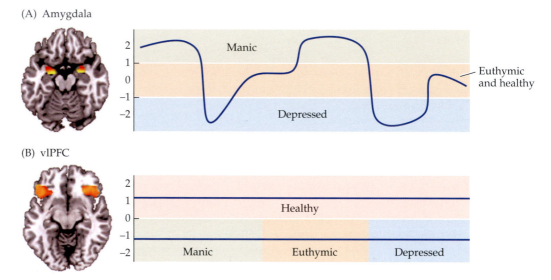

Figure 4.6 (A) Emerging fMRI research in individuals with bipolar disorders reveals state-dependent differences (blue trace) in amygdala activity, with hyperactivity during mania, hypoactivity during depression, and activity equivalent to that seen in healthy participants during euthymic states. (B) In contrast to the state-dependent patterns of amygdala activity, this research reveals state-independent vlPFC hypoactivity throughout manic, depressed, and euthymic states. The two horizontal lines indicate that in all three states, vlPFC activity in those with BD is (1) unchanging and (2) always less than the activity observed in healthy participants. As we will learn in Unit III, these patterns are consistent with abnormal or maladaptive top-down regulation of the amygdala through the prefrontal cortex. Note that 0 represents mean activity in these data. (After Hariri, 2012.)

BD bipolar disorders
vlPFC ventrolateral prefrontal cortex
dlPFC dorsolateral prefrontal cortex

two regions. As we have seen, balance in this dynamic functional circuitry is critical for the expression of behavioral and physiological responses to provocation that are both temporally limited and contextually appropriate. Collectively, the emerging data for BD suggest that the vlPFC may not be adequately capable of regulating amygdala activity, resulting in mania.

If amygdala activity is a state-dependent phenomenon in BD and trait-like hypoactivation of regulatory prefrontal regions creates a permissive environment for the translation of amygdala hyperactivity into manic symptoms, then what could be driving amygdala hypoactivity in the depressed state? Again, the relative functioning of prefrontal regions may be key. During a depressive episode, individuals with BD exhibit increased functional connectivity between the amygdala and vlPFC. This is in contrast to the *decreased* functional connectivity between the amygdala and vlPFC, which can be interpreted as less top-down regulation, observed during manic episodes. Thus, it is possible that the abnormal mood states of BD reflect dysfunctional increases or decreases in connectivity between these two nodes, resulting in inappropriate regulation of the amygdala. The data suggest that these differences, not simply in the activation of brain regions (i.e., the vlPFC is hypoactive across states) but rather in the functional connectivity of distributed regions (i.e., amygdala-vlPFC connectivity is decreased in mania but increased in depression), may be particularly important for understanding changes in mood states characterizing BD.

You have probably noticed that the amygdala hypoactivity observed in individuals with BD during a major depressive episode is in stark contrast to the trait-like amygdala hyperactivity seen in individuals with MDD, which exists even when they are not currently depressed. In several important ways, the pattern of amygdala activity in BD is more consistent with the role of the amygdala in driving reactions to our environment by potentiating arousal and triggering adaptive changes in our physiology and behavior. When the amygdala is hyperactive in BD, individuals experience dramatic increases in their levels of activity and energy and also are more socially engaged (for better or worse) with their friends, family, and colleagues. When the amygdala is hypoactive, individuals with BD experience a loss of energy, are less active, and avoid or lose interest in social interactions. This difference may reflect the important role of anxiety in the development of a major depressive episode in MDD but not in BD. That is, depression in individuals with MDD represents dysfunctional underregulation of an amygdala that is hyperactive to stress and threat, while depression in individuals with BD represents dysfunctional overregulation of otherwise normal amygdala activity. These differences are further reflected in the generally higher levels of trait anxiety, negative emotionality, and comorbid anxiety disorders in MDD relative to BD.

Anxiety Disorders

Anxiety disorders are characterized by sustained mental symptoms including apprehension, fear, and general uneasiness, as well as physical symptoms including dizziness or light-headedness, chest/abdominal pain, nausea, increased heart rate, and even diarrhea. Similar to mood disorders, anxiety disorders involve an exaggerated response or hypersensitivity to threat and stress. However, with anxiety disorders there is a pronounced physical

anxiety disorders Characterized by exaggerated fear responses to perceived threat and stress that, unlike mood disorders, are accompanied by physical as well as emotional distress.

---

dmPFC dorsomedial prefrontal cortex
MDD major depressive disorder

expression of this hypersensitivity not commonly observed in mood disorders. In fact, anxiety disorders are sometimes difficult to recognize because of their many physical symptoms, which result in their treatment only as physical disorders (e.g., irritable bowel syndrome).

The constellation of mental and physical symptoms common across anxiety disorders is clearly consistent with amygdala hyperactivity. This will be readily apparent as we review common forms of these disorders below. However, as with mood disorders, dysfunction in other nodes of the corticolimbic circuit is also present across anxiety disorders and, sometimes, unique to specific forms. The most prevalent forms of anxiety disorders, which we will review below, are panic disorder, generalized anxiety disorder, social anxiety disorder, and specific phobia. We will also review posttraumatic stress disorder, which was historically classified as an anxiety disorder but as of the fifth edition of the *DSM* is now considered under the new category of trauma- and stress-related disorders. We will discuss generalized anxiety disorder in a separate section later in the chapter.

Panic disorder

panic attack Overwhelming experience of fear with severe physical symptoms that can be mistaken for a heart attack.

panic disorder (PD) Characterized by recurring, unpredictable panic attacks.

agoraphobia Fear of places and situations where escape may be difficult.

anticipatory anxiety Fear experienced only in anticipation of a threat, with no actual exposure to the threat.

A **panic attack** is a discrete period of overwhelming fear that comes on abruptly. Panic attacks involve both mental and physical discomfort (with the latter sometimes interpreted by the sufferer as a heart attack because of the intense chest pain). Fortunately, these symptoms typically peak after a few minutes and subside as abruptly as they begin. **Panic disorder (PD)** is characterized by *unexpected and recurrent* panic attacks. The frequency of panic attacks varies from several times a day to only once or twice a year. Although PD specifically is uncommon, the experience of panic attacks is often present in many anxiety disorders, where they may be triggered by specific stimuli or contexts.

Individuals with PD often also have **agoraphobia**, which literally means "fear of the marketplace." More broadly, agoraphobia refers to the experience of marked fear and distress when in a place or a situation that makes escape difficult, embarrassing, or impossible. Agoraphobia typically involves characteristic clusters of situations such as leaving home alone, being in crowds, going over a bridge, and using public transportation. In individuals with agoraphobia, such situations that cause fear are avoided or are endured with intense distress. Over time, individuals with agoraphobia may experience intense fear and even panic attacks when merely thinking about or imagining provocative situations, a condition referred to as **anticipatory anxiety**.

As you can imagine, anticipatory anxiety and agoraphobia make it difficult to conduct fMRI studies in individuals with PD. For these individuals, the mere specter of spending an hour or more inside a large magnet with only a rather small opening can trigger their fears and anxiety. Nevertheless, there have been a small number of fMRI studies in PD. Of note, viewing of emotional facial expressions does not typically produce significantly greater amygdala activity in patients with PD compared with healthy participants. There is, however, evidence for decreased activity of the prefrontal cortex, including the vmPFC, dmPFC, and vlPFC when processing negative emotional information such as threat-related facial expressions, or when undergoing fear learning. These deficits in prefrontal function suggest that PD may reflect abnormalities in the ability to integrate and regulate the bottom-up drive of the amygdala rather than an exaggerated drive directly.

PD   panic disorder
vmPFC   ventromedial prefrontal cortex
dmPFC   dorsomedial prefrontal cortex

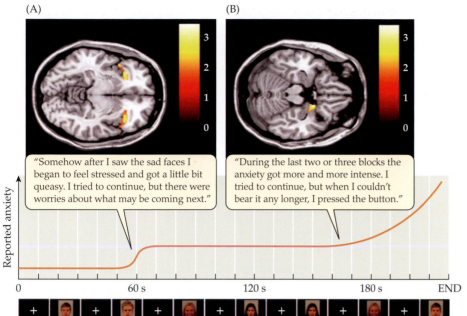

Figure 4.7 One fMRI study captured a panic attack during scanning. Careful analysis of the data revealed an initial increase in the activity of the insula that was related to feelings of discomfort (A) followed by increased activity in the amygdala (B) just before the patient discontinued the scan. (From Dresler et al., 2011.)

More remarkably, a small number of experiments have actually recorded changes in brain function during a panic attack. In the most striking of these studies, a person with specific phobia was able to reconstruct the experience of a panic attack during the scan, which involved viewing emotional facial expressions, allowing the investigators to identify corresponding changes in corticolimbic circuit function. Interestingly, at the first report of feeling both mentally and physically distressed, there was a corresponding increase in insula activity. Subsequently, as this individual's anxiety and fear escalated to the point that the scan was terminated, there was a corresponding increase in amygdala activity (**Figure 4.7**). Such increased activity of the amygdala has been positively correlated with increased heart rate. A general pattern of decreased PFC activity also has been observed during spontaneous panic attacks.

Collectively, these studies suggest that panic attacks may result from an initially increased awareness of changes in our peripheral physiology as registered by the insula, which then leads to amygdala hyperactivity and subsequently further exaggeration of both mental and physical distress. This exaggerated sensitivity may persist because of an inability to integrate and control these changes associated with decreased prefrontal activity. Extending to PD, the above pattern of corticolimbic circuit disorder suggests that amygdala and insula hyperactivity may be a state feature (i.e., occurring only during panic attacks), while PFC hypoactivity may be a trait feature (i.e., occurring always in response to negative emotional information).

Social anxiety disorder

Social anxiety disorder (SAD), also known as **social phobia**, is characterized by persistent fear and avoidance of social or performance situations without apparent justification (i.e., the individuals are not being ridiculed or threatened by others in these situations). The fear of public scrutiny leads individuals with SAD to experience embarrassment, anxiety, and situationally bound panic attacks.

social anxiety disorder (social phobia) Characterized by excessive or unreasonable fear of public scrutiny leading to persistent avoidance of social or performance situations and situationally bound panic attacks.

vlPFC   ventrolateral prefrontal cortex
SAD   social anxiety disorder
PFC   prefrontal cortex

Figure 4.8 Meta-analysis of 30 fMRI and PET studies revealed that relative to healthy participants, amygdala (A) and insula (B) hyperactivity is more pronounced in social anxiety disorder (SAD) and specific phobia than in posttraumatic stress disorder (PTSD). (After Etkin & Wager, 2007.)

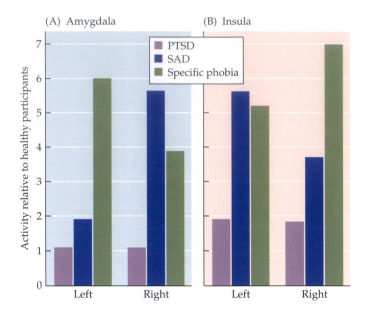

Amygdala hyperactivity has been consistently identified across fMRI studies of SAD (**Figure 4.8A**). In addition, increased activity of the insula is a common observation in theses studies (**Figure 4.8B**). Such hyperactivity is consistent with the exaggerated fear, anxiety, and panic attacks experienced when these individuals encounter or simply anticipate socially provocative situations. This hypersensitivity and hyperresponsiveness may be exacerbated by deficient top-down integration and, possibly, deficient regulation. While there is generally little evidence of decreased activity in the mPFC of individuals with SAD, some studies have reported decreased functional connectivity between the amygdala and vmPFC. Interestingly, the ability to activate regions of the vmPFC during attempts to regulate their social anxiety may decrease the intensity of the distress experienced in these individuals.

Specific phobia

Specific phobia is characterized by excessive or unreasonable fear and avoidance of a place, thing, or situation. As with SAD, individuals with specific phobia often experience panic attacks when confronted by or anticipating exposure to a phobic stimulus. There are several general categories of specific phobia, with multiple exemplars in each category. These include situational phobias, such as when riding public transportation, driving, flying, and traveling through tunnels or across bridges; natural environment phobias with stimuli such as storms, heights, and water; and animal phobias including stimuli such as snakes, spiders, and dogs.

As these examples suggest, specific phobia is the clearest example of an exaggerated fear response that may once have had adaptive value (i.e., in our ancestral environments) but is generally maladaptive in modern contexts. Phobic stimuli generally do represent some form and degree of potential threat (getting bitten by a venomous snake, for example, can certainly result in death). However, they are typically encountered in contexts that effectively eliminate any real danger (e.g., most of us only encounter snakes in zoos,

specific phobia Characterized by excessive or unreasonable fear and avoidance of a specific place, thing, or situation.

SAD   social anxiety disorder
mPFC   medial prefrontal cortex
PTSD   posttraumatic stress disorder

where a thick plate of glass separates us from any real danger). While most of us have some initial fear response to situations and stimuli encompassing some degree of threat or danger, we (like our hiker on the trail) manage to regulate this response and resume our preferred activities. For those with specific phobia, however, such exposure is debilitating.

As we would expect, amygdala hyperactivity is clearly present in individuals with specific phobia. Interestingly, this hyperactivity is generally the largest observed among the anxiety disorders (see Figure 4.8A). While this may reflect actual neurobiological differences between the disorders, it could also be a methodological artifact because fMRI studies of specific phobia confront the patients with the stimuli they most fear (e.g., spiders in individuals with spider phobia), while fMRI studies of other anxiety disorders rely on indirect triggers (e.g., emotional facial expressions that represent conditioned stimuli). Recall from Chapter 3 that the most intense fear learning occurs when there is a perfect match between the conditioned stimulus and unconditioned stimulus. This is often the case in fMRI studies of specific phobia but not of other anxiety disorders. Consistent with this perspective, individuals with specific phobia exhibit faster amygdala activity in response to their phobic stimuli than to generally threatening stimuli.

In addition to hyperactivity of the amygdala, fMRI studies of specific phobia also document increased activity of the insula (see Figure 4.8B) and dmPFC. The former may reflect the intense physical distress experienced by phobic individuals. The latter may reflect attempts by phobic individuals to regulate their fear through top-down inhibition of the amygdala. Given the persistent amygdala hyperactivity, this effortful control is obviously ineffective. Top-down regulation of amygdala hyperactivity may be further limited by deficient integration of bottom-up amygdala drive, as suggested by relatively decreased vmPFC activity in specific phobia.

Allowing individuals to develop a tolerance for their phobic stimuli and the ability to regulate their intense fear is a hallmark of treatment in specific phobia. Such treatment almost always involves exposure therapy, wherein a patient is gradually brought into closer and closer proximity (even contact) with a phobic stimulus under carefully controlled settings where no harm can be done and with directions from the therapist about how to regulate the fear response. For example, a patient with spider phobia may be asked first to look at pictures of spiders, then to look at plastic spiders, then to hold plastic spiders, then to view a real spider in a cage, and finally to hold a real spider. This progression typically occurs slowly over many weeks and involves a great deal of input from the therapist to reassure the patient of his safety, but positive effects have been found after even a single session. Such exposure therapy is one of the most successful treatment approaches, not only in anxiety disorders but in all psychiatric disorders.

Remarkably, exposure therapy in specific phobia produces a striking normalization of the patterns of dysfunctional activity observed in individuals prior to treatment (**Figure 4.9**). Exposure therapy is associated with reductions in hyperactivity of the amygdala as well as the insula and dmPFC, compared with pretreatment levels in individuals with spider phobia. Moreover, decreases in amygdala and insula hyperactivity correspond to a drop in fear and anxiety levels when viewing pictures of spiders. Exposure therapy also has been associated with a relative increase in the activity of the vmPFC, which can be observed after only one treatment session. Collectively, these

dmPFC dorsomedial prefrontal cortex
vmPFC ventromedial prefrontal cortex

(A)

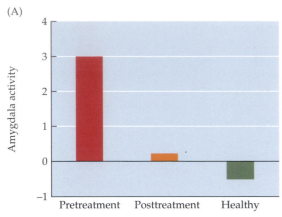

Figure 4.9 (A) Compared with healthy participants, individuals with spider phobia showed amygdala hyperactivity to pictures of spiders before exposure therapy. After 2 weeks of exposure therapy, this hyperactivity significantly decreased and reached levels comparable to those of the healthy participants. (B) There was a positive correlation between amygdala activity in response to spider pictures and phobic symptoms as measured with the Spider Phobia Questionnaire (SPQ). The relative decrease in amygdala hyperactivity posttreatment in comparison to pretreatment is associated with decreased phobia. (C) Treatment-related decreases in amygdala hyperactivity likely reflect increases in regulatory activity of the prefrontal cortex, including the vmPFC, which have been observed after even a single treatment session. Note that 0 represents mean activity in these data. (A,B after Goossens et al., 2007; C from Schienle et al., 2007.)

(B)

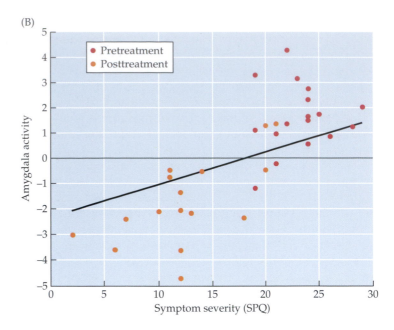

(C)

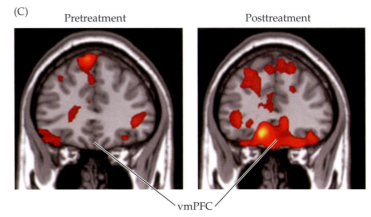

changes in corticolimbic circuit function following exposure therapy are highly consistent with the basic process of fear extinction and reflect the acquired capacity to actively inhibit the fear conditioning associated with the phobic stimulus. Dysfunction of fear extinction appears to be a critical feature of the final specific anxiety disorder we will consider here: posttraumatic stress disorder.

Posttraumatic stress disorder

posttraumatic stress disorder (PTSD) Characterized by a complex pattern of dysfunctional responses following exposure to a discrete, identifiable traumatic event or experience involving threat of death or serious bodily harm.

Posttraumatic stress disorder (PTSD) involves a pattern of dysfunctional responses following exposure to a traumatic event or experience involving threat of death or serious bodily harm. While the threat can be direct (i.e., something happening to you) or indirect (i.e., something you observe happening to another), diagnosis of PTSD follows if a discrete traumatic event or experience (e.g., severe weather such as a hurricane, or violent crime such as a mugging or rape) can be identified. In contrast, it is not a diagnostic necessity (and it

vmPFC   ventromedial prefrontal cortex
PTSD   posttraumatic stress disorder

is often difficult) to identify a specific negative experience that preceded and possibly precipitated one of the other anxiety disorders (e.g., being bitten by a spider precipitating a specific phobia, or being publicly ridiculed precipitating SAD).

Once a traumatic event or experience is identified, the diagnosis of PTSD follows if for 30 days or longer the individual exhibits symptoms from each of four categories. The first category, *re-experiencing*, includes spontaneous memories of the traumatic event, recurrent dreams and/or flashbacks related to the event, and intense or prolonged psychological distress. *Avoidance of people and places* is a reaction to distressing memories, thoughts, feelings, or external reminders of the event. Individuals may suffer persistent and distorted *negative cognitions and mood* and be unable to remember key aspects of the event. This negative cognitive state can manifest in blaming of self or others, estrangement from others, and diminished interest in normal activities. The final category is that of *arousal*, including hypervigilance, sleep disturbances, and aggressive, reckless, or self-destructive behavior.

Many studies of PTSD have observed amygdala hyperactivity in response to both trauma-related imagery and more general threat-related stimuli, such as emotional facial expressions (**Figure 4.10A**; also see Figure 4.9A). This is not surprising given both the importance of the amygdala in driving arousal and subsequent reactions to threat and the hypervigilance found in individuals with PTSD. In fact, the magnitude of amygdala hyperactivity is positively correlated with the severity of PTSD symptoms (**Figure 4.10B**). In addition, studies have noted abnormal activity of the hippocampal formation and a persistent pattern of mPFC hypoactivity in response to negative stimuli including trauma-related imagery in individuals with PTSD.

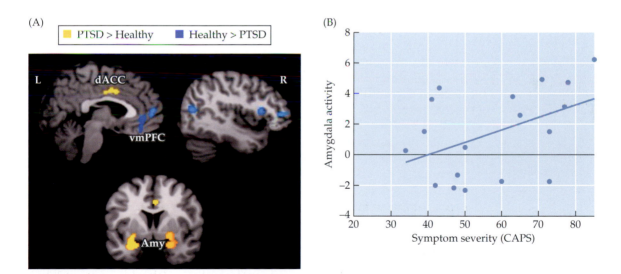

Figure 4.10 (A) Meta-analysis of 26 fMRI studies involving viewing of both trauma-related and trauma-unrelated emotional pictures reveals hyperactivity of the amygdala and dorsal ACC (yellow); and hypoactivity of the vmPFC and vlPFC (blue) in PTSD relative to healthy participants. (B) Amygdala hyperactivity to negative trauma-related imagery predicts symptom severity measured with the Clinician-Administered PTSD Scale for *DSM*-IV (CAPS). Note that 0 represents mean activity in these data. (A from Hayes et al., 2012; B after Browhawn et al., 2010.)

SAD   social anxiety disorder
mPFC   medial prefrontal cortex
dACC   dorsal anterior cingulate cortex

Figure 4.11 (A) Activity of the dmPFC during viewing of threat-related stimuli is associated with decreased PTSD symptom severity measured with the CAPS. (B) Activity of the HF during viewing of trauma-related imagery is similarly associated with decreased CAPS-measured symptoms. Note that 0 represents mean activity in these data. (A after Shin et al., 2005; B after Hayes et al., 2011.)

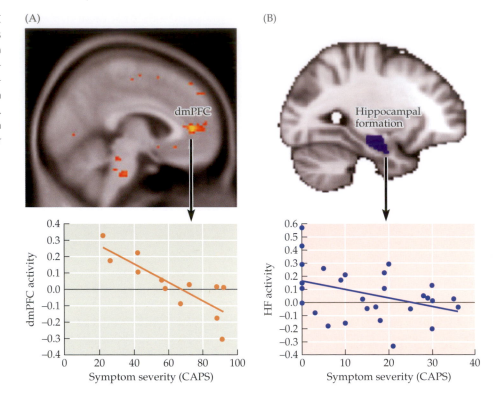

Interestingly, the magnitude of activity in both the HF and dmPFC is inversely correlated with symptom severity (**Figure 4.11**). This suggests that retaining some ability to regulate bottom-up drives associated with amygdala hyperactivity and encode contextual cues may lessen the severity of PTSD symptoms. Collectively, the pattern of relative hyperactivity of the amygdala and hypoactivity in target regions within the corticolimbic circuit, notably the hippocampus and mPFC, is consistent with the trio of diagnostic symptoms in PTSD involving poorly controlled and inappropriate fear responses.

More specifically than this general pattern of corticolimbic circuit dysfunction, the trio of symptoms in PTSD aligns closely with dysfunctional fear learning. In an elegant study published in 2009, Mohammad Milad and colleagues at Harvard University examined the integrity of corticolimbic circuit function during fear learning in individuals with PTSD (**Figure 4.12**). In their landmark study, Milad and colleagues first completed a fear conditioning paradigm in patients with PTSD. Remarkably, there were no differences in either the strength of the fear conditioning or the activation of corticolimbic circuit nodes, including the amygdala, between these individuals and a comparison group of 15 healthy participants who had been exposed to a similar trauma but never developed PTSD or any other disorder. In other words, in patients with PTSD, fear conditioning was normal. Developing a fear response to a traumatic event and the cues and context that were associated with the event (e.g., a specific place where you were mugged or survived a hurricane) is not only normal but also highly appropriate and adaptive. The dysfunction in PTSD occurs when this normal and adaptive

HF   hippocampal formation
dmPFC   dorsomedial prefrontal cortex
PTSD   posttraumatic stress disorder

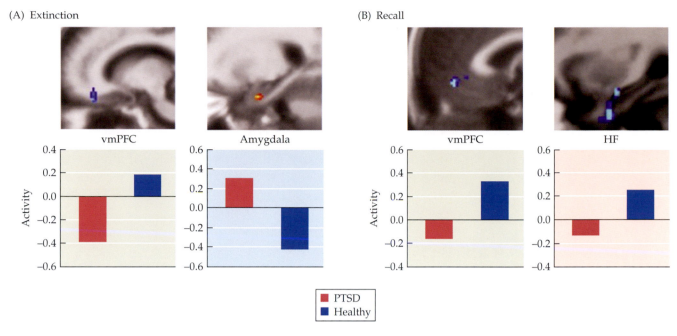

(A) Extinction   (B) Recall

vmPFC   Amygdala   vmPFC   HF

PTSD
Healthy

Figure 4.12 Although fear *conditioning* occurs normally in PTSD, there is impaired fear *extinction* and associated abnormal corticolimbic circuit function. (A) In comparison with trauma-exposed healthy participants, individuals with PTSD show relatively decreased activity in the vmPFC and increased activity in the amygdala when learning that, in a new context, a previously fear-conditioned stimulus no longer predicts a mild electric shock. (B) Individuals with PTSD continue to exhibit corticolimbic circuit dysfunction 24 hours later during fear recall, where they exhibit relatively decreased activity in both the vmPFC and HF. This dysfunctional pattern of corticolimbic activity is consistent with the general inability to distinguish safe from threatening environments and consequent persistent expression of fear characteristic of PTSD. Note that 0 represents mean activity in these data. (After Milad et al., 2009.)

fear response persists for too long and is expressed in inappropriate contexts (e.g., in a different place than where the trauma occurred). In other words, PTSD appears to be a disorder not of fear conditioning but of fear extinction.

In the second component of their fear learning study, Milad and colleagues had their participants perform a fear extinction protocol. In comparison with healthy participants, individuals with PTSD exhibited amygdala hyperactivity, suggesting that there is a failure to extinguish the conditioned fear response in PTSD. In fact, the physiological fear response in PTSD to the CS—a response that should have been extinguished in the safe context—was also greater than that of healthy participants. In addition, there was vmPFC hypoactivity in PTSD, suggesting deficits in integrating bottom-up drive from the amygdala. These patterns are consistent with the persistent fear responses and hypervigilance seen in PTSD even when cues in the environment indicate relative safety and absence of threat.

In the third and final component of their study, Milad and colleagues took fMRI scans of the participants one day following their original fear learning experience. This second-day scan was conducted to measure fear recall—the memory of fear conditioning and extinction learning. On this second day, individuals with PTSD failed to recall extinction and reduce their

CS   conditioned stimulus
vmPFC   ventromedial prefrontal cortex

fear responses in the safe context. This failed extinction recall was manifest in the corticolimbic circuit as hypoactivity of the vmPFC and HF. Thus, key nodes of the corticolimbic circuit supporting the integration of amygdala activity (i.e., the vmPFC) and the formation of memories for specific contextually appropriate fear (i.e., the HF) were impaired in PTSD. Furthermore, the degree of this impairment in both the vmPFC and HF predicted the paucity of fear extinction. These findings support the hypothesis that fear extinction is specifically impaired in PTSD and that this impairment reflects dysfunctional integration (and subsequent regulation) of amygdala activity mediating fear conditioning, rather than dysfunctional conditioning in the first place.

RESEARCH SPOTLIGHT

One of the most important research areas in psychopathology seeks to identify and understand preexisting neurobiological factors that represent predictive markers of who will and who will not develop mental illness over time. There are many ongoing longitudinal neuroimaging studies following at-risk individuals (e.g., those with family history of a mood or anxiety disorder) with the purpose of ultimately looking back in time to identify differences in brain function that predict who will and will not become ill. However, the results of such studies are typically not available until many years after their initiation. In addition, these studies are exceedingly difficult to conduct, because of the costs associated with studying individuals over many years or even decades of life, as well as the uncertainty of successfully bringing individuals back to the laboratory for follow-up studies. Because of the explicit diagnostic requirement of discrete and identifiable exposure to a traumatic event, PTSD represents a unique opportunity to study preexisting neurobiological markers of risk in an accelerated albeit not easy manner. Such studies in PTSD generally focus on populations who are highly likely to experience a traumatic event that can be measured discretely. Military personnel, including soldiers and medics preparing for deployment to a combat zone, represent such a population and have been the focus of several ongoing studies seeking to identify patterns of corticolimbic circuit function that predict relative vulnerability and resilience to combat-related PTSD. In a prospective study of combat paramedics in the Israel Defense Forces, Admon et al. found that higher predeployment amygdala activity predicted greater postdeployment stress symptoms. Moreover, deployment was associated with changes in the functional connectivity of the HF and vmPFC. Interestingly, an increase in functional connectivity between the hippocampus and vmPFC predicted lesser stress symptoms. Thus, amygdala hyperactivity may reflect a predictive

marker of sensitivity to combat-related stress, possibly by impairing the ability of the HF and vmPFC to regulate this activity when facing stressors (**Figure 4.13**). However, none of the paramedics in this study were diagnosed with PTSD, so the relevance of these patterns for predicting clinical disorder remains to be determined.

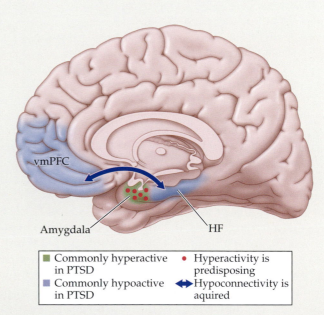

■ Commonly hyperactive in PTSD	• Hyperactivity is predisposing
■ Commonly hypoactive in PTSD	⬌ Hypoconnectivity is aquired

Figure 4.13 Research in military personnel reveals that amygdala hyperactivity prior to combat exposure predicts increased sensitivity to combat-related stress. This increased sensitivity may further reflect impairments in the ability of the HF and vmPFC to effectively regulate this amygdala hyperactivity when facing stressors. (After Admon et al., 2009, 2013.)

---

vmPFC   ventromedial prefrontal cortex
HF   hippocampal formation
PTSD   posttraumatic stress disorder

Generalized anxiety disorder

In contrast to PTSD and the anxiety disorders reviewed above, generalized anxiety disorder (GAD) is characterized by a "free-floating" anxiety not associated with a particular object, event, or situation. In other words, there is no specific trigger resulting in fear, but rather a general and pervasive anxiety ranging from mild nervousness to continuous dread. There also is a higher degree of comorbidity between MDD and GAD than between disorders already reviewed. Interestingly, longitudinal studies suggest that the pervasive anxiety associated with GAD often precedes the development of MDD, particularly in response to stressful life events as discussed above.

As would be expected, given the high comorbidity between GAD and MDD, fMRI studies in individuals with GAD alone or comorbid GAD and MDD have shown amygdala hyperactivity (**Figure 4.14A**). Decreased vmPFC activity and functional connectivity between the amygdala and mPFC have also been noted in GAD. Like amygdala hyperactivity, these patterns are also consistent with those observed in MDD (**Figure 4.14B**). In contrast to these similarities, individuals with GAD or comorbid GAD and MDD show

generalized anxiety disorder (GAD)
Pervasive, "free floating" anxiety not bound to any place, thing, or situation. Highly co-morbid with and often precedes the development of major depressive disorder.

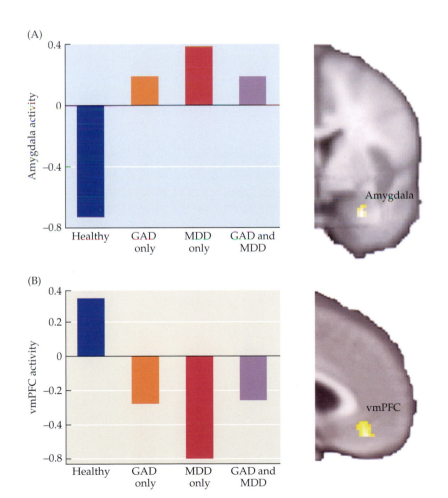

Figure 4.14 (A) During processing of emotional facial expressions, there is evidence for amygdala hyperactivity in patients with GAD only, MDD only, or comorbid for both GAD and MDD, in comparison with healthy participants. (B) The opposite pattern of relative hypo- and hyperactivity is observed for the vmPFC. Note that 0 represents mean activity in these data. (After Etkin & Schatzberg, 2011.)

GAD generalized anxiety disorder
MDD major depressive disorder
mPFC medial prefrontal cortex

decreased activity in the vlPFC not present in those with MDD only. This suggests that the pervasive anxiety that defines GAD may be related specifically to dysfunction of this regulatory region of the prefrontal cortex.

A recent study suggests that another potentially critical difference may exist in GAD in comparison with other anxiety disorders (**Figure 4.15**). Specifically, individuals with GAD exhibit amygdala hyperactivity when only anticipating the appearance of negative pictures but not during the actual viewing of these pictures. Interestingly, these individuals show the same hyperactivity even when the subsequent pictures are neutral. This general hyperactivity when anticipating potentially negative or aversive stimuli (even when it turns out to be neutral) is consistent with the pervasive anxiety characterizing GAD. Importantly, the localization of this hyperactivity was to the dorsal extended amygdala near the bed nucleus of the stria terminalis (BNST). This is also consistent with a general or undefined anxiety that is not in response to specific triggers.

Michael Davis and his colleagues at Emory University have provided compelling evidence that, while the amygdala is critical for fear and anxiety responses provoked by specific stimuli in our environment, the BNST is involved in *maintaining* these responses in the absence of such triggers. As we learned in Chapter 2, the amygdala can potentiate activity in the BNST in response to specific cues. Thus, these lines of evidence suggest the pervasive, nonspecific anxiety in GAD reflects persistent hyperactivity of the BNST (possibly after its initial activation by the amygdala) in the context of deficient prefrontal regulation.

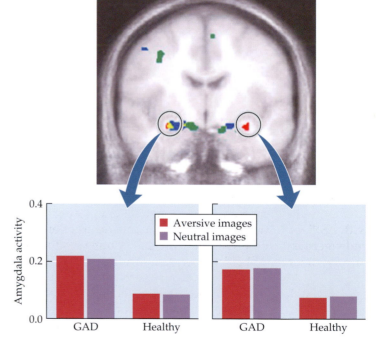

Figure 4.15 In comparison with healthy participants, patients with GAD exhibit amygdala hyperactivity during the anticipation (seen here) but not the actual viewing of either aversive or neutral pictures. The localization of this hyperactivity is in the dorsal extended amygdala near the BNST (black circles). The histograms are the plotted data from these activation clusters. Note that 0 represents baseline activity in these data. (After Nitschke et al., 2009.)

MDD	major depressive disorder
GAD	generalized anxiety disorder
vlPFC	ventrolateral prefrontal cortex
BNST	bed nucleus of the stria terminalis

RESEARCH SPOTLIGHT

Somerville and colleagues at Dartmouth College conducted an fMRI study in healthy participants while they completed a shock anticipation task (**Figure 4.16**). During the task, participants viewed a screen with a scrolling line that constantly fluctuated in its height. When the line breached a specified threshold, the subjects in the study accrued an electric shock that they were to get later. Critically, they never received any shocks during the scan. Thus, the experimenters were able to create a general state of heightened anxiety in the absence of an actual shock. Analyses of the fMRI data revealed that activity in the BNST was positively correlated with the anticipation of accruing later shocks. This anticipatory activity was also present in the insula. However, anticipatory activity in the amygdala and insula was present only in individuals reporting relatively higher levels of trait anxiety and not those reporting lower levels of trait anxiety. These results indicate that the BNST is involved not only in clinically significant anxiety like GAD but also in the broader dimensional expression of anxiety present to varying degrees in us all.

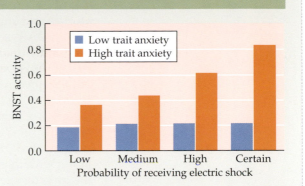

Figure 4.16 Activity in the BNST increases as healthy participants track the probability of receiving a mild electric shock in the future, with the strongest activity occurring when participants are certain that they will subsequently receive a shock. Interestingly, this pattern of anticipatory activity in the BNST only occurs in individuals with relatively high levels of self-reported trait anxiety. Note that 0 represents baseline activity in these data. (After Somerville et al., 2010.)

Disorders of Social Behavior

As the previous sections reveal, corticolimbic circuit dysfunction generally and amygdala hyperactivity specifically manifest as core symptoms of exaggerated sensitivity and maladaptive responses to threat and stress in mood and anxiety disorders. Such dysfunction is also present in psychopathology not commonly categorized as mood and anxiety disorders—that is, in several conditions characterized by abnormal social interactions and behaviors, including inappropriate aggression and social withdrawal, which we will refer to broadly as disorders of social behavior. The specific categorical diagnoses we will review in the context of relative amygdala hyperactivity are antisocial personality disorder, intermittent explosive disorder, and autism spectrum disorders.

Antisocial personality disorder

Antisocial personality disorder (ASPD) is characterized by a blatant disregard for the needs, safety, and well-being of others, as well as an inability to follow moral, societal, or legal rules. ASPD is more often diagnosed in men, and these individuals are generally hypersensitive to threat and respond aggressively when they perceive themselves to be threatened (i.e., they exhibit reactive aggression). Common delinquent and antisocial acts of individuals with ASPD include assault, larceny, arson, destruction of property, reckless endangerment, and other criminal activity often leading to arrest. Although the diagnosis of ASPD is reserved for individuals 18 years of age or older, these individuals typically have a persistent history of delinquent and antisocial behaviors dating to childhood, when such behavior is diagnosed as conduct disorder (CD). A subset of individuals with ASPD also exhibit callous and unemotional (CU) traits, which involve a lack of empathy and remorse, as

antisocial personality disorder (ASPD) Characterized by disregard for the needs, safety, and well being of others, as well as an inability to follow moral, societal, or legal rules.

reactive aggression Anger or violence in response to perceived threat, especially from other individuals.

conduct disorder (CD) Characterized by delinquent and antisocial behavior during childhood and adolescence. When such behavior persists beyond age 18, it may be diagnosed as antisocial personality disorder.

callous and unemotional (CU) traits Lack of empathy and remorse for the suffering of others.

ASPD   antisocial personality disorder
CD   conduct disorder
CU   callous and unemotional

intermittent explosive disorder (IED) Characterized by hypersensitivity to threat leading to episodes of grossly inappropriate (usually violent) reactive aggression.

well as a tendency to rationalize distress inflicted on others. As we will consider later in the chapter, CU traits are also a hallmark feature of psychopaths.

Amygdala hyperactivity has been observed in fMRI studies of ASPD. Some studies reporting amygdala hyperactivity have been conducted in children with CD because they represent those at-risk for later developing ASPD. In addition, there is some evidence for hypoactivity of regulatory regions of the PFC in ASPD and CD. This pattern of corticolimbic dysfunction is consistent with the hypersensitivity of some individuals with ASPD to threat, and their reactive aggression. However, as ASPD represents a heterogeneous set of disordered behaviors, the most useful fMRI studies attempt to isolate corticolimbic circuit dysfunction in specific subsets of individuals with more homogeneous symptoms (e.g., ASPD with or without CU traits). These studies, along with those in psychopaths, will be discussed in the upcoming section on amygdala hypoactivity.

Intermittent explosive disorder

Similar to some individuals with ASPD, those with intermittent explosive disorder (IED) characteristically exhibit hypersensitivity to threat and heightened levels of reactive aggression. Individuals with IED, who are typically men,

RESEARCH SPOTLIGHT

Although the inappropriate and persistent reactive aggression common to ASPD and IED represents an extreme manifestation of amygdala hyperactivity and corticolimbic circuit dysfunction, more modest forms of reactive aggression are expressed to varying degrees across all individuals. This spectrum of reactive aggression and anger more generally can be measured using a variety of self-report instruments such as the State-Trait Anger Expression Inventory (STAXI) or Lifetime History of Aggression. My lab has examined the relationship between amygdala activity in response to emotional facial expressions and self-reported aggression in a normative sample of healthy adults (**Figure 4.17**). Analyses revealed a pattern that was remarkably similar to that reported in individuals with IED. Specifically, amygdala hyperactivity in response to angry but not fearful facial expressions uniquely predicted higher levels of trait anger, and particularly reactive anger, as measured by the STAI. However, this relationship was present only in men who also reported high levels of trait anxiety, as measured by the State-Trait Anxiety Inventory. Amygdala activity was unrelated to trait anger in women regardless of their levels of trait anxiety. Thus, these data are consistent with a role of amygdala hyperactivity in mediating reactive aggression, as only men who were more sensitive to threat (i.e., high in trait anxiety) exhibited higher reactive anger as a function of increased amygdala activity, specifically to explicit displays of threat (i.e., angry facial expressions).

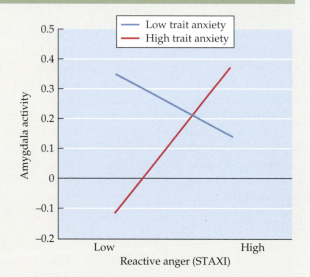

Figure 4.17 For men (but not women), the propensity to experience more or less anger in contexts of reasonable provocation (e.g., when demeaned, criticized, or treated unfairly) is predicted by the magnitude of amygdala activity to angry but not fearful facial expressions. However, this association between amygdala activity and the experience of anger is present only in men who also experience high levels of trait anxiety; it is not found in those with low trait anxiety. This pattern is consistent with the role of threat-related amygdala activity in reactive aggression. Note that 0 represents mean activity in these data. (After Carré et al., 2012.)

CU	callous and unemotional
ASPD	antisocial personality disorder
CD	conduct disorder

PFC	prefrontal cortex
IED	intermittent explosive disorder

may attack others and their possessions, causing bodily injury and property damage that is grossly out of proportion to any precipitating psychosocial stressor. For formal diagnosis, a patient must have exhibited at least three episodes of inappropriate reactive aggression during any time in his life. In contrast to individuals with ASPD, who often rationalize their aggressive behavior, those with IED typically express remorse and experience guilt after episodes of aggression.

Not surprisingly, fMRI studies of individuals with IED have shown amygdala hyperactivity as well as decreased functional connectivity between the amygdala and vmPFC. Interestingly, amygdala hyperactivity appears to be specific for stimuli that signal threat, namely angry facial expressions, and the magnitude of this hyperactivity is correlated with the number of aggressive acts committed by individuals with IED. Amygdala hyperactivity also may exist to neutral facial expressions, which may subsequently be interpreted by individuals with IED as threatening. Thus, the inappropriate reactive aggression in IED reflects a hyperactive response of the amygdala to signals of threat or potential threat, followed by a failure to effectively regulate this response through the PFC.

Autism spectrum disorders

Autism spectrum disorders (ASD) refers to a group of disorders, including autism and Asperger's syndrome, characterized by varying degrees of social, emotional, and cognitive dysfunction. ASD is more commonly diagnosed in boys and encompasses a paucity or significant delay in the development of verbal and nonverbal language; marked social disengagement, including poor eye contact and flattened affect; stereotypical behaviors; and a hypersensitivity to sensory input. Most prominent in this constellation of symptoms in the context of corticolimbic circuit dysfunction are the deficits in social and emotional behavior that are present across the spectrum.

Many early theories suggested that ASD, and autism in particular, reflected blunting of emotional responsiveness and hyposensitivity to social input. However, recent evidence from fMRI and psychophysiological studies has led to a reconceptualization of ASD as reflecting hyperresponsiveness to social and emotional stimulation. In turn, this hyperresponsiveness leads individuals with ASD to avoid social interactions and withdraw into stereotypical patterns of familiar, nonthreatening behaviors. Consistent with this model, Temple Grandin, an accomplished research scientist who has autism and is a vocal advocate for increased understanding of ASD, describes herself as having "the nervous system of a prey species," experiencing fear as a dominant emotional state. Such insight is uniquely valuable, as many individuals with the diagnosis, particularly autism, are cognitively low functioning and unable to articulate their internal states and experiences.

Interestingly, early fMRI studies of ASD appeared consistent with the blunted affect and social hyposensitivity models. In these studies, which required that subjects make simple perceptual decisions about objects or faces, there was a notable lack of difference in amygdala activity between healthy participants and individuals with ASD or there was significantly decreased amygdala activity in ASD. However, these early studies were critically limited by a failure to account for one of the core deficits in ASD: poor eye contact.

One of the more consistent deficits observed in ASD is gaze aversion, where patients avert their gaze from the eyes of faces and toward the mouths

autism spectrum disorders (ASD) A group of disorders, including autism and Asperger's syndrome, characterized by varying degrees of intellectual dysfunction, including delayed or deficient verbal and nonverbal language skills, with persistent deficits in social and emotional behavior.

vmPFC ventromedial prefrontal cortex
ASD autism spectrum disorders

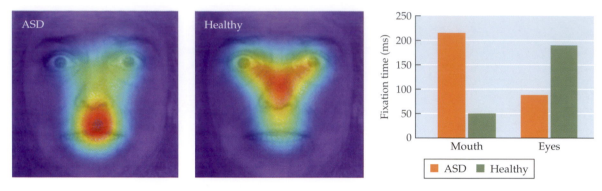

Figure 4.18 Unlike healthy individuals, who focus their attention on the eyes of a face, individuals with ASD focus their attention on the mouth. (After Neumann et al., 2006.)

(**Figure 4.18**). As we learned in Chapter 3, the amygdala is particularly responsive to the eyes and, moreover, the subtle differences in the presentation of the sclera associated with different emotional facial expressions. Normally, we focus our gaze on the eyes of faces, and this attentional bias contributes to eliciting amygdala activity. In the absence of this gaze bias toward the eyes, there is little to no amygdala activity. Because early fMRI studies failed to account for eye gaze, which is generally low in ASD, these studies observed a relative decrease or no difference in amygdala activity in comparison with healthy participants.

Recent studies either have worked to carefully control for differences in eye gaze between individuals with ASD and healthy participants, or the studies have employed tasks that minimize these differences. These studies consistently observe amygdala hyperactivity in those with ASD. In the first of such studies, Kim Dalton and colleagues at the University of Wisconsin found that the magnitude of amygdala activity was positively correlated with the percent of time that gaze was fixated on the eyes of facial stimuli. As expected, individuals with ASD spent less time fixating on the eyes than did

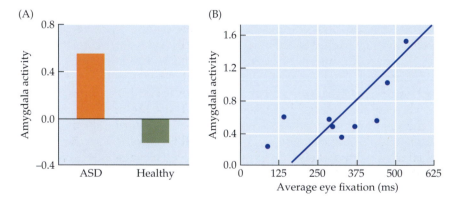

Figure 4.19 (A) Amygdala activity is greater in individuals with ASD in comparison to healthy participants when they attend to the eyes of face stimuli. (B) The magnitude of amygdala activity is positively correlated with the amount of time individuals with ASD attend to the eyes. Note that 0 represents mean activity in (A) and baseline activity in (B). (After Dalton et al., 2005.)

ASD autism spectrum disorders

(A)
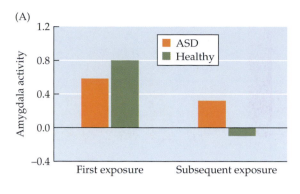

(B)
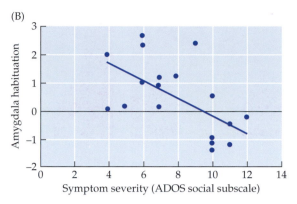

Figure 4.20 (A) Amygdala activity to faces habituates upon repeated exposure in healthy participants but not individuals with ASD. (B) The lack of amygdala habituation (lower scores on *x*-axis) is associated with greater social deficits in individuals with ASD assessed using the social subscale of the Autism Diagnostic Observation Schedule (ADOS). Note that 0 represents mean activity in these data. (After Kleinhans et al., 2009.)

the healthy participants. However, when Dalton and colleagues examined fMRI data only from faces where patients with ASD did fixate their gaze on the eyes, they found evidence for amygdala hyperactivity (**Figure 4.19A**). In fact, the magnitude of amygdala activity was positively correlated with the amount of time patients spent gazing at the eyes of the stimuli (**Figure 4.19B**). Additional fMRI studies in ASD have noted similar amygdala hyperactivity or amygdala activity equivalent to that of healthy participants. As would be suggested by their amygdala hyperactivity, individuals with ASD are faster in processing emotional facial expressions and have higher levels of social anxiety.

In addition to observing amygdala hyperactivity in ASD, recent studies have detected hypoactivity in the vmPFC, as well as decreased amygdala-vmPFC functional connectivity. Consistent with this pattern, there is also evidence for decreased habituation of amygdala activity in ASD, and this failure to habituate is associated with greater severity of social deficits (**Figure 4.20**).

These patterns of corticolimbic circuit dysfunction are highly consistent with the emerging model of ASD as representing a hypersensitivity to challenges we face from our environment. Poorly regulated amygdala hyperactivity leads to a generally anxious and fearful state, which individuals with ASD attempt to reduce by shifting their attention away from specific triggers, such as eyes, and by avoiding novel or unfamiliar places and people, which they experience as highly aversive. These biases further manifest as stereotypical or rigid patterns of behavior, which work to limit exposure to anxiety-producing and fearful contexts and triggers. A specific aversion to social interactions likely exacerbates delayed language and other cognitive abilities in individuals with ASD.

Amygdala Hypoactivity

Although far less commonly observed than amygdala hyperactivity, hypoactivity of the amygdala also occurs and leads to specific symptoms

vmPFC ventromedial prefrontal cortex

of psychopathology. As would be expected, psychopathology associated with amygdala hypoactivity manifests as generally blunted affect and hyporesponsiveness to threat as well as diminished sensitivity to fear or distress expressed by others. Dysfunction in the broader corticolimbic circuit, particularly the mPFC, may also be observed in parallel with amygdala hypoactivity.

Importantly, such dysfunction does not manifest as different, nonoverlapping disorders. Rather, amygdala hypoactivity and related circuit dysfunction manifest as specific symptoms or response biases within disorders already discussed above. This is not only an indication of the substantial heterogeneity that exists within categorical diagnoses and the need to map disorder in brain circuit function onto specific symptoms or features of psychopathology, but also a critical illustration of the need to consider the stimuli and paradigms used with fMRI to probe variability in circuit function.

Major depressive disorder

Several fMRI studies of individuals with MDD have observed amygdala hypoactivity. Interestingly, this hypoactivity is often observed in individuals who also exhibit amygdala hyperactivity. The critical difference is to what stimuli the relative hyper- and hypoactivity of the amygdala occur. As reviewed above, amygdala hyperactivity in MDD is generally to facial expressions conveying threat such as anger and fear. This hyperactivity, which is poorly regulated by hypoactive prefrontal regions, manifests as an exaggerated sensitivity to threat, stress, and other negative experiences. There is also evidence of amygdala hyperactivity in response to facial expressions of sadness, which may reflect a mood-congruent attentional bias or sensitivity to stimuli signaling negative emotional states or social interactions. In contrast, amygdala hypoactivity has been observed to stimuli conveying positive emotion, namely, happy facial expressions (**Figure 4.21**).

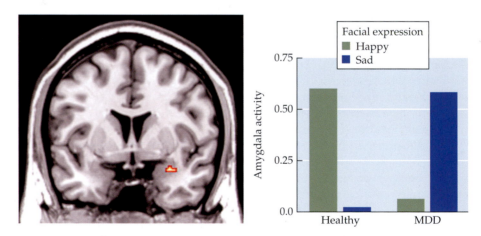

Figure 4.21 Individuals with MDD can exhibit differential amygdala hyper- and hypoactivity to specific emotional expressions. In this study, individuals with MDD exhibited relative hypoactivity to happy facial expressions but hyperactivity to sad facial expressions. The opposite pattern was found in healthy participants. The pattern of expression-specific amygdala hypo- and hyperactivity in MDD may reflect mood-congruent biases during an MDE (i.e., high levels of sadness and low levels of happiness). Note that 0 represents mean activity in these data. (After Suslow et al., 2010.)

mPFC   medial prefrontal cortex
MDD   major depressive disorder
MDE   major depressive episode

Moreover, the magnitude of amygdala activity in response to happy expressions is negatively correlated with the severity of depressive symptoms, suggesting that the ability to trigger responses to positive social stimuli may protect against deepening depression. Thus, in MDD there may be a specific failure to generate arousal, attention, and subsequent interest in stimuli that represent positive changes in our environment (e.g., the arrival of a close friend). This amygdala hypoactivity specifically to happy facial expressions is likely related to the anhedonia commonly experienced by individuals with MDD. While amygdala hypoactivity may contribute to anhedonia, the core dysfunction associated with this symptom is in the corticostriatal circuit and will be discussed in Unit II.

Bipolar disorders

As noted above, amygdala hypoactivity in BD is a state-dependent phenomenon, observed only when individuals experience a major depressive episode (see Figure 4.6A). This state-dependent hypoactivity appears to emerge through dysfunctional overregulation of what is otherwise normal amygdala activity, as indicated by the state-dependent increase in amygdala-vlPFC connectivity observed only during an MDE. This overall pattern of dysfunction is consistent with the lethargy, apathy, and lack of interest in social interactions that define an MDE in individuals with BD.

Antisocial personality disorder

Amygdala hyperactivity is consistent with the general pattern of reactive aggression characteristic of ASPD and its developmental precursor, conduct disorder. However, amygdala hypoactivity has been observed when studies carefully work to reduce the heterogeneity of symptoms and features of ASPD. In particular, amygdala hypoactivity emerges in studies of antisocial individuals, particularly children and adolescents, who are also high in CU traits (Figure 4.22A). In addition, the amygdala activity that does exist in such individuals does not appear to properly drive activity in the vmPFC, and this diminished functional connectivity predicts greater severity of CU traits, including deficits in recognizing expressions of distress—specifically sadness and fear—and feeling less fear and less empathy for victims of aggression. Individuals high in CU traits also demonstrate reduced eye gaze, particularly to fearful facial expressions (Figure 4.22B).

Curiously, reduced eye gaze is also seen in ASD, which differs markedly with respect to both amygdala activity and social behaviors from ASPD with high CU traits. It is possible that in ASD amygdala hyperactivity leads to excessive anxiety and fear, which is counteracted through averting gaze from the eyes and social withdrawal. In contrast, the amygdala hypoactivity in individuals high in CU traits may actually lead to a failure to gaze at the eyes, an inability to recognize the emotions of others, a hyposensitivity to threat, and diminished fear. These features culminate in general callousness and antisocial behavior in the absence of guilt or remorse in ASPD.

Psychopathy

Amygdala hypoactivity and diminished amygdala-mPFC functional connectivity are observed in the most extreme form of antisocial, callous, and unemotional behavior, referred to as pyschopathy. Although no longer recognized in the *DSM*, psychopathy can be formally identified using an

anhedonia Diminished interest in and inability to experience pleasure from common activities.

psychopathy Characterized by extreme callousness, selfishness, narcissism, and remorseless use of others and a persistent pattern of unstable relationships and antisocial behavior, including instrumental (proactive) aggression.

BD bipolar disorders
vlPFC ventrolateral prefrontal cortex
ASPD antisocial personality disorder
vmPFC ventromedial prefrontal cortex
CU callous and unemotional
ASD autism spectrum disorders

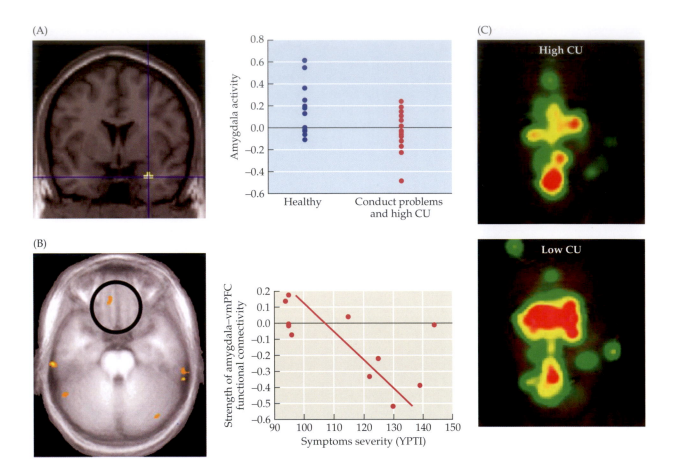

Figure 4.22 (A) Boys with conduct problems who also have high levels of callous and unemotional (CU) traits exhibit decreased amygdala activity to fearful facial expressions in comparison with healthy boys. (B) Decreased functional connectivity between the amygdala and vmPFC while viewing fearful facial expressions is associated with higher scores on the Youth Psychopathic Traits Inventory (YPTI), which includes the presence of CU traits. (C) In comparison with adolescents low in CU traits, adolescents with high levels of CU traits spend significantly less time attending to the eyes of fearful facial expressions. Note that 0 represents mean activity (A) and mean connectivity (B) in these data. (A from Jones et al., 2009; B after Marsh et al., 2008; C from Dadds et al., 2008.)

instrumental (proactive) aggression The purposeful and premeditated use of violence to achieve a personal goal and (unlike reactive aggression) not in response to provocation.

interview-based procedure that establishes high degrees of callousness, selfishness, narcissism, and remorseless use of others, as well as a persistent pattern of unstable relationships and antisocial behavior, established through review of case histories. Fortunately, few individuals are identified as psychopaths. The very few who are typically display instrumental, or proactive, aggression in addition to the reactive aggression commonly found in ASPD. **Instrumental aggression** involves the purposeful and premeditated use of violence to achieve a personal goal and is not in response to provocation.

Interestingly, a common feature of psychopaths is a failure to acquire conditioned fear responses (**Figure 4.23**). This deficit exists even in the presence of an explicit awareness of CS-US pairings, which is consistent with

ASPD	antisocial personality disorder	**CU**	callous and unemotional
CS	conditioned stimulus	**vmPFC**	ventromedial prefrontal cortex
US	unconditioned stimulus		

(A)

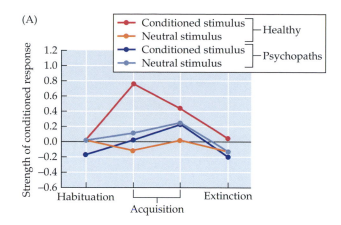

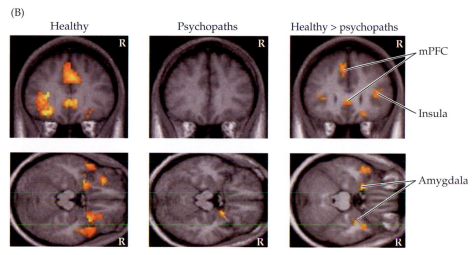

(B)

Figure 4.23 (A) In contrast to their failure to develop a conditioned fear response as measured through changes in peripheral physiology (here, sweating), psychopaths did consciously learn which of two stimuli was paired with painful pressure (the conditioned stimulus) and rated the CS as more aversive. Note that 0 represents the baseline in these data. (B) Consistent with the failure to acquire a conditioned fear response, there was significantly decreased activity in the amygdala, mPFC, and insula of psychopaths in comparison with healthy participants. (After Birbaumer et al., 2005.)

the generally high level of cognitive functioning in psychopaths. Thus, there may be relatively preserved cognitive function but impaired emotional function in psychopathy. This impaired fear conditioning is reflected in relative hypoactivity of the amygdala and interconnected corticolimbic circuit nodes, including the mPFC and insula. Collectively, the emerging data in psychopathy suggests that corticolimbic circuit dysfunction leads to deficits in the ability to recognize signals of distress, such as fearful facial expressions, and to learn conditioned fear responses. In the absence of recognizing these signals, which function to promote empathy and social affiliation as well as help us avoid danger, the intact cognitive processes in psychopaths emerge as persistent antisocial behavior and instrumental aggression.

mPFC   medial prefrontal cortex

RESEARCH SPOTLIGHT

While psychopaths represent a very small fraction of the population, psychopathic traits such as callousness and antisocial behavior are dimensional constructs that exist to varying degrees across us all. As in the earlier study of reactive aggression, my lab examined the relationships between the spectrum of psychopathic traits and amygdala activity in 200 young adult students. Psychopathic traits were assessed using the Self-Report of Psychopathy (SRP) short form questionnaire (**Figure 4.24**). Amygdala activity to angry and fearful facial expressions was assessed using fMRI. Amygdala hypoactivity specifically to fearful expressions was associated with greater levels of remorseless and

callous exploitation of others. This is consistent with the failure to recognize distress in others that is found in psychopaths. In contrast, amygdala hyperactivity, specifically to angry expressions, was associated with greater levels of challenging authority, dangerous activities, and reckless behavior, including promiscuity. This is consistent with the reactive aggression seen in ASPD broadly, particularly in the absence of high CU traits. Thus, across the entire spectrum of psychopathic traits, we can observe both amygdala hypo- and hyperactivity, depending on the nature of the stimulus or trigger, which is expressed as different forms of antisocial behavior.

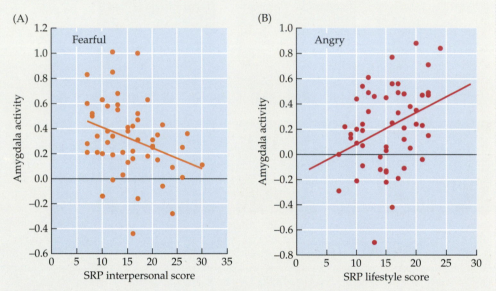

Figure 4.24 (A) Amygdala hypoactivity, specifically to fearful facial expressions, is associated with greater levels of remorseless and callous exploitation of others as measured by the Self-Report of Psychopathy (SRP) interpersonal score. (B) Amygdala hyperactivity to angry facial expressions is associated with greater levels of challenging authority, dangerous activities, and reckless behavior, including promiscuity as measured by the SRP lifestyle score. Note that 0 represents mean activity in these data. (After Carré et al., 2012.)

Williams Syndrome

Williams syndrome A developmental disorder resulting from a partial deletion of chromosome 7. Associated with multiple physical and mental symptoms that include distinct patterns of disordered social and emotional behavior, notably social disinhibition and fearlessness of others.

Although not formally a psychiatric disorder and generally reflecting multiple physical and mental symptoms, **Williams syndrome** includes distinct patterns of disordered social and emotional behaviors that warrant consideration in the context of corticolimbic circuit dysfunction. Most notably, individuals with Williams syndrome (which results from the partial deletion of chomosome 7) typically exhibit a marked social *dis*inhibition and fearlessness of others. This pattern of gregarious and often indiscriminate social behavior is in stark contrast to that characterizing autism spectrum disorders, even though generally low intellectual functioning is shared by Williams syndrome and ASD.

ASD   autism spectrum disorders
ASPD   antisocial personality disorder
CU   callous and unemotional

This divergence in social behavior is mirrored in the patterns of amygdala activity to facial expressions in individuals with Williams syndrome (**Figure 4.25**). As expected, there is amygdala hypoactivity in response to social stimuli, including facial expressions conveying threat. Interestingly, amygdala hypoactivity in response to threat predicts the degree of social fearlessness, often measured as the willingness to trust and approach strangers, in Williams syndrome. In contrast, there is evidence for amygdala hyperactivity to stimuli signaling positive emotion, such as happy facial expressions.

Critically, this fearlessness to engage in social interactions does not generalize to other stimuli. In fact, patients with Williams syndrome often exhibit higher levels of anxiety and fears, including specific phobias, than are observed in the general population, or even in other developmental disorders. Here again, the differential activity of the amygdala closely matches this aspect of the syndrome. Specifically, while there is amygdala hypoactivity in response to social threats (i.e., angry or fearful facial expressions), there is hyperactivity in response to nonsocial threats such as spiders, snakes, and snarling dogs (**Figure 4.26**).

Studies of functional connectivity in Williams syndrome suggest that the stimulus-specific patterns of amygdala hypo- and hyperactivity reflect abnormal patterns of top-down

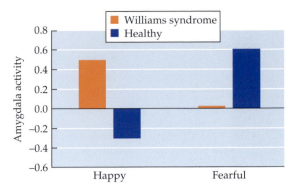

Figure 4.25 Individuals with Williams syndrome exhibit relative amygdala hyperactivity to happy facial expressions but marked hypoactivity to fearful facial expressions. Note that 0 represents mean activity in these data. (After Haas et al., 2009.)

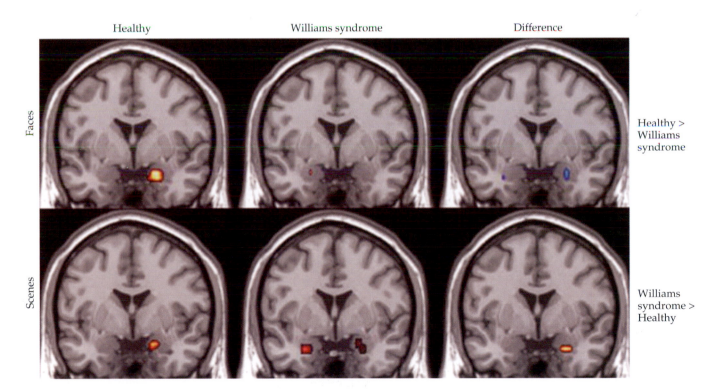

Figure 4.26 In comparison with healthy participants, individuals with Williams syndrome exhibit amygdala hypoactivity to social threat (angry and fearful facial expressions in this study) but hyperactivity to nonsocial threat (snakes, spiders, and dogs in this study). (From Meyer-Lindenberg et al., 2005.)

regulation of the amygdala by regions of the PFC. Specifically, there appears to be too little top-down regulation to nonsocial threat and too much to social threat. This pattern is consistent with the highly elaborative nature of social and emotional language seen in Williams syndrome. Such linguistic function is highly preserved in comparison not only to other developmental disorders (e.g., Down syndrome), but also to other functions (e.g., visuospatial skills) in Williams syndrome. When individuals with Williams syndrome engage in their unique and elaborate linguistic processing of social stimuli and situations, there is likely increased prefrontal activity, which could mediate top-down inhibition of otherwise heightened amygdala activity and lead to disinhibited or gregarious social behavior. The absence of such linguistic elaboration for nonsocial stimuli, in contrast, does not engage these top-down regulatory processes in the PFC, thereby allowing the expression of relatively increased amygdala activity as anxiety and fear.

Summary

Corticolimbic circuit dysfunction, manifesting as amygdala hyper- or hypoactivity, commonly emerges as psychopathology associated with mood and anxiety disorders as well as disorders of social behavior. While there are symptoms and features unique to each categorical disorder reviewed above, a shared or core dysfunction across all of these disorders is maladaptive behavioral and physiological reactions to challenges present in our environment.

Disorders characterized by heightened sensitivity to threat and stress (e.g., major depressive disorder, social anxiety disorder, specific phobia) emerge when there is amygdala hyperactivity, which is typically associated with hypoactivity of the ventromedial and dorsomedial prefrontal cortex, leading to deficient top-down integration and regulation. In contrast, disorders characterized by lessened sensitivity to threat and stress (e.g., antisocial personality disorder with callous and unemotional traits, psychopathy) emerge when there is amygdala hypoactivity, which can be associated with hyperactivity of these prefrontal regions and thus excessive top-down inhibition. Unique features of these disorders likely reflect subtle differences in the nature of dysfunctional prefrontal regulation (e.g.,

state-like in major depressive disorder, but trait-like in bipolar disorders) or the precise locus of dysregulated activity (e.g., amygdala in social anxiety disorder and specific phobia, but bed nucleus of the stria terminalis in generalized anxiety disorder).

Moreover, unique features also emerge as a function of differential amygdala activity in response to specific stimuli (e.g., hyperactivity in response to threatening and sad facial expressions, but hypoactivity to happy facial expressions in major depressive disorder), which likely reflect abnormal learning of specific associations between cues and outcomes. The form of such aberrant learning also contributes to the emergence of disorder-specific features (e.g., abnormal fear extinction but not fear conditioning in posttraumatic stress disorder, but abnormal fear conditioning in psychopathy).

Finally, while there is ample evidence for shared dysfunction of the corticolimbic circuit that maps onto specific symptoms across disorders, the underlying cellular, molecular, and even genetic factors ultimately leading to the observed dysfunction at the circuit level may differ considerably between disorders. While beyond the scope of this text, such unique features of disorders may be critical in the relative responsiveness of each to either pharmacological or behavioral treatment.

Literature Cited & Further Reading

Admon, R., Lubin, G., Stern, O., Rosenberg, K., Sela, L., Ben-Ami, H., & Hendler, T. (2009). Human vulnerability to stress depends on amygdala's predisposition and hippocampal plasticity. *Proceedings of the National Academy of Science USA*, 106: 14120–14125.

Admon, R., Milad, M. R., & Hendler, T. (2013). A causal model of post-traumatic stress disorder: Disentangling predisposed from acquired neural abnormalities. *Trends in Cognitive Sciences*, 17: 337–347.

Altshuler, L., & 9 others. (2005). Increased amygdala activation during mania: A functional magnetic resonance imaging study. *American Journal of Psychiatry*, 162: 1211–1213.

Anand, A., Li, Y., Wang, Y., Gardner, K., & Lowe, M. J. (2007). Reciprocal effects of antidepressant treatment on activity and connectivity of the mood regulating circuit: An fMRI study. *Journal of Neuropsychiatry & Clinical Neurosciences*, 19: 274–282.

Anderson, N. E., & Kiehl, K. A. (2012). The psychopath magnetized: Insights from brain imaging. *Trends in Cognitive Science*, 16: 52–60.

Bellugi, U., Lichtenberger, L., Jones, W., Lai, Z., & St. George, M. (2000). The neurocognitive profile of Williams syndrome: A complex pattern of strengths and weaknesses. *Journal of Cognitive Neuroscience*, 12, Supplement 1: 7–29.

Birbaumer, N., Veit, R., Lotze, M., Erb, M., Hermann, C., Grodd, W., & Flor, H. (2005). Deficient fear conditioning in psychopathy. *Archives of General Psychiatry*, 62: 799–805.

Blair, R. J., & Viding, E. (2008). Psychopathy. Chapter 51, pp. 852–863 in Rutter et al. (ed.) *Rutter's Child and Adolescent Psychiatry, 5th Edition*. New York: John Wiley & Sons.

Brohawn, K. H., Offringa, R., Pfaff, D. L., Hughes, K. C., & Shin, L. M. (2010). The neural correlates of emotional memory in posttraumatic stress disorder. *Biological Psychiatry*, 68: 1023–1030.

Carré, J. M., Fisher, P. M. Manuck, S. B., & Hariri, A. R. (2012). Interaction between trait anxiety and trait anger predict amygdala reactivity to angry facial expressions in men but not women. *Social Cognitive & Affective Neuroscience*, 7: 213–221.

Coccaro, E. F., McCloskey, M. S., Fitzgerald, D. A., & Phan, K. L. (2007). Amygdala and orbitofrontal reactivity to social threat in individuals with impulsive aggression. *Biological Psychiatry*, 62: 168–178.

Coulston, C., & 9 others. (2013). Is coping well a matter of personality? A study of euthymic unipolar and bipolar patients. *Journal of Affective Disorders*, 145: 54–61.

Critchley, H. D., & 10 others. (2000). The functional neuroanatomy of social behaviour: Changes in cerebral blood flow when people with autistic disorder process facial expressions. *Brain*, 123: 2203–2212.

Dadds, M. R., El Masry, Y., Wimalaweera, S., & Guastella, A. J. (2008). Reduced eye gaze explains "fear blindness" in childhood psychopathic traits. *Journal of the American Academy of Child & Adolescent Psychiatry*, 47: 455–463.

Dalton, K. M., Nacewicz, B. M., Johnstone, T., Schaefer, H. S., Gernsbacher, M. A., Goldsmith, H. H., Alexander, A. I., & Davidson, R. J. (2005). Gaze fixation and the neural circuitry of face processing in autism. *Nature Neuroscience*, 8: 519–526.

Davis, M., Walker, D. L., Miles, L., & Grillon, C. (2010). Phasic versus sustained fear in rats and humans: Role of the extended amygdala in fear versus anxiety. *Neuropsychopharmacology*, 35: 105–135.

DeRubeis, R. J., Siegle, G. J., & Holton, S. D. (2008). Cognitive therapy versus medication for depression: Treatment outcomes and neural mechanisms. *Nature Reviews Neuroscience*, 9: 788–795.

Dresler, T., Guhn, A., Tupak, S. V., Ehlis, A.-C., Herrmann, M. J., Fallgater, A. J., Deckert, J., & Domschke, K. (2013). Revise the revised? New dimensions of the neuroanatomical hypothesis of panic disorder. *Journal of Neural Transmission*, 120: 3–29.

Drevets, W. C., Videen, T. O., Price, J. L., Preskorn, S. H., Carmichael, S. T., & Raichle, M. E. (1992). A functional anatomical study of unipolar depresssion. *The Journal of Neuroscience*, 12: 3628–3641.

Dykens, E. M. (2003). Anxiety, fears, and phobias in persons with Williams syndrome. *Developmental Neuropsychology*, 23: 291–316.

El Khoury-Malhame, M., & 13 others. (2011). Amygdala activity correlates with attentional bias in PTSD. *Neuropsychologia*, 49: 1969–1973.

Etkin, A., & Schatzberg, A. F. (2011). Common abnormalities and disorder-specific compensation during implicit regulation of emotional processing in generalized anxiety and major depressive disorders. *American Journal of Psychiatry*, 168: 968–978.

Etkin, A., & Wagner, T. D. (2007). Functional neuroimaging of anxiety: A meta-analysis of emotional processing it PTSD, social anxiety disorder, and specific phobia. *American Journal of Psychiatry*, 164: 1476–1488.

Finger, E. C., & 13 others. (2012). Impaired functional but preserved structural connectivity in limbic white matter tracts in youth with conduct disorder or oppositional defiant disorder plus psychopathic traits. *Psychiatric Research*, 202: 239–244.

Goossens, L., Sunaert, S., Peeters, R., Griez, E. J. L., & Schruers, K. R. J. (2007). Amygdala hyperfunction in phobic fear normalizes after exposure. *Biological Psychiatry*, 62: 1119–1125.

Groenewold, N. A., Opmeer, E. M., de Jonge, P., Aleman, A., & Costafreda, S. G. (2013). Emotional valence modulates brain functional abnormalities in depression: Evidence from a meta-analysis of fMRI studies. *Neuroscience & Biobehavioral Reviews*, 37: 152–163.

Haas, B. W., Hoeft, F., Searcy, Y. M., Mills, D., Bellugi, U., & Reiss, A. (2010). Individual differences in social behavior predict amygdala response to fearful facial expressions in Williams syndrome. *Neuropsychologia*, 48: 1283–1288.

Haas, B. W., Mills, D., Yam, A., Hoeft, F., Bellugi, U., & Reiss, A. (2009). Genetic influences on sociability: Heightened amygdala reactivity and event-related responses to positive social stimuli in Williams syndrome. *The Journal of Neuroscience*, 29: 1132–1139.

Hamilton, J. P., Etkin, A., Furman, D. J., Lemus, M. G., Johnson, R. F., & Gotlib, I. H. (2012). Functional neuroimaging of major depressive disorder: A meta-analysis and new integration of baseline activation and neural response data. *American Journal of Psychiatry*, 169: 693–703.

Hariri, A. R. (2012). The highs and lows of amygdala reactivity in bipolar disorders. *American Journal of Psychiatry*, 169: 780–783.

Hayes, J. P., LaBar, K. S., McCarthy, G., Selgrade, E., Nasser, J., Dolcos, F., VISN 6 Mid-Atlantic MIRECC workgroup, & Morey, R. A. (2011). Reduced hippocampal and amygdala activity predicts memory distortions for trauma reminders in combat-related PTSD. *Journal of Psychiatric Research*, 45: 660–669.

Hayes, J. P., Hayes, S. M., & Mikedis, A. M. (2012). Quantitative meta-analysis of neural activity in posttraumatic stress disorder. *Biology of Mood & Anxiety Disorders*, 2: 9.

Herpertz, S. C., & 8 others. (2008). Emotional processing in male adolescents with childhood-onset conduct disorder. *Journal of Child Psychology and Psychiatry*, 49: 781–791.

Johansen-Berg, H., Gutman, D. A., Behrens, T. E. J., Matthews, P. M., Rushworth, M. F. S., Katz, E., Lozano, A. M., & Mayberg, H. S. (2008). Anatomical connectivity of the subgenual cingulate regions targeted with deep-brain stimulation for treatment-resistant depression. *Cerebral Cortex*, 18: 1374–1383.

Jones, A. P., Laurens, K. R., Herba, C. M., Barker, G. J., & Viding, E. (2009). Amygdala hypoactivity to fearful faces in boys with conduct problems and callous-unemotional traits. *American Journal of Psychiatry*, 166: 95–102.

Kendler, K. S., Kuhn, J., & Prescott, C. A. (2004). The interrelationship of neuroticism, sex, and stressful life events in the prediction of episodes of major depression. *American Journal of Psychiatry*, 161: 631–636.

Killgore, W. D. S., & 9 others. (2013). Cortico-limbic responses to masked affective faces across PTSD, panic disorder, and specific phobia. *Depression & Anxiety*, Wiley Online Library, DOI 10.1002/da.22156.

Kleinhans, N. M., Johnson, L. C., Richards, T., Mahurin, R., Greenson, J., Dawson, G., & Aylward, E. (2009). Reduced neural habituation in the amygdala and social impairments in autism spectrum disorders. *American Journal of Psychiatry*, 166: 467–475.

Klin, A., Jones, W., Schultz, R., Volkmar, F., & Cohen, D. (2002). Visual fixation patterns during viewing of naturalistic social situations as predictors of social competence in individuals with autism. *Archives of General Psychiatry*, 59: 809–816.

Larson, C. L., Schaefer, H. S., Siegle, G. J., Jackson, C. A., Anderle, M. J., & Davidson, R. J. (2006). Fear is fast in phobic individuals: Amygdala activation in response to fear-relevant stimuli. *Biological Psychiatry*, 60: 410–417.

Lieberman, M. D., Eisenberger, N. I., Crockett, M. J., Tom., S. M., Pfeifer, J. H., & Way, B. M. (2007). Putting feelings into words: Affect labeling disrupts amygdala activity in response to affective stimuli. *Psychological Science*, 18: 421–428.

Markram, K., & Markram, H. (2010). The intense world theory: A unifying theory of the neurobiology of autism. *Frontiers of Human Neuroscience*, 4: 224.

Marsh, A. A., & 9 others. (2008). Reduced amygdala response to fearful expressions in children and adolescents with callous-unemotional traits and disruptive behavior disorders. *American Journal of Psychiatry*, 165: 712–720.

Matthews, S. C., Strigo, I. A., Simmons, A. N., Yang, T. T., & Paulus, M. P. (2008). Decreased functional coupling of the amygdala and supragenual cingulate is related to increased depression in unmedicated individuals with current major depressive disorder. *Journal of Affective Disorders*, 111: 13–20.

Meyer-Lindenberg, A., Hariri, A. R., Munoz, K. E., Mervis, C. B., Mattay, V. S., Morris, C. A., & Berman, K. F. (2003). Neural correlates of genetically abnormal social cognition in Williams syndrome. *Nature Neuroscience*, 8: 991–993.

Milad, M. R., & 9 others. (2009). Neurobiological basis of failure to recall extinction memory in posttraumatic stress disorder. *Biological Psychiatry*, 66: 1075–1082.

Moffitt, T. E., Harrington, H., Caspi, A., Kim-Cohen, J., Goldberg, D., Gregory, A. M., & Poulton, R. (2007). Depression and generalized anxiety disorder: cumulative and sequential comorbidity in a birth cohort followed prospectively to age 32 years. *Archives of General Psychiatry*, 64: 651–660.

Monk, C. S., & 8 others. (2010). Neural circuitry of emotional face processing in autism spectrum disorders. *Journal of Psychiatry & Neuroscience*, 35: 105–114.

Neumann, D., Spezio, M. L., Piven, J., & Adolphe, R. (2006). Looking you in the mouth: Abnormal gaze in autism resulting from impaired top-down modulation of visual attention. *Social Cognitive & Affective Neuroscience*, 1: 194–202.

Nitschke, J. B., Sarinopoulos, I., Oathes, D. J., Johnstone, T., Whalen, P. J., Davidson, R. J., & Kalin, N. H. (2009). Anticipatory activation in the amygdala and anterior cingulate in generalized anxiety disorder and prediction of treatment response. *American Journal of Psychiatry*, 166: 302–310.

Paul, B. M., Snyder, A. Z., Haist, F., Raichle, M. E., Bellugi, U., & Stiles, J. (2009). Amygdala response to faces parallels social behavior in Williams syndrome. *Social Cognitive & Affective Neuroscience*, 4: 278–285.

Pierce, K., Haist, F., Sedaghat, F., & Courchesne, E. (2004). The brain response to personally familiar faces in autism: Findings of fusiform activity and beyond. *Brain*, 127: 2703–2716.

Schienle, A., Schäfer, A., Hermann, A., Rohrmann, S., & Vaitl, D. (2007). Symptom provocation and reduction in patients suffering from spider phobia: An fMRI study on exposure therapy. *European Archives of Psychiatry & Clinical Neuroscience*, 257: 486–493.

Schultz, R. T., & 9 others. (2000). Abnormal ventral temporal cortical activity during face discrimination among individuals with autism and Asperger syndrome. *Archives of General Psychiatry*, 57: 331–340.

Seara-Cardoso, A., & Viding, E. (2014). Functional neuroscience of psychopathic personality in adults. *Journal of Personality*, DOI 10.1111/jopy.12113.

Shin, L., & 13 others. (2005). A functional magnetic resonance imaging study of amygdala and medial prefrontal cortex responses to overtly presented fearful faces in posttraumatic stress disorder. *Archives of General Psychiatry*, 62: 273– 281.

Somerville, L. H., Whalen, P. J., & Kelley, W. M. (2010). Human bed nucleus of the stria terminalis indexes hypervigilant threat monitoring. *Biological Psychiatry*, 68: 416–424.

Stuhrmann, A., Suslow, T., & Dannlowski, U. (2011). Facial emotion processing in major depression: A systematic review of neuroimaging findings. *Biology of Mood & Anxiety Disorders*, 1: 10.

Suslow, T., & 12 others. (2010). Automatic mood-congruent amygdala responses to masked facial expressions in major depression. *Biological Psychiatry*, 67: 155–160.

Swartz, J. R., Wiggins, J. L, Carrasco, M., Lord, C., & Monk, C. S. (2013). Amygdala habituation and prefrontal functional connectivity in youth with autism spectrum disorders. *Journal of the American Academy of Child and Adolescent Psychiatry*, 52: 893.

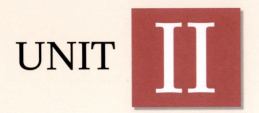
The Corticostriatal Circuit for Motivation and Action

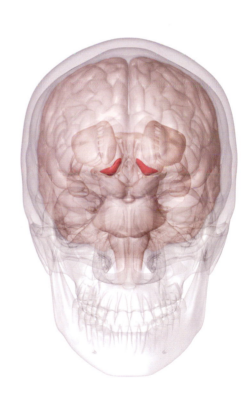

5 Anatomy

Much as the corticolimbic circuit supports the life-sustaining functions of recognition and reaction, the corticostriatal circuit supports equally critical functions and behaviors. In the case of the corticostriatal circuit, these functions and behaviors can broadly be categorized as *motivation* and *action*. In this chapter, we will review the general anatomy of the corticostriatal circuit and identify how the key nodes of this circuit interact to shape what we need, want, and like in our continually changing worlds (i.e., generate motivation to achieve or obtain what we find rewarding) and then coordinate our behaviors to achieve these goals (i.e., generate an appropriate action).

As specific actions begin to satisfy specific motivations consistently over time, the corticostriatal circuit represents the neuroanatomical foundation for learning about the cues in our environment that predict these associations. Thus, the corticostriatal circuit helps us anticipate and proactively respond to our worlds in a manner that maximizes our rewards. This key role of the corticostriatal circuit in normal reward-related learning and goal-directed behaviors will be highlighted in Chapter 6. Then, in Chapter 7, we will see how disorder within the corticostriatal circuit leads to dysfunctional reward learning and the emergence of pathological motivations and maladaptive actions.

The corticostriatal circuit (**Figure 5.1**) is comprised of the following interconnected structures:

1. Striatum
2. Thalamus
3. Amygdala
4. Hippocampal formation
5. Ventral pallidum
6. Hypothalamus
7. Prefrontal cortex
8. Dorsal pallidum
9. Motor cortices
10. Midbrain

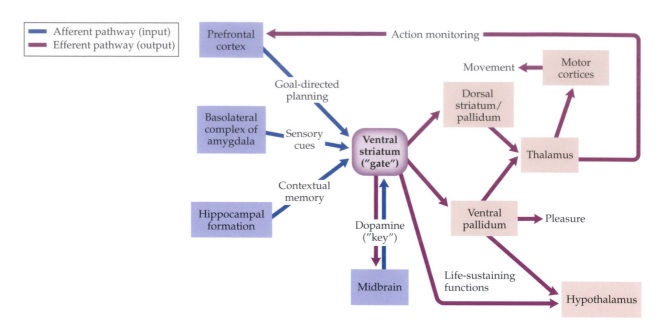

Figure 5.1   Overview of the corticostriatal circuit. The ten key circuit nodes and basic interconnections that support the core circuit functions of motivation and action, as well as reward learning.

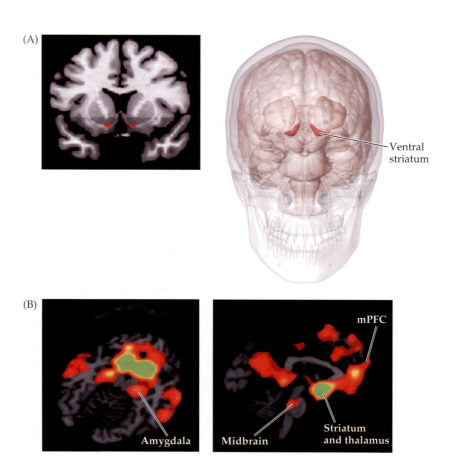

Figure 5.2   There is extensive functional connectivity between the ventral striatum (A) and distributed nodes of the corticostriatal circuit (B), including the medial prefrontal cortex, dorsal striatum, thalamus, midbrain, and amygdala. (fMRIs from Cauda et al., 2011.)

Through a network of connections between these subcortical, cortical, and brainstem structures (**Figure 5.2**), the corticostriatal circuit mediates the translation of our motivations into goal-directed actions resulting in rewarding experiences and life-sustaining functions

The Striatum

The striatum as a whole is a bilaterally symmetrical subcortical structure adjacent to the lateral ventricles of the cerebrum at approximately the cerebrum's center of mass (**Figure 5.3A**). The striatum was named for its striated, or striped, appearance. These striations reflect the passing of the internal capsule (a large bundle of myelinated axons, or white matter, providing afferent and efferent communication between the central and peripheral nervous systems) through the major dorsal and ventral subregions of the striatum, which are comprised primarily of neurons (gray matter).

The dorsal subregion of the striatum—the dorsal striatum (DS)—is further divided into two distinct gray matter structures: the caudate nucleus and the putamen. The ventral subregion of the striatum, or ventral striatum (VS), is primarily comprised of the nucleus accumbens (NAcc), which is further subdivided into the shell and core (**Figure 5.3B**). There are several important anatomical and functional distinctions between the shell and core of the NAcc that are beyond the scope of our introductory coverage. Within the corticostriatal circuit for motivation and action, the shell is of greater importance because it possesses critical connections with other circuit nodes not present in the core. However, because the neuroimaging techniques used in human studies lack sufficient spatial resolution to discriminate between these subregions, studies in humans commonly refer to activity in the VS broadly. Unless otherwise noted, we have used the broader term, ventral striatum, throughout

(A)

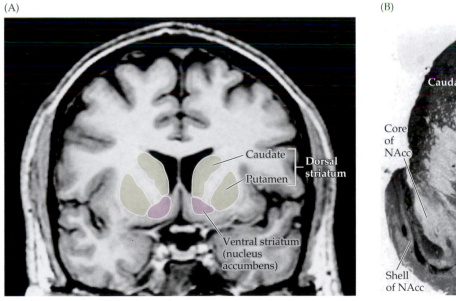

(B)

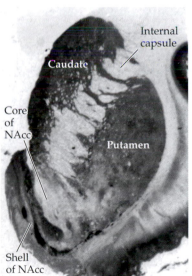

Figure 5.3 The two major structural divisions of the striatum seen in the cross-sectional (coronal) plane from a structural MRI (A) and a postmortem dissection (B). (A from Haber and Knutson, 2010; B from Groenewegen, 2007.)

DS   dorsal striatum
VS   ventral striatum
NAcc nucleus accumbens

the rest of our exploration of the anatomy, behaviors, and psychopathology of the corticostriatal circuit.

The VS represents the functional hub of the corticostriatal circuit. Anthony Grace at the University of Pittsburgh usefully conceptualizes the hub function of the VS as a "gate" through which our motivations are translated into actions. As we will see below, information from varied sources of both intrinsic (e.g., hunger) and extrinsic (e.g., food) motivation converges at this circuit hub, and when conditions allow, the VS gate opens to shape our actions through feedforward activation of downstream circuit nodes (e.g., taking a bite of a delicious hamburger). Over time, the VS gate opens in anticipation of a reward when we detect a cue in our environment that we have learned predicts the reward (e.g., McDonald's Golden Arches).

The Thalamus

As we saw in the corticolimbic circuit, the thalamus (see Figure 2.4) represents a critical multimodal sensory relay structure connecting key brain regions to information streaming in from the world outside. While specific thalamic nuclei such as the pulvinar serve this sensory relay function, other nuclei in the thalamus provide important relay functions between cortical and subcortical structures, including the striatum and prefrontal cortex.

The midline and medial intralaminar thalamic nuclei relay signals from the medial prefrontal cortex to the striatum broadly, with some fibers reaching the VS specifically. More importantly, these nuclei, particularly the dorsomedial nucleus, relay information from the VS back to the PFC in the service of monitoring our actions. Other nuclei of the thalamus connect the striatum, primarily the caudate and putamen in the DS, to cortical regions responsible for motor behaviors (e.g., movement). Of particular importance, the ventral anterior and ventral lateral nuclei function as critical relays through which the DS can ultimately influence goal-directed movement through motor cortices. Thus, connections between thalamic nuclei and the striatum function to coordinate execution and monitoring of our actions in the service of our motivation. Curiously, the sensory nuclei of the thalamus do not project to the striatum directly. Rather, information about specific sensory cues is provided through the amygdala.

The Amygdala

Of specific importance to corticostriatal circuit anatomy and function is the basolateral complex of the amygdala (BLA), which as we saw in Chapter 2 receives afferent input from auditory, visual, gustatory, and somatosensory cortices, as well as sensory nuclei of the thalamus. In the context of the corticolimbic circuit, the BLA relays sensory information to the central nucleus of the amygdala (CeA), which subsequently coordinates a host of downstream changes that help us recognize and react to challenges in our environments, such as threat. As it turns out, the BLA also projects to the VS, allowing multimodal sensory input to reach the VS gate of the corticostriatal circuit. In the context of the corticostriatal circuit, however, the detailed sensory input from the BLA will ultimately contribute to learning about specific cues in the environment (e.g., the Golden Arches) that predict when specific actions will satisfy specific motivations.

VS	ventral striatum	BLA	basolateral complex of the amygdala
PFC	prefrontal cortex	CeA	central nucleus of the amygdala
DS	dorsal striatum		

RESEARCH SPOTLIGHT

A major limitation in neuroscience research is the establishment of cause and effect through experimentation. Quite simply, the vast majority of research (and almost all of that conducted in humans) establishes only that one variable (e.g., brain activity) is correlated statistically with another variable (e.g., behavior). Seldom have neuroscientists been able to demonstrate that one variable causes an effect on another. Over the last decade, however, the revolutionary technique of optogenetics has allowed for many such cause-and-effect links to be established in animal models. Briefly, *optogenetics* refers to a genetic manipulation (hence *genetics*) that allows control over the activity of specific neurons using concentrated beams of light (hence *opto*), and subsequent recording/observation of the effects of the genetically marked neurons' activity on other neurons, as well as on behavior. In one study, Stuber and colleagues demonstrated that optogenetic stimulation of glutamatergic neurons in the BLA drives activity in the NAcc of living rats (**Figure 5.4**). Remarkably, stimulation of this pathway between the BLA and NAcc not only led the rats to consume more sugar water—a natural reward rats love—but also reinforced a behavior (poking their nose into a small opening) that resulted in even greater stimulation of this pathway. This reinforcement of behavior or learning was dependent on the release of dopamine in the NAcc at the time of optogenetic stimulation. We will return to the critical importance of dopamine in modulating the VS gate of the circuit later in this chapter.

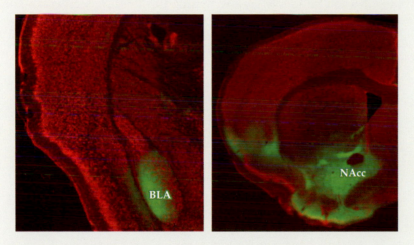

Figure 5.4 Optogenetic studies in rats reveal the presence of direct connections between neurons in the BLA and neurons in the NAcc. (From Stuber et al., 2011.)

The Hippocampal Formation

As it does in the corticolimbic circuit, the hippocampal formation (HF) provides important information about the context of our experiences (i.e., the where, when, what, and whom). Input from the HF to the VS initially contributes to learning about the context in which a specific motivation was satisfied by a specific action (e.g., my hunger was satisfied by eating a hamburger at the McDonald's in my hometown when I was a kid). Experiencing the same

HF   hippocampal formation
NAcc nucleus accumbens

motivation-action association repeatedly in the same context (or in similar contexts, such as a McDonald's in another town) furthers this learning, and eventually this contextual input from the HF helps to properly operate the VS gate. When you are in the appropriate context (a McDonald's), the input from the HF helps to open the VS gate, allowing a specific action to occur in the service of satisfying a specific motivation (ordering a hamburger because you're hungry). However, when you are in an inappropriate context (e.g., a doctor's office), this HF input is absent and the VS gate is less likely to open, even when the motivation may exist (you're not going to order a hamburger in a doctor's office, even if you're hungry). Thus, while input from the BLA regulates the VS gate by signaling information about specific cues that predict rewarding stimuli or experiences, the HF does so also, by signaling information about the broader context in which motivations (as well as cues) occur.

The Ventral Pallidum

endogenous opioids Neuro-modulators produced in response to reward and associated with the subjective experience of pleasure.

Until now, we have largely considered the varying inputs to the VS that help us learn associations between specific cues (from the BLA) and contexts (from the HF), as well as thalamic nuclei relaying information between the striatum and cortical regions. We have seen that as the hub of the corticostriatal circuit, the VS functions as a gate regulating when it is and is not appropriate to translate our motivations into actions. However, the VS gate largely operates indirectly, through an adjacent rostral region known as the ventral pallidum (VP). More specifically, the VS projects to neurons in the VP, which in turn drive activity of downstream regions to facilitate goal-directed behaviors (**Figure 5.5**). In fact, in fMRI studies of human reward-related and goal-directed behaviors, the BOLD signal from this region likely represents activity of neurons not only in the VS but also in the VP.

Of particular importance, the VP contains cholinergic neurons that project to the PFC. Thus, the VS gate can indirectly increase responsiveness of prefrontal neurons through these VP cholinergic pathways, thereby selectively tuning or focusing our attention on signals that help us coordinate actions that satisfy our motivations. This indirect pathway for increasing the activity of prefrontal neurons is very similar to the one between the amygdala and nucleus basalis of Meynert in the corticolimbic circuit for recognition and reaction, which we reviewed in Unit I. In fact, the VP is located adjacent to the NBM and was historically considered by anatomists as part of the broader substantia innominata.

The VP also serves as a key relay through which activity of the VS gate can be communicated to the PFC via thalamic nuclei. Specifically, information from the VS is first communicated to the VP, which then feeds forward to the midline and medial intralaminar thalamic nuclei (e.g., dorsomedial nucleus). These thalamic nuclei, in turn, forward information to regions of the PFC, including the ventromedial prefrontal cortex (vmPFC) and dorsolateral prefrontal cortex (dlPFC).

Finally, the VS can drive specific neurons in the VP that contain **endogenous opioids**. The activation of these

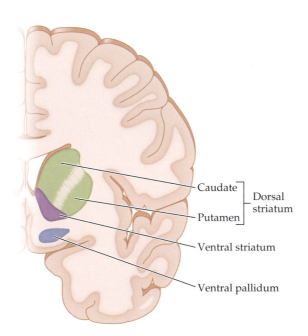

Caudate ⎤
Dorsal striatum
Putamen ⎦

Ventral striatum

Ventral pallidum

Figure 5.5 Location of the ventral pallidum in the human brain, seen in coronal section through the striatum.

HF	hippocampal formation	**VP**	ventral pallidum
VS	ventral striatum	**PFC**	prefrontal cortex
BLA	basolateral complex of the amygdala	**NBM**	nucleus basalis of Meynert

endogenous opioid-releasing VP neurons is responsible for generating **hedonic tone**, or how much we subjectively enjoy our experiences and like stimuli we encounter. Growing evidence suggests that such hedonic tone, or "liking" things, is anatomically distinct from "wanting" things, as well as from learning associations between specific motivations and specific actions (i.e., how to get what we want). While these latter two processes of wanting and learning are also mediated through the corticostriatal circuit and the VS gate, they are shaped not by opioid signaling but by that of dopamine, which we will consider in detail when we discuss the midbrain (see p. 102).

hedonic tone General level of pleasure an individual experiences from stimuli and activities they find rewarding. Endogenous opioids increase hedonic tone.

RESEARCH SPOTLIGHT

Research conducted by Kent Berridge and colleagues at the University of Michigan has been particularly important for understanding the neuroanatomical basis of "liking" versus "wanting." In a series of studies using rodent models, Berridge and his colleagues have identified subregions within the VP that appear to signal liking of rewards. You may be asking how, if at all, one can measure pleasure, or liking, and its opposite, "disliking," in animals such as rats? As it turns out, many animals, including humans, exhibit a highly conserved facial response to tastes they like or dislike. With sweet tastes (which nearly all animals like), there is a consistent pattern of facial expressions, including tongue protrusions, while with bitter tastes that most animals dislike there are other facial expressions, such as mouth gapes (**Figure 5.6**). By looking for these facial expressions when rats with specific lesions were given sweet-tasting foods, Berridge and colleagues identified specific subregions of the VP, VS, and brainstem that generate "like" responses and named these "hedonic hot spots" (**Figure 5.7**).

Further work revealed that these hedonic hot spots contain neurons that synthesize endogenous opioids. Experimentally adding opioids to these hot spots intensified the liking expressions when rats were given sweets. Thus, subregions of the VP, which receives input from the VS, code the hedonic quality, or pleasure, we derive from rewarding stimuli, and this function is mediated by opioid signaling in these subregions.

Figure 5.7 Hedonic hot spots in the rat brain are found in the ventral striatum, ventral pallidum, and parabrachial nucleus of the brainstem, regions where opioids cause amplification of core "liking" reactions to sweetness. (After Berridge, 2009.)

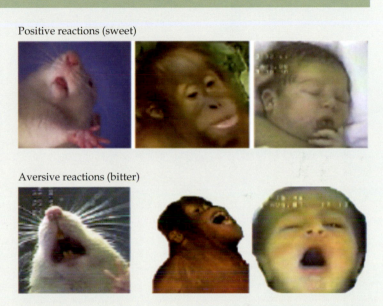

Positive reactions (sweet)

Aversive reactions (bitter)

Figure 5.6 Taste reactions. Positive "liking" reactions to pleasant sweet tastes shared by human newborn, young orangutan, and adult rat (tongue protrusion; top), and aversive "disliking" reactions to unpleasant bitter tastes (mouth gape; bottom). (From Berridge, 2009.)

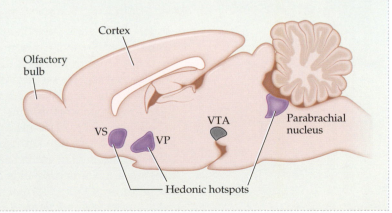

| PFC | prefrontal cortex | dlPFC | dorsolateral prefrontal cortex |
| vmPFC | ventromedial prefrontal cortex | VTA | ventral tegmental area |

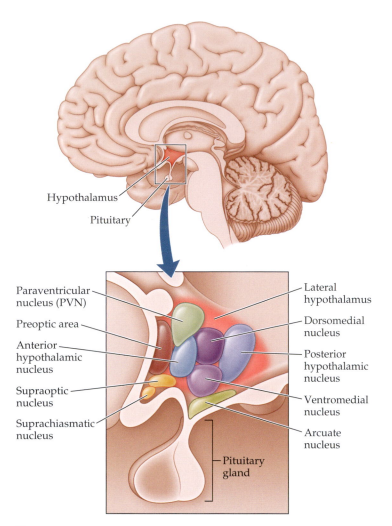

Figure 5.8 The core nuclei of the hypothalamus. The ventral striatum can gate the activity of hypothalamic nuclei, including the lateral hypothalamus and medial preoptic area, which are responsible for life-sustaining activities such as feeding, drinking, and copulation.

structural dimorphism When the same structure exists in distinctively different sizes in males and females of the same species.

conflict monitoring Process of detecting when an outcome deviates from an expectation, which helps generate changes to plans so the desired outcome is achieved. Supported by activity in the dACC.

The Hypothalamus

At a primal level, goal-directed behaviors maintain life-sustaining functions such as obtaining food or water to nourish our bodies and finding mates to perpetuate our genetic lineage. The VS gate supports these life-sustaining functions by either directly or indirectly (via the VP) driving activity of core regions in the hypothalamus (**Figure 5.8**). One such hypothalamic target of the VS is the lateral hypothalamus, which regulates feeding and drinking behaviors. Another hypothalamic target of the VS is the medial preoptic area (PO), which regulates sexual behaviors, including copulation. Interestingly, the medial PO of the hypothalamus is one of the few brain regions in humans that exhibit significant sexual dimorphism, with larger volumes observed in men than in women. This **structural dimorphism** is further reflected in the output of the PO, including as it functions in downstream signaling through the VS gate, contributing to pronounced differences in the sexual behaviors of men and women.

The Prefrontal Cortex

The VS has extensive reciprocal connections with the prefrontal cortex, particularly regions of the medial PFC. As with the corticolimbic circuit, the mPFC functions to systematically integrate converging bottom-up and top-down information to better shape adaptive responses to our environments. First, the ventromedial PFC (vmPFC) is the region where bottom-up sensory information from the thalamus and cortex, interoceptive (internal) information from the insula, and contextual information from the HF are integrated with motivational information from the VS. In this manner, the vmPFC contributes to awareness of hunger by integrating signals from your growling stomach and watering mouth (through input from the insula) and, furthermore, awareness that you are near a McDonald's (through input from the HF) and, thus, have the opportunity to eat.

The vmPFC also serves as the junction through which top-down information from lateral and dorsal regions of the PFC can inform, direct, and regulate the motivational signals generated by the VS. Of particular importance, complex behavioral plans necessary to satisfy our motivations are communicated from the dlPFC to the VS through the vmPFC. This indirect input from the dlPFC is another critical factor in opening the VS gate and subsequently putting our plans into action via the DS and motor cortices. The dorsal anterior cingulate cortex (dACC) functions to monitor conflict between our expectations and actual outcomes. This **conflict monitoring**, or error detection, in the

VS	ventral striatum	**mPFC**	medial prefrontal cortex
VP	ventral pallidum	**vmPFC**	ventromedial prefrontal cortex
PO	preoptic area	**HF**	hippocampal formation

dACC is relayed to the dlPFC, which allows for real-time control and correction of our actions to achieve our goals. We will consider in detail the anatomy and function of the dlPFC when we discuss executive control in Unit III on the corticohippocampal circuit.

Working across these regions, we find that the vmPFC communicates our motivational state as well as related sensory, interoceptive, and contextual information to the dlPFC, which initiates a plan of action (i.e., goal-directed behavior). Using the example from above, this information loop would result in the generation of a plan to head over to the nearby McDonald's, go up to the counter, and place an order for a hamburger. Execution of this plan, however, requires the vmPFC to relay these top-down "instructions" to the VS gate, which opens to drive activity in the DS and motor cortices, ultimately leading you to satisfy your hunger by eating a delicious hamburger.

Conflict monitoring is supported by the dACC much the same way as it is within the corticolimbic circuit. In the context of the corticostriatal circuit, the dACC signals conflict between your goal-directed plans and the effectiveness of your actions. If you take a wrong turn on your way to McDonald's, the dACC would signal this conflict back to the dlPFC, allowing for a new set of plans to be executed until you finally arrive at your destination and eat your hamburger. In Chapter 6, we will further consider the critical importance of dynamic interactions between these prefrontal regions and the VS in shaping our actions to satisfy our motivations for stimuli and experiences we find rewarding. In Chapter 7 we will consider how dysfunction between these particular nodes of the corticostriatal circuit contributes to maladaptive motivations and actions.

The Dorsal Pallidum

Much like the ventral pallidum, which relays signals from the ventral striatum gate supporting motivation, the dorsal pallidum (DP) relays signals from the DS to target regions supporting goal-directed actions—namely the motor cortices we will describe next. The DP is comprised of the external and internal segments of the globus pallidus (**Figure 5.9**), which along with the caudate and putamen of the dorsal striatum are commonly referred to as the **basal ganglia**. Importantly, neurons from the DP do not directly innervate those of the motor cortices. Rather, axons from the DP relay onto neurons of the ventral anterior and ventral lateral thalamic nuclei, which in turn project to the motor cortices.

The Motor Cortices

The goal-directed behaviors planned via the dlPFC and gated through the VS ultimately emerge as patterns of movement through the premotor and primary motor cortices (via the dorsal striatum, dorsal pallidum, and thalamus). The primary motor cortex is comprised largely of **pyramidal neurons** (see Chapter 10) whose axons descend via the corona radiata (a "crown" of radiating axons below the cortex) and internal capsule into the brainstem and spinal cord to ultimately provide direct innervation of our skeletal muscles

basal ganglia Anatomical circuit consisting of the globus pallidus together with the caudate and putamen of the dorsal striatum. Important for the proper execution and coordination of movement.

pyramidal neurons Excitatory glutamatergic neurons named for their pyramid-shaped central cell body. These neurons are found throughout the cortex and are preeminent in the generation of sensory, motor, affective, and cognitive processes.

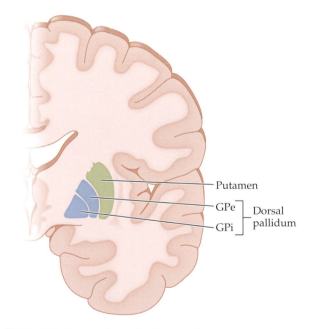

Figure 5.9 The basal ganglia. Cross section showing external (GPe) and internal (GPi) segments of the globus pallidus, which together comprise the dorsal pallidum.

---

dlPFC	dorsolateral prefrontal cortex	dACC	dorsal anterior cingulate cortex
DP	dorsal pallidum	GP	globus pallidus
DS	dorsal striatum		

via neuromuscular junctions. The premotor cortex functions to coordinate the specific sequence of movements directed by the primary motor cortex. Working together, these two motor cortices allow the corticostriatal circuit to generate and regulate voluntary goal-directed movement.

The Midbrain

dopamine (DA) Neuromodulator produced in the VTA and substantia nigra of the midbrain. Important for modulating the gating function of the ventral striatum in support of motivation and action.

The last node of the corticostriatal circuit may, in fact, be the most important. We have seen that the VS functions as a gate allowing our motivations to be translated into actions. Signals from the midbrain, however, determine whether the VS gate ultimately opens to generate goal-directed behaviors linking motivations and rewards. These signals arise specifically from a region of the midbrain called the ventral tegmental area. The VTA consists primarily of neurons that synthesize the neuromodulator **dopamine (DA)** and release it in multiple downstream targets, including the VS and PFC (**Figure 5.10**). In contrast, an adjacent region of the midbrain, the substantia nigra, contains dopamine-synthesizing (dopaminergic) neurons that project primarily to the DS and DP. Dopamine released from the substantia nigra into the DS and DP functions to regulate motor output, and it is these dopaminergic neurons that are primarily affected in Parkinson's disease.

Within the corticostriatal circuit for motivation and action, DA release from the VTA into the VS is necessary for opening of the gate. Thus, it is useful to think of DA as the "key" of the corticostriatal circuit. Simply, the VS gate does not open without the DA key. In the context of goal-directed behaviors, DA release in the VS initially signals the experience of stimuli or actions we find intrinsically rewarding, such as drinking water when thirsty or eating food when hungry. Over time, DA signals occur in response to cues that predict intrinsic rewards (e.g., the Golden Arches) and no longer to the rewards directly (e.g., the hamburger). When this DA release occurs in the VS, all the various inputs and outputs are reinforced to strengthen a particular goal-directed behavior. In this way, DA signaling in the VS drives learning of associations between cues and rewarding outcomes, as well as reinforcing the behaviors that allow us to successfully experience rewarding outcomes. Thus, the DA "key" opens the VS "gate" and enables us to translate our motivations into goal-directed actions that result in a rewarding experience.

When a reward (the hamburger) coincides with a specific set of cues (the Golden Arches) and motivational states (hunger), we begin to learn what exactly predicts this rewarding experience. We then shape our behaviors accordingly to increase the chances it will happen again in the future (going to a McDonald's). If there is no rewarding experience, however, there is no DA release and the specific set of inputs and outputs of the VS are not reinforced and may in fact be weakened. In this way, the absence of DA signaling in the VS works to keep the gate closed and prevents us from executing actions that have not satisfied our motivations in the past and are unlikely to do so in the future.

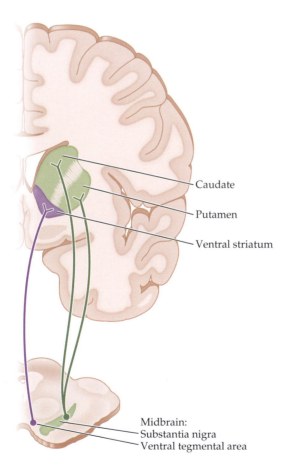

Caudate

Putamen

Ventral striatum

Midbrain:
Substantia nigra
Ventral tegmental area

Figure 5.10 Midbrain VTA and substantia nigra and their dominant projections to the ventral and dorsal striatum, respectively.

VS	ventral striatum	DP	dorsal pallidum
PFC	prefrontal cortex	VTA	ventral tegmental area
DS	dorsal striatum	DA	dopamine

RESEARCH SPOTLIGHT

Our current understanding of how dopamine functions as a key to open the VS gate is largely based on the work of Wolfram Schultz. Beginning in the early 1990s, Schultz and his colleagues conducted a series of studies in awake, behaving monkeys that defined the critical roles of DA signaling in reinforcement learning and reward-related behaviors. First they demonstrated that DA is released from the VTA when a monkey unexpectedly receives a rewarding stimulus. In Schultz's experiments, this was a squirt of juice in the monkey's mouth when it was sitting in a chair and not performing any behaviors. The DA signal always occurred as long as the monkey was not expecting the juice (i.e., the reward occurred randomly; **Figure 5.11A**).

In this context, DA release from the VTA serves a role similar to that of the CeA and NBM in the corticolimbic circuit: it generates broad increases in attention to help identify those stimuli in the environment that are associated with what is happening to us. With the corticostriatal circuit, the focus is on identifying cues that predict a reward in the future. In fact, VTA neurons send projections to the PFC as well as to the VP and NBM, allowing DA signaling to directly increase the activity of neurons supporting attention and exploration. This is the general role of DA when it comes to unpredicted or unexpected rewards.

If, however, a cue is presented before the monkey receives the juice, then the DA release occurs in step with the cue (a light) that predicts the later reward and not the reward itself (the juice; **Figure 5.11B**). This shift in timing of DA release is critical for the learning of goal-directed behaviors. Rather than generally increasing the monkey's attention and processing of environmental stimuli, DA release in response to the cue predicting reward reinforces whatever inputs and outputs were co-occurring in the VS at the time of DA release. This reward prediction signal helps us (and monkeys) learn what specific cues (and subsequent actions, such as sucking on a straw through which juice is delivered) result in reward.

Finally, Schultz and colleagues demonstrated that if the reward is withheld after a monkey has learned that a cue predicts a reward, there is a decrease in DA release at the time the reward would normally be experienced (**Figure 5.11C**). This decrease in DA release results in a weakening of the reward learning that has occurred in the VS, and it allows the monkey to explore alternative strategies (such as looking for other cues or trying different behaviors) in an effort to receive the reward. In this way, the decrease in DA release serves as a reward-prediction error signal that helps the monkey break out of a now unsuccessful pattern and go in search of new avenues of success. Thus, Schultz's studies demonstrated that the presence or absence of DA release from the VTA functions, respectively, to strengthen goal-directed behaviors that consistently result in reward and to weaken those that do not.

(A) **Unpredicted reward occurs**

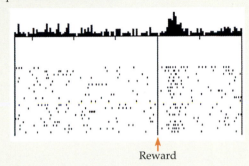

Reward

(B) **Predicted reward occurs**

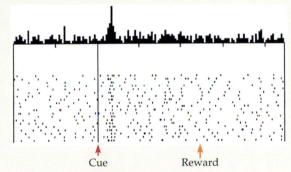

Cue   Reward

(C) **Predicted reward does not occur**

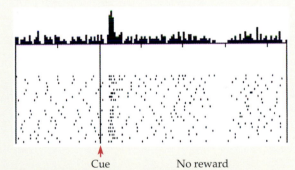

Cue   No reward

Figure 5.11 (A) Activity of DA neurons increases in response to an unpredicted, unexpected reward. (B) When a cue such as a light reliably predicts a reward over time, this increase in activity shifts from the reward to the cue. (C) When a cue predicts a reward but the reward fails to occur, there is a decrease in DA activity at the time when the reward would have occurred. (From Schultz et al., 1997, by permission of AAAS.)

VP   ventral pallidum
CeA   central nucleus of amygdala
NBM   nucleus basalis of Meynert

Summary

The corticostriatal circuit, through a network of connections between subcortical, cortical, and brainstem structures, mediates the translation of our motivations into actions resulting in rewarding experiences and life-sustaining functions. The ventral striatum serves as the hub or "gate" of this circuit where incoming information about cues (via the basolateral complex of the amygdala) and contexts (via the hippocampal formation) is integrated with our subjective experiences (via the ventromedial prefrontal cortex) and goal-directed plans (via the dorsolateral prefrontal cortex) to generate actions (via the dorsal striatum) that ultimately satisfy our motivations. This gating function of the ventral striatum is critically controlled by dopamine signaling (via the ventral tegmental area of the midbrain) occurring in response to intrinsically rewarding stimuli as well as the cues predicting these stimuli. Thus, when the dopamine "key" coincides with convergent bottom-up and top-down signaling, the ventral striatum "gate" opens and our motivations are translated into actions.

Literature Cited & Further Reading

Baxter, M. G., & Murray, E. A. (2002). The amygdala and reward. *Nature Reviews Neuroscience*, 3: 563–573.

Berridge, K. C. (2009). 'Liking' and 'wanting' food rewards: Brain substrates and roles in eating disorders. *Physiology & Behavior*, 97: 537–550.

Breedlove, S. M., and Watson, N. V. (2013). *Biological psychology: An introduction to behavioral, cognitive, and clinical neuroscience, 7th Ed.* Sunderland, MA: Sinauer Associates.

Cauda, F., Cavanna, A. E., D'agata, F., Sacco, K., Duca, S., & Geminiani, G. C. (2011). Functional connectivity and coactivation of the nucleus accumbens: A combined functional connectivity and structure-based meta-analysis. *Journal of Cognitive Neuroscience*, 23: 2864–2877.

Grace, A. A. (2000). Gating of information flow within the limbic system and the pathophysiology of schizophrenia. *Brain Research Reviews*, 31: 330–341.

Groenewegen, H. J. (2007). The ventral striatum as an interface between the limbic and motor systems. *CNS Spectrums*, 12: 887–892.

Haber, S. N., & Knutson, B. (2010). The reward circuit: Linking primate anatomy and human imaging. *Neuropsychopharmacology*, 35: 4–26.

Schultz, W., Dayan, P., & Montague, P. R. (1997). A neural substrate of prediction and reward. *Science*, 275: 1593–1599.

Stuber, G. D. & 10 others. (2011). Excitatory transmission from the amygdala to nucleus accumbens facilitates reward seeking. *Nature*, 475: 377–380.

6

Order

In this chapter, we will first consider how the corticostriatal circuit mediates the broader functions of motivation and action through the specific process of reward learning. We focus on reward learning because this process allows us to dissect the critical functions of the circuit nodes described in Chapter 5. As we did with the corticolimbic circuit, we will then broaden our lens to consider different types of stimuli that engage or trigger the corticostriatal circuit, particularly its hub—the ventral striatum—as well as specific behaviors that are supported by circuit function. In Chapter 7, we will consider how disorder within the corticostriatal circuit emerges as specific forms of psychopathology revolving around maladaptive expressions of these processes.

Reward Learning

Much of our current understanding of the corticostriatal circuit stems from studies of how animals learn to anticipate, respond to, and actively pursue rewards in their environment. Such reward learning and the goal-directed behaviors that emerge in its service generally fall under two broad types or categories: classical conditioning and operant conditioning. We will first consider classical conditioning and the specific corticostriatal circuit nodes supporting this form of reward learning.

Classical conditioning

In the context of reward learning, classical conditioning entails the development of a basic (often physiological) response to a cue predicting a reward. With classical conditioning, the individual does not need to first learn and then express a specific behavior in response to the cue in order to receive the reward. In other words, the reward always follows the cue regardless of what the individual does or does not do. Thus, classical conditioning can be considered a passive or reflexive form of learning. In fact, fear learning, as we described in Unit I, is a form of negative classical conditioning. During fear conditioning, the animal is shocked after a cue regardless of what behaviors it does or does not express (e.g., freezing in response to the cue doesn't prevent the shock). Similarly, during extinction, the shock never follows the cue, regardless of what the animal is or is not doing. With reward or positive classical conditioning, the animal always receives a reward following a cue, regardless of its explicit behavior.

(A)

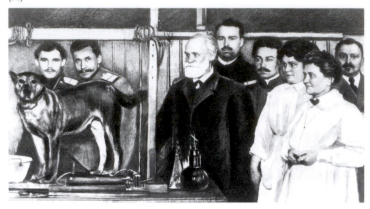

(B)

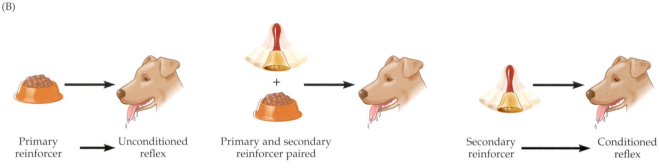

Primary reinforcer → Unconditioned reflex

Primary and secondary reinforcer paired

Secondary reinforcer → Conditioned reflex

Figure 6.1 (A) This photograph from Ivan Pavlov's lab shows the setup for his famous conditioning experiments (Pavlov is in the center, with the white beard). (B) Cartoon depicting the general experimental methodology employed by Pavlov to demonstrate classical, or Pavlovian, conditioning. Food was the primary reinforcer; food provokes salivation (the unconditioned reflex). When food is consistently paired with a secondary reinforcer such as the ringing of a bell, over time the secondary reinforcer alone will elicit the same response (the conditioned reflex) as the primary reinforcer.

classical conditioning Passive process of learning that a previously neutral stimulus predicts a reward. Aslo known as Pavlovian conditioning.

primary reinforcer A stimulus that is inherently rewarding because it satisfies basic needs like hunger, thirst, and sex.

secondary reinforcer A neutral stimulus (such as a sound) that over time reliably predicts a primary reinforcer through classical or operant conditioning.

Most of us are familiar with **classical conditioning** through the seminal studies of the Russian psychologist Ivan Pavlov (**Figure 6.1A**). In fact, the term "Pavlovian conditioning" is sometimes used interchangeably with classical conditioning, although the latter encompasses many other forms of simple learning. Beginning in 1901, Pavlov and his colleagues systematically described the "conditioned or conditional reflex" in dogs. In Pavlov's experiments, salivation in dogs was measured when they were given food in parallel with the presentation of an unrelated stimulus—most famously the ringing of a bell (**Figure 6.1B**). Over time, the dogs began to salivate in response to the sound of the bell, even in the absence of food. The dogs had learned that ringing of the bell predicted food, and appropriate physiological responses followed (i.e., salivating in preparation for chewing and swallowing the food).

In these experiments, the food is the **primary reinforcer**, something that in and of itself is of value to the animal's survival and triggers a coordinated physiological response (i.e., salivation related to feeding and digestion). Such primary reinforcers include food, water, and sex, all of which increase dopamine signaling in the corticostriatal circuit. Although the evidence is less clear, several aspects of social behavior in humans (e.g., joy, laughter, empathy) may also act as primary reinforcers.

Returning to the experiments of Pavlov, the ringing bell became a **secondary reinforcer** by virtue of being consistently paired with food. Critically, the dogs were never required to perform any behaviors (e.g., barking or sitting) for the food to be delivered when the bell was rung. Nevertheless, the physiological response of salivation (the conditional reflex), which is a form of basic learning, emerged over successive pairings of the food with the bell. We now turn to the contributions of specific corticostriatal circuit nodes to classical conditioning.

The ventral striatum and classical conditioning

The ventral striatum serves as the neural substrate for reward learning in classical conditioning (**Figure 6.2**). This function of the VS is analogous to that of the amygdala in learning associations (e.g., tone-shock) in the context of fear or threat, and it reflects the coordinated convergence of multiple inputs to the VS gate. In experiments like those of Pavlov and colleagues, information about the secondary reinforcer (the ringing bell) is communicated to the VS from the BLA. Simultaneously, the hippocampal formation communicates information regarding broader context in which the secondary reinforcer appears (the laboratory kennel). The most critical input, however, comes from the midbrain VTA when the dog is given the primary reinforcer (food). The release of dopamine from the VTA into the VS strengthens the convergent inputs from the BLA and HF and results in the opening of the VS gate. This is a fundamental example of how DA functions as the key for the VS gate.

With classical conditioning, opening of the VS gate results in downstream activation of circuit nodes mediating basic physiological and general attentional changes. In Pavlov's dogs, the VS gate opens and drives activity in the ventral pallidum. In turn, neurons in the VP drive those in the lateral hypothalamus, which initiates feeding reflexes, including salivation. Some neurons in the VS directly project to the lateral hypothalamus, further driving these reflexes. These pathways control the basic physiological

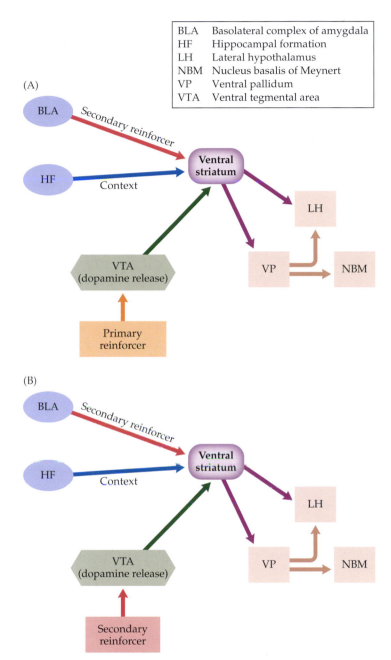

BLA	Basolateral complex of amygdala
HF	Hippocampal formation
LH	Lateral hypothalamus
NBM	Nucleus basalis of Meynert
VP	Ventral pallidum
VTA	Ventral tegmental area

Figure 6.2 Basic corticostriatal circuitry for classical conditioning. (A) Initially, the primary reinforcer drives the ventral tegmental area and subsequent release of the dopamine key to open the VS gate. This is represented in the top panel of the original work by Schultz et al. described in Figure 5.11. (B) Over repeated pairings, the secondary reinforcer comes to drive the VTA and subsequent release of dopamine. This shift is represented in the middle panel of Figure 5.11.

VS	ventral striatum	DA	dopamine
VTA	ventral tegmental area	VP	ventral pallidum
BLA	basolateral complex of the amygdala	NBM	nucleus basalis of Meynert
HF	hippocampal formation		

response to food and, over repeated pairings of the food and ringing bell to the conditioned reflex to the bell alone.

In addition to the conditioned reflex, the corticostriatal circuit mediates more general increases in attention and activity associated with classical conditioning. This broader effect is mediated through projections from the VP to the nucleus basalis of Meynert, as well as cholinergic neurons within the VP. These cholinergic projections generate activity in distributed cortical structures, including the prefrontal cortex. Thus, opening of the VS gate also increases the capacity to process sensory and spatial information and helps to broaden attention in search of additional information related to the current rewarding experience. For Pavlov's dogs, this may have been learning about other features of their environment (e.g., the presence of Pavlov or one of his research assistants) that predicted the imminent arrival of food.

Operant conditioning

operant conditioning Active process of learning that a previously neutral stimulus results in a reward only if an appropriate action is performed.

operant response Actions or behaviors performed with the goal of producing a reward.

In contrast to classical conditioning, the second broad category of reward learning, operant conditioning, *does* require an explicit behavioral response to a cue in order to receive a reward. After all, we seldom have it as easy as Pavlov's dogs and typically must work for our rewards.

As the name implies, in operant conditioning an animal must "operate" on its environment in some specific manner for a cue to be translated into a reward. In animal models, the operant response, or behavior performed to produce a reward, typically involves pressing a small lever built inside the testing chamber (a lever press) or poking the nose through a small opening in the chamber (a nose poke). For example, a mouse can be conditioned to press a lever for a food pellet when a light is turned on in its chamber. The pairing of the light and the food is identical to that observed in classical conditioning, but now the mouse must perform a specific behavior (press a lever) to receive the food reward. Because the mouse's *motivation* for food is only satisfied through its *action*, operant conditioning is an ideal experimental strategy for studying the full dynamics of corticostriatal circuit.

Moreover, operant conditioning requires that the mouse learn what specific action is successful in obtaining the food reward and what actions are unsuccessful. Because a multitude of behavioral responses may exist (e.g., typically a mouse has the option of either a lever press or a nose poke in the same testing chamber), the mouse effectively uses a process of trial and error to eventually learn what operant response is successful under what specific conditions. For example, one experiment may require the mouse to respond with a lever press for food when a light is turned on but with a nose poke for food when a loud tone is played (many different secondary reinforcers can be presented in typical test chambers). In such a scenario, the mouse first must learn that two independent cues predict reward (i.e., there are two secondary reinforcers). More importantly, to receive the food reward (every time), the mouse must then learn that each of the cues requires a specific response. Depending on the nature of the study population (e.g., mouse, monkey, or man), the complexity of the associations is nearly limitless with operant conditioning. Thus, operant conditioning also allows us to more fully explore the contributions of the corticostriatal circuit to reward learning and the gradual emergence of specific goal-directed behaviors. Our quest for a hamburger at McDonald's, because it requires explicit goal-directed behaviors on our part, more closely aligns with the complexity of operant

VP   ventral pallidum
VS   ventral striatum
PFC prefrontal cortex

conditioning than with the simplicity of classical conditioning. As we will see in the next section, the operant response requires the recruitment of extended corticostriatal circuit nodes, most notably the PFC.

Prefrontal cortex and operant conditioning

The basic corticostriatal circuitry described above for classical conditioning also operates during operant conditioning. The VS gate translates input from the BLA and HF into alterations in physiological responses through hypothalamic nuclei either directly or indirectly via the VP. Parallel pathways through the VP and NBM further allow the VS to drive cholinergic output to cortical regions, thereby increasing processing of sensory information. This cholinergic drive also reaches the PFC, where it functions to broaden our attentional spotlight.

While this bottom-up process is similar in both classical and operant conditioning, it is the critical top-down contributions of the prefrontal cortex that uniquely distinguishes the latter. As outlined in Chapter 5, the role of the PFC within the corticostriatal circuit is twofold. First, the vmPFC functions to simultaneously integrate bottom-up sensory, interoceptive, and contextual input with our motivational states, thereby generating subjective awareness of our internal and external worlds. The vmPFC also functions as a relay between the VS and the dorsolateral prefrontal cortex, which is responsible for the second critical function of the PFC in the corticostriatal circuit: action planning (**Figure 6.3**).

Top-down behavioral plans or programs to help us satisfy our motivations and obtain rewards are generated through the dlPFC. The generation of an action plan or behavioral program by the dlPFC (and analogous brain regions in animals like the mouse) is necessary for operant conditioning. It is this top-down programming that eventually emerges as a lever press or a nose poke in our mouse looking for food in response to a specific cue. While the top-down behavioral programs and action plans initially emerge randomly (i.e., the mouse will "try" all possible operant responses available in its testing chamber), these will be pruned down to only those resulting in the receipt of the food reward.

As with classical conditioning, the release of DA from the midbrain VTA in response to a primary reinforcer is critical for this pruning process and the emergence of successful goal-directed behaviors and reward learning. With operant conditioning, however, this DA release strengthens not only the basic reward learning but also the specific pattern of top-down behavioral programming from the dlPFC as well as the behavioral output through the dorsal striatum and motor cortices. Thus, in operant conditioning the DA key opens the VS gate through which specific goal-directed behaviors are implemented in the service of obtaining predicted rewards. With our mouse, the release of DA upon receiving food after a lever press following a light, or after a nose poke following a tone, is responsible for reinforcing the association between the primary and secondary reinforcers, as well as the successful top-down program and goal-directed behavior. Similarly, the absence of DA release when the incorrect behavior is performed (i.e., nose poke to light, or lever press to tone) weakens the associated unsuccessful top-down program, resulting in a gradual process of refining our goal-directed behaviors to consistently produce **adaptive responses** (i.e., successful and accurate) to cues.

adaptive response Any constellation of changes in behavior or physiology that increases an individual's survival.

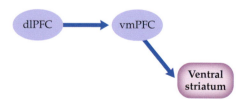

Figure 6.3 Goal-directed planning begins in the dorsolateral prefrontal cortex and is relayed to the VS gate via the ventromedial prefrontal cortex.

BLA	basolateral complex of the amygdala
HF	hippocampal formation
NBM	nucleus basalis of Meynert
vmPFC	ventromedial prefrontal cortex

dlPFC	dorsolateral prefrontal cortex
DA	dopamine
VTA	ventral tegmental area

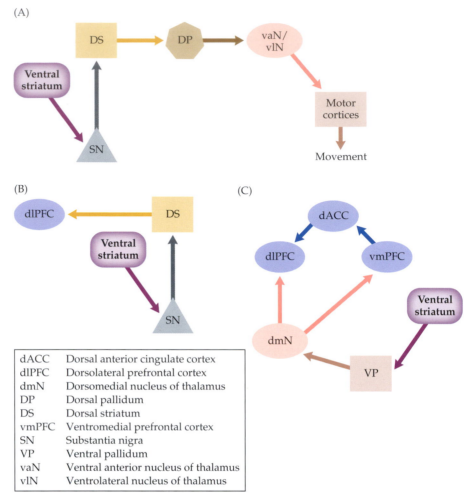

(A)

(B)

(C)

dACC	Dorsal anterior cingulate cortex
dlPFC	Dorsolateral prefrontal cortex
dmN	Dorsomedial nucleus of thalamus
DP	Dorsal pallidum
DS	Dorsal striatum
vmPFC	Ventromedial prefrontal cortex
SN	Substantia nigra
VP	Ventral pallidum
vaN	Ventral anterior nucleus of thalamus
vlN	Ventrolateral nucleus of thalamus

Figure 6.4 (A) Goal-directed action pathway. The VS gate opens to generate motor behaviors and drive actions through this pathway, culminating in activity of the motor cortices. (B,C) Action monitoring pathways. (B) Actions are monitored through this pathway from the VS to the dlPFC via the SN and DS. (C) Actions are also monitored through a pathway from the VS to multiple regions of the PFC via the VP and the dorsomedial nucleus of the thalamus.

The execution of the top-down behavioral programs or action plans generated by the dlPFC as goal-directed behaviors requires opening of the VS gate and downstream activation of the DS and motor cortices (**Figure 6.4A**). The control of motor behavior specifically occurs through indirect pathways from the VS to the DS via a second population of midbrain dopaminergic neurons known as the substantia nigra (SN). Of note, the DA-releasing neurons of the SN are largely distinct from those of the VTA, which release DA in response to a primary or secondary reinforcer. Once stimulated by input from the SN, the DS communicates via the dorsal pallidum to the ventral anterior and ventral lateral thalamic nuclei, which project onto the motor cortices to effect direct control of skeletal muscles.

This motor output through the VS gate is also communicated to the PFC through multiple parallel pathways, which allows for monitoring of the

SN	substantia nigra	DS	dorsal striatum	dlPFC	dorsolateral prefrontal cortex
DA	dopamine	VS	ventral striatum	VP	ventral pallidum
VTA	ventral tegmental area	PFC	prefrontal cortex		

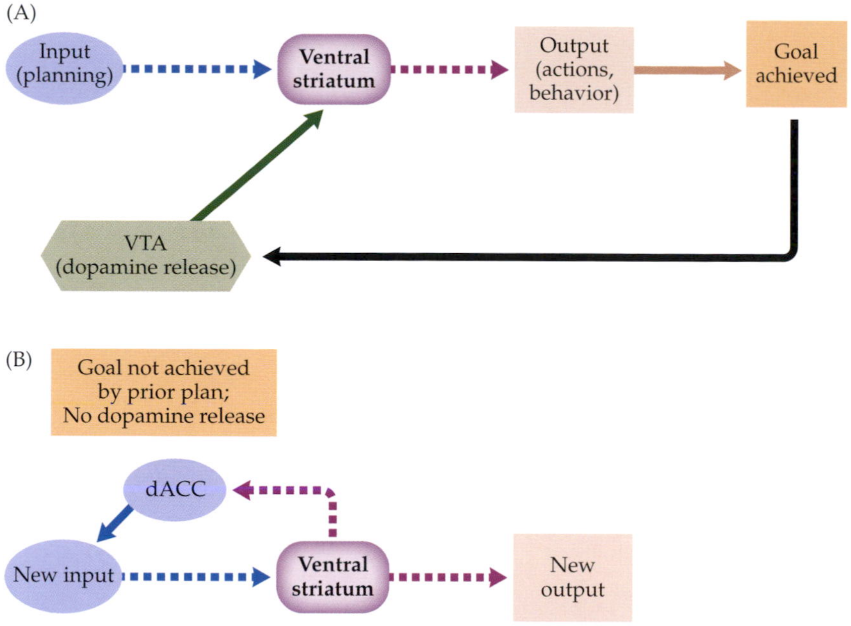

(A)

(B)

Figure 6.5 (A) Successful goal-directed plans result in DA release from the VTA, which strengthens the connections or pathways mediating the goal-directed plan. (B) When goal-directed plans fail, no DA is released and the pathways and connections for that plan are not reinforced. This failure is registered through the monitoring loops described in Figures 6.4B and 6.4C, particularly the dACC, which relays information to the dlPFC so that a new plan can be initiated.

relative success of our actions and subsequent refinement of our behavior. In one pathway, the VS communicates with the dlPFC indirectly via the DS (**Figure 6.4B**). Here again, the link between the VS and DS is largely through midbrain dopaminergic neurons in the SN. In a second pathway, the VP acts as relay between the VS and the dorsomedial thalamic nucleus, which in turn projects to both the dlPFC and vmPFC (**Figure 6.4C**).

Through these parallel pathways of information processing, the PFC—most importantly the dorsal anterior cingulate cortex and dlPFC—can monitor the output of the VS gate, and goal-directed behaviors can be refined (**Figure 6.5**). When the execution of a specific action plan (e.g., a lever press in response to light) results in a reward (e.g., a food pellet), the associated input and output pathways are reinforced through the release of DA in the VS gate. When the execution of a specific action plan (e.g., lever press in response to tone) does not result in reward, the input and output pathways are not reinforced, as there is no DA release in the VS. This unsuccessful result is brought to our (or the mouse's) awareness through the processing of convergent information in the vmPFC. The vmPFC also relays this information to the dACC, which functions to monitor our behavior and register conflict between our goals and the outcome. When the dACC relays information regarding the presence of conflict forward to the dlPFC, an alternate action plan (e.g., a nose poke) can be generated and then executed through the VS gate. Thus, alternate behavioral plans can be "tested" until a goal is achieved, at which point the successful plan is reinforced and expressed as reward learning.

dACC   dorsal anterior cingulate cortex
vmPFC   ventromedial prefrontal cortex

RESEARCH SPOTLIGHT

Our current understanding of how connections between nodes of the corticostriatal circuit support goal-directed actions and reward learning has come about in large part thanks to the detailed anatomical studies of Suzanne Haber and colleagues at the University of Rochester. These connections were identified by injecting tracer chemicals into neurons in various nodes of the corticostriatal circuit in monkeys (**Figure 6.6**). From the site of injection, these tracers move forward (anterograde), backward (retrograde), or bidirectionally along the connections of the injected neurons. After several days, the pathways along which the tracers traveled from their injection site can be visualized using immunocytochemistry. Thus, Haber and her colleagues were able to define the anatomical connections between key nodes of the corticostriatal circuit, revealing the flow of information supporting reward learning.

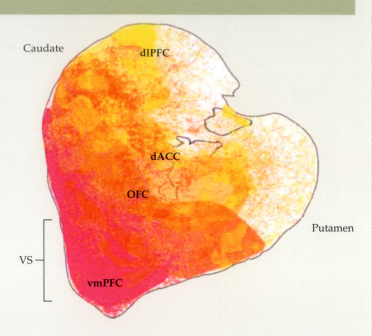

Figure 6.6 Anatomical tracing studies by Haber and colleagues have revealed discrete patterns of connections between nodes of the corticostriatal circuit. Here different colors overlaid on the DS (caudate and putamen) and VS represent the unique connections of each region with specific subregions of the prefrontal cortex. (From Haber & Knutson, 2010.)

Beyond Reward Learning

Regardless of whether or not an operant response is necessary to obtain a reward, the establishment of associations between primary and secondary reinforcers forms the backbone of reward learning and goal-directed behavior. This is clearly evident in fMRI studies of corticostriatal circuit function, which highlight the myriad triggers—whether unconditioned or conditioned stimuli, primary or secondary reinforcers—of the VS gate and extended circuitry. Because of the ventral striatum's critical role as the hub of the corticostriatal circuit, much of the fMRI literature, as well as our review of this literature in the following sections, focuses on reward-related activity of the VS. When possible, we will further consider fMRI evidence supporting other corticostriatal circuit nodes in responding to various reinforcing stimuli and goal-directed behaviors. We will first review the fMRI evidence for primary reinforcers as triggers of the VS.

Primary reinforcers

Multiple fMRI studies have revealed that primary reinforcers like water, food, and psychoactive drugs (i.e., those drugs that affect our behavior) trigger a robust response in the VS and adjacent regions, including the VP and DS (**Figure 6.7**). Typically, fMRI studies of primary reinforcers involve direct delivery of the rewarding stimulus to the participant through a series of tubes, valves, and pumps. For example, during fMRI, water, juice, or even milkshake can be

VS	ventral striatum	dACC	dorsal anterior cingulate cortex
DS	dorsal striatum	OFC	orbitofrontal cortex
VP	ventral pallidum	vmPFC	ventromedial prefrontal cortex
dlPFC	dorsolateral prefrontal cortex		

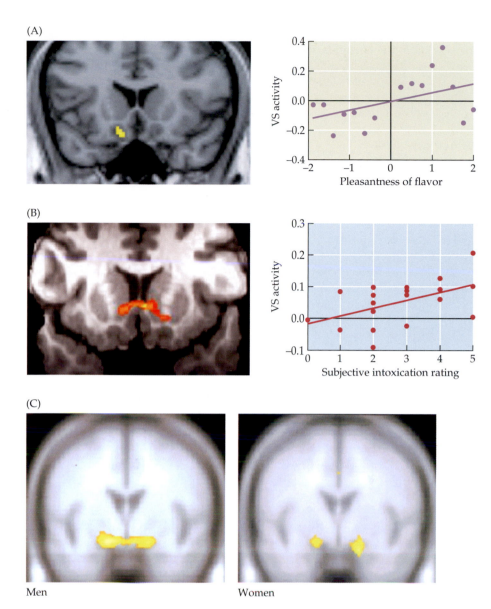

(A)

(B)

(C)

Men   Women

Figure 6.7 (A) The magnitude of VS activity in response to milkshakes predicts subjective pleasantness of the flavor. (B) The magnitude of VS activity in response to alcohol predicts subjective intoxication. Note that 0 represents mean activity in both graphs. (C) In both men and women, VS activity increases while viewing erotic film excerpts. (A from Grabenhorst et al., 2010; B from Gilman et al., 2012; C from Karama et al., 2002.)

pumped directly into the mouths of participants, while drugs can be delivered intravenously or through the air supply for inhalation.

MMM, MMM, GOOD! Delivery of food or drink, particularly when participants are thirsty or hungry, triggers robust VS activity. This activity is consistent with the role of these substances as primary reinforcers with direct value for our survival (i.e., calories for fuel). This VS activity likely reflects the release of DA, and in fact some fMRI studies have reported activity in the midbrain VTA in response to these primary reinforcers. Interestingly, activity in not

DA   dopamine
VTA   ventral tegmental area

only the VS but also the vmPFC correlates with how subjectively pleasant or enjoyable the participants find these substances. The correlation with VS as well as adjacent VP likely reflects the activation of "hedonic hot spots," while that with vmPFC likely reflects the convergent processing of sensory, interoceptive, contextual, and other information with motivational states during the administration.

THE RUSH OF A HIGH   Very similar if not identical effects have been observed for many different drugs of abuse. Typically, drugs of abuse such as alcohol, cocaine, marijuana, and nicotine are delivered intravenously, allowing for careful control of dosing. Of note, most of these studies are conducted in habitual drug users or addicts, because of the ethical considerations related to administering controlled substances to drug-naïve participants. All of these drugs elicit strong activity in the VS. Much like the correlations observed with foods, the subjective pleasantness of drugs also correlates with activity in the VS and vmPFC. We will consider the effects of drugs on the corticostriatal circuit in greater detail in Chapter 7 when discussing addiction.

ADAM AND EVE   Given the paramount role of sex in our survival as a species, it should come as no surprise that sexual stimuli and the sexual arousal they predict are associated with strong activity of the VS. There are a few rather exceptional neuroimaging studies documenting the corticostriatal circuit response to direct sexual stimulation resulting in orgasm. These studies typically involve self-stimulation during imaging. Because of the movement involved, these studies have measured regional cerebral blood flow using positron emission tomography (PET) rather than fMRI because PET is less sensitive to motion. Generally, these studies have found strong activation in the striatum broadly, as well as in the midbrain, hypothalamus, amygdala, PFC, and sensory cortices.

Viewing sexually erotic videos also elicits strong activity in the VS and extended corticostriatal circuit. Even black-and-white pictures of attractive (but not of unattractive) members of the opposite sex elicit VS activity. This likely reflects the subjective value and interest in pursuing a sexual relationship with the potential partner. While the response of the corticostriatal circuit to such sexual stimulation and stimuli is generally the same for men and women, a noteworthy difference has been reported in the hypothalamus, where men show greater activity than women when viewing pornographic videos. As described in Chapter 5, the hypothalamus contains the medial preoptic area, which exhibits pronounced sexual dimorphism. Thus, the functional difference between men and women observed with fMRI parallels this structural dimorphism, and these differences could be related to those we observe in our sexual behaviors, including greater subjective sexual arousal in men than women when viewing erotic images or films.

LADY GAGA, THE ROLLING STONES, AND BEETHOVEN WALK INTO A BAR...   While the response of the corticostriatal circuit to primary reinforcers such as food, drugs, and sex appears to be largely conserved across all mammals (e.g., mouse, monkey, man), there are some circuit triggers that appear to act as primary reinforcers uniquely in humans. The first of these is music. Most people have what appears to be an intrinsic positive response to music. While the genre and style may differ wildly between individuals and, certainly, generations,

VS	ventral striatum	VP	ventral pallidum
vmPFC	ventromedial prefrontal cortex	PFC	prefrontal cortex

RESEARCH SPOTLIGHT

Recent neuroimaging studies have begun to reveal interesting contributions of the corticostriatal circuit to the development of musical preference and the subjective appreciation of music. Using a combination of fMRI to measure activity and PET to measure DA release, V. N. Salimpoor and colleagues at McGill University found that when individuals listen to their favorite songs, there is increased activity of the VS gate as well as increased DA release into the VS and DS (**Figure 6.8A**). Moreover, both the amount of activity and the release of DA in the VS predicted how subjectively pleasurable each person found the music, and also how many "chills" they experienced when anticipating hearing a favorite song clip. In a subsequent study, the same authors found that

the amount of VS activity occurring in response to a new song clip predicted how much money a person would later spend to buy the music (**Figure 6.8B**). The strength of the activity in the VS also correlated with activity in other corticostriatal circuit nodes, including the vmPFC and amygdala, as well as the auditory cortices (**Figure 6.8C**). These findings suggest that music we find intrinsically rewarding results in release of the DA key, opening of the VS gate, and downstream activation of circuit nodes involved in generating our subjective emotional states (i.e., the vmPFC), in executing goal-directed behavior (i.e., the DS), and even in mapping our sensory experience (i.e., auditory cortices).

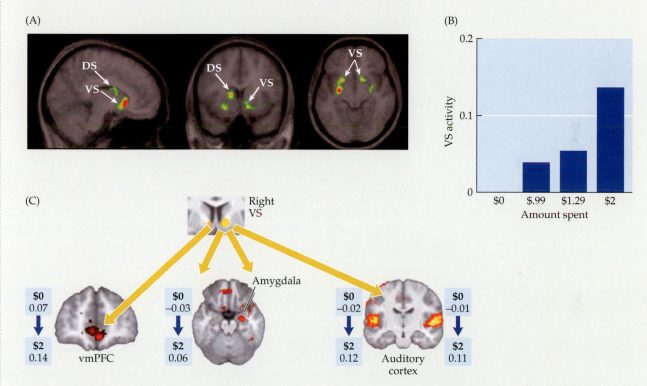

Figure 6.8 (A) Evidence for dopamine release in the VS and DS while listening to pleasurable music compared with listening to neutral music. (B) Greater VS activity during the processing of desirable (amount spent > $0) as opposed to undesirable ($0) music. Note that 0 represents baseline activity. (C) There are robust increases in connectivity between the VS and other corticostriatal circuit nodes, including the vmPFC and amygdala as well as the auditory cortices, when individuals hear music they consider highly desirable compared with music they do not want to hear again. The boxes show changes in connectivity between the VS and each region as a function of amount spent to purchase the desirable music. (A after Salimpoor et al., 2011; B,C after Salimpoor et al., 2013.)

most of us have extensive discographies of music we find enjoyable. Some music in personal discographies likely represents conditioned stimuli, having been paired with some otherwise rewarding experience or unconditioned stimuli, such as the song that was playing when you had your first kiss, or

DS   dorsal striatum
DA   dopamine

Figure 6.9 There is greater VS activity when participants view cartoons that they subjectively find to be funny in comparison to those they do not find funny. Note that 0 represents baseline activity in these data. (After Mobbs et al., 2003.)

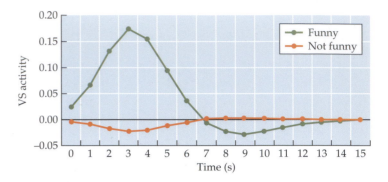

the lullaby your parents sang to you at bedtime. However, much, and likely most, music in our personal discographies has no obvious reward learning history. Rather, this music appears to be intrinsically rewarding.

Music, however, is not the only abstract stimulus that functions as a primary reinforcer uniquely in humans. Another is humor. Again, there is much diversity in what each of us does and does not find funny. I for one am a great admirer of cartoons, particularly those of Gary Larson's "The Far Side," which are not only humorous but also informative. I do accept the sad reality that not all of you find "The Far Side" as funny as I do. To each his own with comedy (as with most things in life). This said, fMRI studies are beginning to reveal that, although what we find funny varies from person to person, the contributions of the corticostriatal circuit to this process appear relatively consistent. Much as with the music we enjoy, what tickles our funny bone—be it a cartoon, a one-liner, or a stand-up comedian—elicits activity in the VS and midbrain VTA as well as other circuit nodes, including the PFC, DS, and even the hypothalamus (**Figure 6.9**). And, as with music, how subjectively funny we find something is correlated with the magnitude of activity in the VS. Thus, activity of the VS gate and the extended corticostriatal circuit helps shape not only basic physiological processes necessary for survival but also aspects of our nature that make us uniquely human.

Secondary reinforcers

As exemplified by both classical and operant conditioning, the corticostriatal circuit plays a critical role in helping us learn the value of otherwise neutral stimuli in predicting rewarding outcomes. Neuroimaging studies have revealed that myriad conditioned stimuli or secondary reinforcers trigger strong activity in the VS gate and extended corticostriatal circuit. Included among these triggers are images of palatable foods, and drug paraphernalia such as lighters, ashtrays, packs of cigarettes, pipes, and bongs. Such images and objects are fairly obvious conditioned stimuli, which have a clear history of predicting primary reinforcers. There are, however, some less obvious secondary reinforcers or conditioned stimuli. For example, a recent study found that tasting the flavor of beer in a solution absent of alcohol elicited the release of DA in the VS; it also resulted in greater craving for beer. We will consider the role of such secondary reinforcers or conditioned stimuli in greater detail in Chapter 7, where we describe how disorder within the corticostriatal circuit contributes to addiction.

DA release in the striatum broadly as well as the vmPFC also predicts how hard an individual will work—measured as the willingness to press a lever 100 times in 21 seconds with the pinky finger of the nondominant hand!—to

VS	ventral striatum	**DS**	dorsal striatum
VTA	ventral tegmental area	**DA**	dopamine
PFC	prefrontal cortex		

(A)

(B)

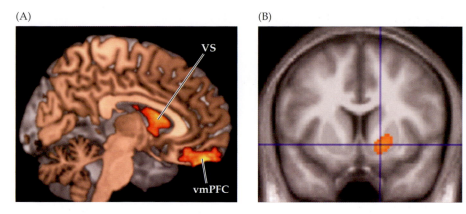

VS

vmPFC

Figure 6.10 (A) Dopamine release in the VS and vmPFC is correlated with the willingness to expend greater effort for larger rewards, particularly when probability of reward receipt is low. (B) Similarly, VS activity (cross hairs) increases as the effort required to receive a reward increases. (A from Treadway et al., 2012; B from Schmidt et al., 2012.)

receive a reward (**Figure 6.10A**). In another study, VS activity was positively correlated with increasing difficulty in squeezing a response ball to achieve a reward (**Figure 6.10B**). Interestingly, there was also greater positive connectivity between the VS and motor cortices during trials requiring more effortful squeezing. Thus, activity of the VS gate and extended corticostriatal circuit in response to conditioned stimuli is associated with changes in motivational states as well as the expression of goal-directed behavior. However, unlike with primary reinforcers; VS activity in response to secondary reinforcers is generally related to wanting rather than liking of stimuli.

"I DON'T CARE TOO MUCH FOR MONEY, MONEY CAN'T BUY ME LOVE" While this famous Beatles stanza is surely right about love, money can and does buy most everything else—including all of the aforementioned primary reinforcers. Thus, there may be no more important and powerful secondary reinforcer for humans than money. Consistent with money's unique role as a secondary reinforcer, the majority of fMRI studies of reward learning and goal-directed behavior involve some form of monetary incentive. Generally, these tasks involve games requiring individuals to perform specific operations for the chance to win varying amounts of money. These operations can range from the mundane, like pressing a button in response to a flashing stimulus (**Figure 6.11A**) or guessing the number on the back of a playing card, to the extraordinary, like shopping for online bargains (see Research Spotlight on the next page). In many fMRI studies, these tasks are presented in a manner that can isolate the corticostriatal circuit response during two critical phases: when you're waiting to play the game for money (i.e., anticipation), and when you're receiving money (i.e., outcome).

Through this design, most monetary incentive tasks closely mirror the original reward paradigms employed by Wolfram Schultz and colleagues (see Chapter 5) to identify the role of DA release in reward learning. Not surprisingly, the activities of the VS and midbrain VTA during monetary incentive tasks also mirror the results of Schultz and colleagues. Namely, activity in both the VS gate and midbrain VTA is strongest during the anticipation of money (that is, during the time period a player is waiting to play a game that

DA	dopamine		DA	dopamine
vmPFC	ventromedial prefrontal cortex		VTA	ventral tegmental area
VS	ventral striatum			

Figure 6.11 The monetary incentive delay (MID) task is one of the most widely used fMRI tasks for studying corticostriatal circuit function. (A) Participants are first presented with a cue that signifies the magnitude of money they will be playing for during the trial. There is then a brief delay during which participants are anticipating the upcoming trial. After the delay, they are presented with a target to which they must respond as quickly as possible with a button press. After the target presentation, participants are informed of the outcome of their response, which is either "correct," that is, their response to the target was fast enough to receive money, or "incorrect," that is, their response was too slow and they do not receive money. (B) The greatest activity in the vmPFC, VS, and VTA is observed during the anticipation phase (delay) of the MID. (A after Knutson et al., 2001; B after Knutson et al., 2005.)

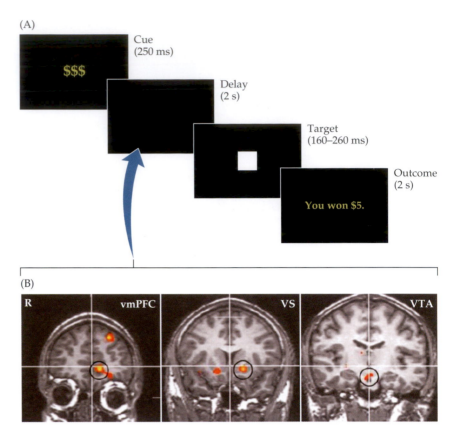

could result in winning money; **Figure 6.11B**). In contrast, there is relatively little involvement of the VS or VTA during the outcome phase (after the player has played and, if successful, receives the money). Rather, this second phase is characterized by activity in prefrontal regions, including the vmPFC, dlPFC, and dACC, associated with our subjective motivational states as well as the evaluation and refinement of our goal-directed behavior. The latter is

RESEARCH SPOTLIGHT

While the majority of fMRI studies of corticostriatal circuit function use very simple games of chance, some recent research has attempted to model more complex behaviors related to money and reward. In one such study, Brian Knutson and colleagues at Stanford University asked participants to "shop" for common goods and products much like we all do in our everyday lives (**Figure 6.12**). Specifically, Knutson and colleagues first showed participants an image of a common product, such as a box of Godiva chocolates, for 4 seconds. During this time, participants could consider how much they wanted the product and how much they would be willing to pay for it. Then, the price of the product was presented for another 4 seconds. After this time, the participants had a final 4 seconds to choose whether they did

or did not want to buy the product. Participants completed this three-step "shopping" task for 40 products.

A neat twist to the experiment was that each participant was given $20 at the beginning of the study and was able to spend that money to purchase one of the products they selected, which was shipped to them later. This final manipulation deepened the realistic nature of the experiment and furthered the value of the resulting patterns of activation in the corticostriatal circuit associated with each of the three steps. Activity of the VS gate was most prominent during the first and second steps, when participants were considering their preference for a product as well as the price.

(Continued on next page)

VS	ventral striatum	**dlPFC**	dorsolateral prefrontal cortex
VTA	ventral tegmental area	**dACC**	dorsal anterior cingulate cortex
vmPFC	ventromedial prefrontal cortex	**MID**	monetary incentive delay

RESEARCH SPOTLIGHT (*continued*)

Activity of the VS gate was strongest for products that participants later purchased and weakest for those products they did not purchase. This is consistent with the role of the VS gate in learning the reward value of stimuli and mediating goal-directed behavior to obtain a reward. That is, activity in the VS gate increases in response to product images, which function as conditioned stimuli because of the rewarding experiences we've had with those products in the past, (e.g., the pleasure of a delicious and creamy truffle from a box of Godiva chocolates). Opening of the VS gate is subsequently associated with purchasing the products we prefer. The second step of the shopping task, when participants considered the price of the product, was also associated with activity in the vmPFC. Again, this activity increased for products subsequently

purchased and decreased for those declined. This pattern is consistent with the role of the vmPFC in the subjective evaluation of our experiences as well as the integration of sensory, interoceptive, and motivational information, which appears particularly strong for things we prefer. The third phase of the shopping task, when participants actually chose whether or not to purchase a product, was associated with activity in the insula.

Interestingly, however, there was greater *insula* activity in response to products that were not purchased, suggesting that interoceptive signals contribute to decisions to avoid things we don't want. There may after all be something to the notion of "following your gut" when making decisions.

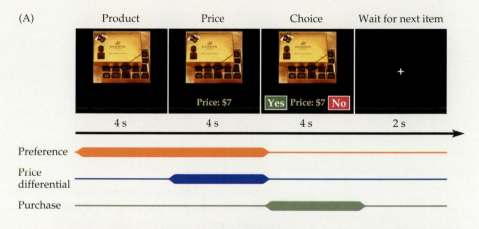

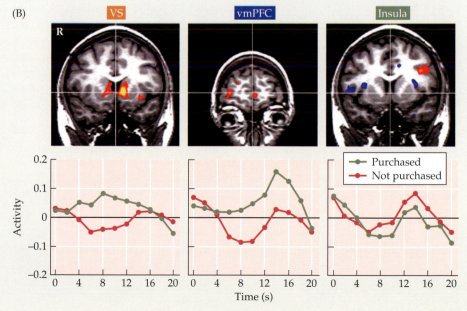

Figure 6.12 When participants were asked to spend money on a variety of common goods (here a box of Godiva chocolates), activity in the VS increased when viewing images and associated prices for products that were subsequently purchased and decreased for those not purchased. Activity in the vmPFC increased specifically when participants were considering the price of products they subsequently purchased, and decreased for those not purchased. In contrast to activity in the VS and vmPFC, activity in the insula increased only when making the decision to *not* buy a product. Note that 0 represents baseline activity in these data. (After Knutson et al., 2007.)

particularly important if the player was unsuccessful on the previous attempt and thus needs to alter their behavior (e.g., respond faster to a cue) to win on the next attempt.

This pattern of corticostriatal circuit activity associated with anticipation and outcome likely reflects the established value of money as a conditioned stimulus, which has faithfully predicted unconditioned stimuli (e.g., food or drugs) in the past. It appears, in fact, that for most of us (at least in Western industrialized nations) money functions as a primary reinforcer to which we generate DA release in the VS and opening of the VS gate to mediate goal-directed behavior through the other circuit nodes. (Translation: We act in a manner that gets us more money.) By virtue of their effectiveness in eliciting distinct aspects of corticostriatal circuit function, monetary incentive tasks are an effective and widely used tool for understanding both normal and abnormal reward learning and goal-directed behavior.

I've Got Your Back!

A growing body of research has highlighted the importance of the corticostriatal circuit for another critical aspect of human behavior: learning who you can and cannot trust. We are an exceptionally social species, and our survival depends very much on the aid of other humans. Thus, we quickly learn either through direct experience or indirect social transmission (e.g., gossip) who in our sphere of influence is and is not trustworthy. This form of social reciprocity is in and of itself rewarding because it helps us overcome challenges and survive. Several fMRI studies have established that activity in the VS gate increases when another individual is kind or generous to us in the context of a social interaction. Moreover, this VS activity serves as a foundation for learning whom we can and cannot trust.

Generally, this VS activity emerges when a fictional partner in a game responds to a decision we have made in a manner resulting in our benefit. For example, in some games we are asked to give money to a partner who can, in turn, make two decisions. The partner can either invest it in a manner that yields more money for each of us (i.e., cooperate) or keep it for himself (i.e., act selfishly, or not cooperate), in which case we lose our initial investment. When our fictional partner decides to cooperate and we both end up making more money, there is an increase in our VS activity (**Figure 6.13**). In contrast, VS activity decreases when a partner betrays our trust and acts selfishly. These differential patterns of VS activity in response to cooperation and selfishness help us learn which partners to trust over time. Interestingly, when these partners are given faces (i.e., partners' decisions are paired with pictures

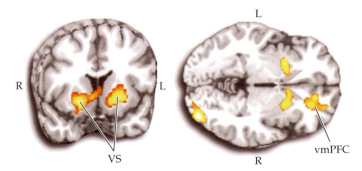

Figure 6.13 Greater activity in the VS (left) and vmPFC (right) when trust is reciprocated versus when trust is violated. (From Phan et al., 2010.)

DA	dopamine
VS	ventral striatum
vmPFC	ventromedial prefrontal cortex

RESEARCH SPOTLIGHT

On the opposite end of the spectrum of human social behavior from trust and reciprocity lies *schadenfreude*: taking pleasure in the suffering of others. A rather clever recent study suggests that the corticostriatal circuit is also involved with this more sinister aspect of human behavior. In this study, Cikara and colleagues at Princeton University took advantage of the common and often intense experience of sports rivalries wherein there is often as much pleasure taken in the failure of the rival team as in the success of the favored team (**Figure 6.14**). To maximize this effect, Cikara and colleagues selected fans from two teams that have arguably the fiercest rivalry in all of sport: the New York Yankees and Boston Red Sox. The investigators made certain of participants' fanatical support by requiring them to ace a test of historical knowledge about their favored team. They then presented a number of different virtual game scenarios involving the success or failure of their favored team and their rival team. Not surprisingly, there was activity in regions of the striatum when the favored team was successful. However, there was also activity in these regions when the rival team failed. This was true even if the rival's loss was in a game with a third team. Although the striatal activity observed was near but not within the VS, the findings nevertheless support the importance of the corticostriatal circuit in reward learning and goal-directed behavior when we take pleasure in the success of our favored team or in the failure of our rival team (i.e., *schadenfreude*). In contrast, activity in the dACC and insula increased with the failure of the favored team and success of the rival team, which is consistent with the high degree of conflict and even physical distress some fans experience when their team fails or their rivals succeed. Interestingly, activity in the striatum predicted the degree of pleasure experienced not only when watching the favored team succeed, but also when watching the rival team fail. More ominously, this activity also predicted the amount of rival-specific harm participants endorsed on a questionnaire. Although there appears to be little to no value in such fanatical behavior in the modern world, it is possible that in our distant past this form of reward learning and associated goal-directed behavior functioned to maintain and deepen the social bonds of members *within* small clans while weakening those *between* clans when fighting over the limited resources necessary for survival.

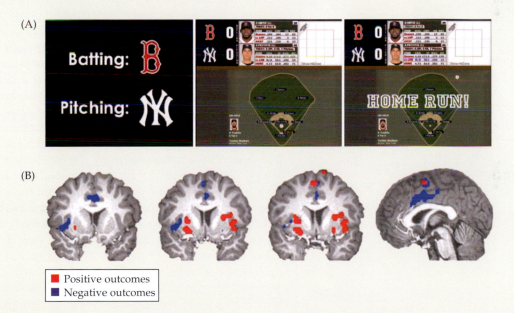

Figure 6.14 (A) Avid fans of either the Red Sox or of the Yankees viewed baseball plays while undergoing fMRI. This example is of a trial in which the Red Sox hit a home run against the Yankees. The first screen designated the participating teams. Then, participants saw the field, the pitcher, and the batter (the background was created from screenshots of televised broadcasts of actual games). The play began when the ball moved from the pitcher's mound to home plate, where the player hit the ball. The final screen designated the outcome of the play. (B) There was greater activity near the VS (middle panels) associated with both success of the favored team and failure of the rival's team (i.e., positive outcomes). There was greater activity in the insula and dACC (left and right panels, respectively) associated with the failure of the favored team or the success of the rival's team (i.e., negative outcomes). (From Cikara et al., 2011.)

dACC   dorsal anterior cingulate cortex

"prisoner's dilemma" Game in which participants are variously rewarded/punished for cooperation versus betrayal of another participant. When iterated (played over and over with the same participants), the game is designed to examine the factors that shape cooperation among individuals.

impulsivity The general tendency to act without full consideration of the possible consequences.

of individuals who consistently cooperate or not), the activity of the VS in response to the faces alone maps faithfully onto our partner-specific prior experiences, with decreased activity in response to faces of selfish partners and increased activity with cooperators. Similar results have been observed with variations of the game involving decisions to cooperate or not in the context of avoiding punishment (e.g., iterated "prisoner's dilemma"). Thus, the VS gate of the corticostriatal circuit serves a critical role in establishing trust between individuals, reinforcing relationships characterized by reciprocity and weakening those characterized by selfishness.

Impulsivity

In the same way that dimensional measures of anxiety are particularly effective at capturing the general functioning of the corticolimbic circuit, comparable measures of impulsivity usefully capture the general functioning of the corticostriatal circuit. Impulsivity broadly refers to our ability to control our goal-directed behavior. Those higher in impulsivity generally act without full consideration of the consequences of their actions. For example, impulsive individuals are more likely to leave for a trip on a whim, not seek medical attention even for serious illness, and fail to plan for the future by saving. In contrast, those lower in impulsivity show considerable forethought and plan diligently for their futures. People who are not impulsive, for example, tend to plan trips months in advance, undergo annual medical and dental checkups, and maximize their annual contributions to retirement plans. In other words, our degree of impulsivity captures our capacity to "think before we act," "look before we leap," and "keep our eyes on the prize."

Like anxiety, impulsivity is a dimensional measure that exhibits considerable variability between individuals and that can be readily measured with a variety of research instruments, including self-report questionnaires and behavioral tests. Regardless of the specific measure used, higher levels of impulsivity are typically associated with greater activity of the VS (**Figure 6.15**) and midbrain VTA in response to common reward-related triggers (e.g., money, food, drugs). In contrast, higher levels of impulsivity are associated with less activity in regulatory regions of the PFC, including the dlPFC and dACC, as well as reduced functional connectivity between the VS and these prefrontal regions in response to these same triggers. Thus, impulsivity usefully reflects the balance between bottom-up (e.g., the VS and VTA) and top-down (e.g., the dlPFC and dACC) components of the corticostriatal circuit. When these circuit

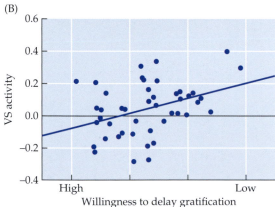
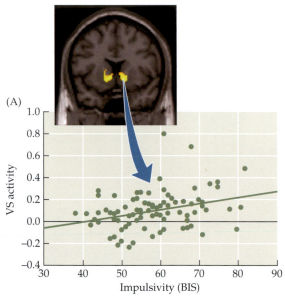

Figure 6.15 Reward-related VS activity predicts (A) higher levels of self-reported impulsiveness as measured using Barrett's Impulsiveness Scale (BIS) and (B) lower willingness to delay receiving a monetary reward measured using a computerized delay discounting test. Note that 0 represents mean activity in these data. (A after Forbes et al., 2009; B after Hariri et al., 2006.)

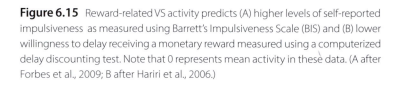

VS	ventral striatum	dlPFC	dorsolateral prefrontal cortex
VTA	ventral tegmental area	dACC	dorsal anterior cingulate cortex
PFC	prefrontal cortex		

components are in balance, there is expression of appropriate or adaptive goal-directed behaviors (e.g., using your monthly income to pay rent and utilities *and* contribute to your savings). When these components are out of balance, however, there is expression of inappropriate or maladaptive goal-directed behavior (e.g., spending all your income on alcohol and drugs). As we will observe in Chapter 7, high levels of impulsivity are a common shared dimensional feature of psychopathology associated with disorder of the corticostriatal circuit.

RESEARCH SPOTLIGHT

A construct closely related to impulsivity, delayed gratification is the capacity of a person to forgo a reward available immediately in favor of a future larger reward. The importance of delayed gratification is perhaps most clearly (and deliciously) portrayed in the seminal research of Walter Mischel of Columbia University. Mischel and his colleagues famously asked a group of young children to choose between eating right away the one marshmallow that was on a plate in front of them, or waiting a few minutes for two marshmallows. As you might imagine, resisting a delicious treat in easy reach is quite difficult for kids. But some of the kids managed to do just that, delaying their gratification, for the larger future reward of two marshmallows.

That some children are better than others in resisting temptation is not very surprising; however, the long-term predictions of this difference have been remarkable. By keeping track of their study participants over time, Mischel and colleagues discovered that those who were able to delay their gratification have led more successful, productive lives characterized by good grades, good jobs, good health, and good relationships in comparison to the kids who could not resist temptation.

While it has been repeatedly demonstrated that the ability to delay gratification early in life predicts later success, more recent studies have considered that the decision to delay gratification may not always be optimal. For example, when there is a history of a child not being given what was promised, the child is more likely to eat the one marshmallow in front of him than to take the chance on waiting for two marshmallows that may never materialize (**Figure 6.16A**). In other words, if there is a pattern of mistrust, the safer (and likely more adaptive) choice is the immediate reward.

A similar pattern has been observed in adults where the likelihood of waiting for a larger reward from someone depends on that person's reputation as being trustworthy or not (**Figure 6.16B**). Regardless of these nuances, the corticostriatal circuit is clearly involved in these processes, with fMRI studies that use a variety of rewards (most often, differing amounts of money now or later) generally finding that greater VS activity predicts lesser ability to delay gratification. In contrast, greater activity in the PFC, particularly dlPFC, typically predicts greater capacity to resist temptation and delay gratification. This is consistent with the role of the VS gate in mediating goal-directed behaviors. As we will discuss in detail in Unit III, this is also consistent with the role of the dlPFC in integrating current and future needs in the service of formulating more complex and adaptive plans of action.

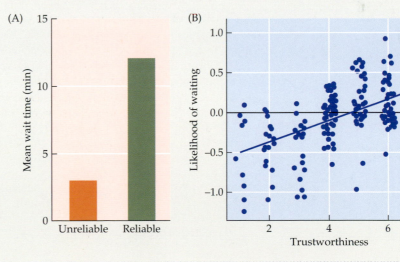

Figure 6.16 (A) Children are more likely to delay gratification for a marshmallow reward if their prior interactions with the adult offering the treat have been reliable (i.e., the adult followed through with prior promises). (B) Adults also are more willing to delay gratification, in this case for money, if they perceive the giver as trustworthy. Note that 0 represents the mean likelihood of waiting in these data. (A after Kidd et al., 2013; B after Michaelson et al., 2013.)

Summary

As exemplified by the experimental protocols of classical and operant conditioning, the corticostriatal circuit functions to register the experience of stimuli we find intrinsically rewarding (i.e., primary reinforcers) and to learn specific goal-directed behaviors, often in response to cues (i.e., secondary reinforcers), that allow us to reliably experience these rewards. The corticostriatal circuit is also important for learning complex and nuanced social relationships involving trust and reciprocity, as well as experiencing uniquely human emotions such as *schadenfreude*. While these more elaborate processes are interesting, it is through the core functions of motivation and action that the corticostriatal circuit becomes critical for survival. The expression of adaptive motivations and actions depends on normal functioning of the circuit, particularly the balance between the ventral striatum, ventral tegmental area, and prefrontal cortex. Imbalance or disorder between these critical circuit nodes results in many maladaptive responses, which we will consider in the next chapter.

Literature Cited & Further Reading

Bray S., & O'Doherty, J. (2007). Neural coding of reward-prediction error signals during classical conditioning with attractive faces. *Journal of Neurophysiology*, 97: 3036–3045.

Cikara, M., Botvinick, M., & Fiske, S. T. (2011). Us versus them: Social identity shapes neural responses to intergroup competition and harm. *Psychological Science*, 22: 306–313.

Filbey, F. M., Schacht, J. P., Myers, U. S., Chavez, R. S., & Hutchison, K. E. (2009). Marijuana craving in the brain. *Proceedings of the National Academy of Science USA*, 106: 13016–13021.

Forbes, E. E., Brown, S. M., Kimak, M., Ferrell, R. E., Manuck, S. B., & Hariri, A. R. (2009). Genetic variation in components of dopamine neurotransmission impacts ventral striatal reactivity associated with impulsivity. *Molecular Psychiatry*, 14: 60–70.

Gilman, J. M., Ramchandani, V. A., Crouss, T., & Hommer, D. W. (2012). Subjective and neural responses to intravenous alcohol in young adults with light and heavy drinking patterns. *Neuropsychopharmacology*, 37: 467–477.

Grabenhorst, F., Rolls, E. T., Parris, B. A., & d'Souza, A. (2010). How the brain represents the reward value of fat in the mouth. *Cerebral Cortex*, 20: 1082–1091.

Haber, S. N., & Knutson, B. (2010). The reward circuit: Linking primate anatomy and human imaging. *Neuropsychopharmacology*, 35: 4–26.

Hariri, A. R., Brown, S. M., Williamson, D. E., Flory, J. D., de Wit, H., & Manuck S. B. (2006). Preference for immediate over delayed rewards is associated with magnitude of ventral striatal activity. *The Journal of Neuroscience*, 26: 13213–13217.

Karama, S., Lecours, A. R., Leroux, J.-M., Bourgouin, P., Beaudoin, G., Joubert, S., & Beauregard, M. (2002). Areas of brain activation in males and females during viewing of erotic film excerpts. *Human Brain Mapping*, 16: 1–13.

Kidd, C., Palmeri, H., & Aslin, R. N. (2013). Rational snacking: Young children's decision-making on the marshmallow task is moderated by beliefs about environmental reliability. *Cognition*, 126: 109–114.

Knutson, B., Adams, C. M., Fong, G. W., & Hommer, D. (2001). Anticipation of increasing monetary reward selectively recruits nucleus accumbens. *The Journal of Neuroscience*, 21(16): RC159.

Knutson, B., Taylor, J., Kaufman, M., Peterson, R., & Glover, G. (2005). Distributed neural representation of expected value. *The Journal of Neuroscience*, 25: 4806–4812.

Knutson, B., Rick, S., Wimmer, G. E., Prelec, D., & Loewenstein, G. (2007). Neural predictors of purchases. *Neuron*, 53: 147–156.

Michaelson, L., de la Vega, A., Chatham, C. H., & Munakata, Y. (2013). Delaying gratification depends on social trust. *Frontiers in Psychology*, 4: 275.

Mobbs., D., Greicius, M. D., Abdel-Azim, E., Menon, V., & Reiss, A. L. (2003). Humor modulates the mesolimbic reward centers. *Neuron*, 40: 1041–1048.

Moffitt, T. E., & 12 others. (2011). A gradient of childhood self-control predicts health, wealth, and public safety. *Proceedings of the National Academy of Science USA*, 108: 2693–2698.

Oberlin, B. G, Dzemidzic, M., Tran, S. M., Soeurt, C. M., Albrecht, D. S., Yoder, K. K., & Kareken, D. A. (2013). *Neuropsychopharmacology*, 38: 1617–1624.

Phan, K. L., Sripada, C. S., Angstadt, M., & McCabe, K. (2010). Reputation for reciprocity engages the brain reward center. *Proceedings of the National Academy of Science USA*, 107: 13099–13104.

Salimpoor, V. N., Benovoy, M., Larcher, K., Dagher, A., & Zatorre, R. J. (2011). Anatomically distinct dopamine release during anticipation and experience of peak emotion to music. *Nature Neuroscience*, 14, 257–262.

Salimpoor, V. N., van den Bosch, I., Kovacevic, N., McIntosh, A. R., Dagher, A., & Zatorre, R. J. (2013). Interactions between the nucleus accumbens and auditory cortices predict music reward value. *Science*, 340, 216–219.

Schmidt, L., Lebreton, M., Clery-Melin, M.-L., Daunizeau, J., & Pessiglione, M. (2012). Neural mechanisms underlying motivation of mental versus physical effort. *PLoS Biology*, 10(2): e1001266.

Schultz, W., Dayan, P., & Montague, P. R. (1997). A neural substrate of prediction and reward. *Science* 275: 1593–1599.

Treadway, M. T., & 9 others. (2012). Dopaminergic mechanisms of individual differences in human effort-based decision making. *The Journal of Neuroscience*, 32: 6170–6176.

In Chapter 5 we established the neuroanatomical basis for the cortico-striatal circuit and reviewed basic functional interactions between key circuit nodes. In Chapter 6 we saw how the orderly processing of information through this circuit generates the pursuit of rewarding stimuli through goal-directed behaviors (i.e., motivation and action). We now consider how disorder within the corticostriatal circuit manifests as psychopathology characterized by maladaptive reward seeking and lack of behavioral control, as well as an inability to experience pleasure. Although corticostriatal circuit dysfunction is most commonly linked with symptoms of externalizing disorders such as substance use disorders and attention deficit hyperactivity disorder, there is considerable involvement of this circuit in internalizing disorders such as depression.

Although we will again adopt the perspective of mapping corticostriatal circuit dysfunction within traditional categorical disorders, a strong emphasis on the specific relationships between circuit dysfunction and the emergence of core symptoms (e.g., impulsivity) that cut across disorders will continue. The importance of understanding the neural basis of these dimensional symptoms rather than categorical differences between groups of individuals with or without a disorder will be brought into stark relief as we encounter several of the same disorders presented for the corticolimbic circuit in Unit I. Here, however, we will focus on the symptoms related to dysfunctional processing of reward rather than threat. As we do so, it should become readily apparent that most disorders are effectively amalgamations of specific symptoms rooted in dysfunction of specific circuits rather than categorical differences in general brain structure and function. Thus, for example, while a categorical approach reveals dysfunction of both the corticolimbic and corticostriatal circuits in depression, the dimensional approach reveals that dysfunction in one circuit—the corticolimbic—maps onto the severity of depressed mood related to abnormalities in recognition and reaction to threat, while dysfunction in the other—the corticostriatal—maps onto the severity of anhedonia related to abnormalities in motivation and action.

As the hub of the corticostriatal circuit, the ventral striatum (VS) "gate" will serve as the entry point for our study of how dysfunction within the broader circuit emerges as disordered behavior or psychopathology. This VS-centric approach, like that adopted with the amygdala for the corticolimbic circuit, is not simply one of convenience; rather it recognizes the critical role of the VS as the gate through which motivation is translated into action. Psychopathology associated with disorder of the VS gate is quintessentially one of maladaptive goal-directed behaviors (i.e., actions) in response to rewarding stimuli (i.e., motivations). It has been observed, however, that disorder of the VS gate can reflect dysfunction in other circuit nodes, most notably the midbrain ventral tegmental area and prefrontal cortex, and the failure of these interconnected circuit nodes to effectively regulate and integrate goal-directed behaviors through the VS. When possible, we will consider how such dysfunction in other nodes of the corticostriatal circuit contributes to disorder of the VS gate and related psychopathology.

Consistent with the approach defined in Unit I on the corticolimbic circuit, we consider relative changes in VS activity in individuals with specific categorical disorders in comparison with individuals with no known psychopathology (i.e., "healthy participants"). Throughout, however, we will emphasize how alterations in VS activity relate to changes in specific symptoms, some of which cut across disorders. We begin by considering decreased activity, or hypoactivity, of the VS gate, which is less common than increased activity and typically is associated with decreased motivation for rewards and goal-directed behavior, as well as deficits in reward learning. We then turn to more commonly observed increased activity, or hyperactivity, of the VS gate, which typically manifests as increased motivation for stimuli not commonly associated with reward, and maladaptive goal-directed behaviors. For psychopathology already described in detail in Unit I (major depressive disorder, bipolar disorders, posttraumatic stress disorder, and antisocial personality disorder), we will provide only a cursory overview of the clinical diagnosis before delving quickly into specific symptoms associated with disorder of the corticostriatal circuit. A more detailed description of several disorders encountered here for the first time (attention deficit hyperactivity disorder, eating disorders, and substance use disorder) will be provided before we consider specific associations between corticostriatal circuit dysfunction and their symptomatology.

Ventral Striatum Hypoactivity

Given the critical importance of the corticostriatal circuit in mediating goal-directed behaviors (i.e., translating motivation into action), hypoactivity of the VS gate is associated with a pronounced blunting of not only seeking rewarding stimuli, but also deriving pleasure from these stimuli. As we saw in Unit I, such inability to both experience and seek pleasure is a hallmark symptom of mood disorders, most notably major depressive disorder. Decreased VS activity is also present in psychopathology where there is difficulty in reward learning and in tailoring goal-directed behaviors to appropriate reward-related cues, as is observed in bipolar disorders and attention deficit hyperactivity disorder.

Major depressive disorder

major depressive disorder (MDD) Commonly referred to simply as depression; characterized by typically recurring major depressive episodes (MDEs), with no occurrence of manic or hypomanic episodes.

Recall that **major depressive disorder (MDD)**, more commonly known as depression, is characterized by experiencing at least one major depressive episode, which must include either depressed mood or markedly diminished interest or pleasure in all, or almost all, activities most of the day, nearly every day for at least 2 weeks. To date, studies of corticolimbic circuit disorder have dominated research on the pathophysiology of MDD and other mood disorders. However, a growing number of recent studies have shifted their focus

VS   ventral striatum
MDD   major depressive disorder

to the relative functioning of the corticostriatal circuit. This shift reflects a deepening appreciation for the need to better understand the biological basis of anhedonia or the loss of interest or pleasure in nearly all activities, which is a core symptom in MDD. In contrast, studies of the corticolimbic circuit primarily address depressed mood, another core symptom, as well as risk factors associated with the development of MDD, namely high trait anxiety and hyperresponsiveness to threat and stress.

Several studies of corticostriatal circuit disorder in MDD (**Figure 7.1**) have employed the monetary incentive delay (MID) tasks described in Chapter 6. An advantage of the MID is its ability to isolate circuit responses, particularly VS activity, during two important stages of reward processing: anticipation and outcome. Although two early studies found no difference between affected and healthy participants in VS activity during reward anticipation, a third, later study found evidence for decreased activity in affected individuals. Interestingly, the relative VS hypoactivity in this third study normalized (i.e., increased to levels in controls) after a 6-week course of treatment with a selective serotonin reuptake inhibitor (SSRI). Moreover, pretreatment VS hypoactivity was associated with greater anhedonic symptoms, while the magnitude of posttreatment increase in VS activity predicted the level of overall improvement in depressive symptoms. Similarly, decreased VS activity has been observed in MDD relative to healthy participants during the outcome stage of the MID task, where all participants learn that they have won money, although it is unclear whether this outcome-related hypoactivity is associated with symptom severity.

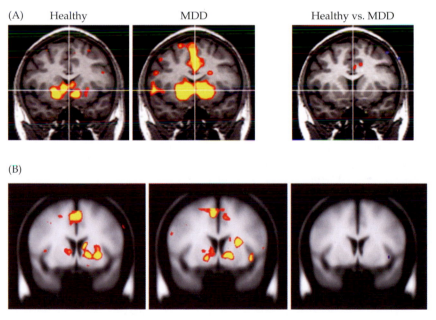

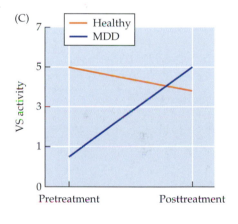

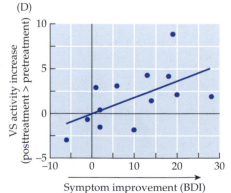

Figure 7.1 (A,B) Some studies have not found evidence for VS hypoactivity during the anticipation of reward in MDD. (C,D) Another study found that treatment with an SSRI increased VS activity to levels seen in healthy participants (C) and that the magnitude of this increase predicted improvements in symptoms measured using the Beck Depression Inventory (BDI). Note that 0 represents baseline activity in C and mean activity in D. (A after Knutson et al., 2008; B after Pizzagalli et al., 2009; C,D after Stoy et al., 2011.)

MID   monetary incentive delay
SSRI   selective serotonin reuptake
        inhibitors

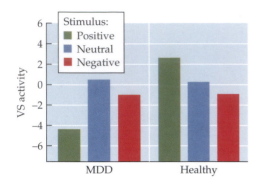

Figure 7.2 Relative to healthy participants, individuals with MDD demonstrate significantly less VS activity to positive stimuli. Responses to neutral and negative stimuli are similar in both groups. Note that 0 represents mean activity in these data. (After Epstein et al., 2006.)

VS hypoactivity has also been reported for individuals with MDD when they are processing nonmonetary cues. In one particularly interesting study, VS activity was measured in both depressed and healthy participants while they viewed a series of words conveying positive emotion (e.g., *success, heroic, admired*), negative emotion (e.g., *worthless, bleak, burden*), or no specific emotion (e.g., *transfer, fasten, trunk*). These broad categories of emotion-conveying words were chosen because individuals suffering from MDD often strongly identify with self-referential negative, but not positive, words (i.e., think poorly of themselves and have low self-worth). Consistent with this negative self-schema, in comparison with healthy participants, those with MDD exhibited decreased VS activity to positive words specifically (**Figure 7.2**). There was no difference in VS activity between affected and healthy participants to either negative or neutral words. Critically, the magnitude of VS activity to positive words was negatively correlated with anhedonic symptoms.

Additional evidence for the importance of the VS gate in depression comes from surgical studies targeting this circuit hub with deep brain stimulation, or DBS (**Figure 7.3**). As is true for DBS treatment of MDD targeting the ventromedial PFC, this procedure is used in individuals with a chronic history of MDD who have not responded to any other treatments, including SSRIs and electroconvulsive therapy. A small but growing number of studies demonstrate that DBS of the VS results in increased activity in not only this circuit hub but also interconnected nodes, including the amygdala and regions of the PFC. Moreover, DBS targeting the VS results in an almost instantaneous

(A)

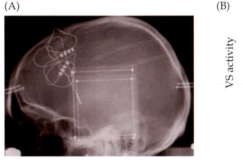

(B)

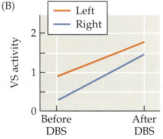

(C)

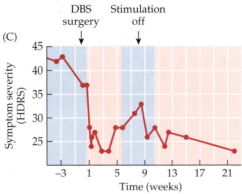

Figure 7.3 (A) X-ray showing the location of electrode leads in the VS for deep brain stimulation treatment in a patient with MDD. (B) VS activity, measured with positron emission tomography, increased in both left and right hemispheres one week after treatment began. (C) Depression severity as measured by the Hamilton Depression Rating Scale (HDRS) decreased immediately after DBS surgery and stayed low as long as the DBS was active. Note that 0 represents baseline activity in these data. (After Schlaepfer et al., 2008.)

VS	ventral striatum	**DBS**	deep brain stimulation
MDD	major depressive disorder	**SSRI**	selective serotonin reuptake inhibitors

RESEARCH SPOTLIGHT

Recent studies in my lab have demonstrated the importance of corticostriatal circuit function in maintaining positive affect ("upbeat mood") in the face of normal stress. In one study of a large sample of healthy college students, we found that the magnitude of VS activity to reward predicted self-reported positive affect in the face of stressful life events (**Figure 7.4**). Specifically, we found that college students who experienced more stressors in the past year (such as a death in the family, relationship breakups, or struggling with their courses) reported lower levels of positive affect than students not experiencing these stressors. However, this association between stress and low positive affect was only present for students also having relatively low levels of reward-related VS activity. If VS activity was relatively high, students reported higher positive affect, especially if they also experienced greater stress.

In other words, high VS activity to reward appears to confer relative stress resiliency in the form of high positive affect despite the experience of stressful life events. Thus, reward-related VS activity impacts not only the core symptom of anhedonia in MDD, but also the ability to more generally experience positive affect, particularly in the face of life's challenges.

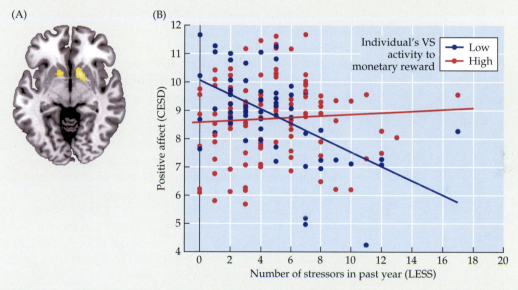

Figure 7.4 (A) Reward-related VS activity in a large sample of college students. (B) Only if this VS activity is relatively low do students report lower levels of positive affect (as measured by the Center for Epidemiologic Studies Depression scale, or CESD) if they have also experienced a greater number of stressors in the past year as measured by the Life Events Scale for Students (LESS). (After Nikolova et al., 2012.)

improvement in depressive symptoms, including anhedonia. Importantly, it is not yet clear whether DBS targeting the VS or DBS targeting the vmPFC works better to relieve depression in severe cases; clinical trials are under way to compare the two strategies directly. It is possible that DBS targeting the vmPFC may be more effective for individuals who suffer from stress-related depressed mood, while DBS targeting the VS may be more effective for those suffering primarily from anhedonia.

Bipolar disorders

Much as is the case with the corticolimbic circuit, relatively few studies of corticostriatal circuit dysfunction have been conducted in individuals with **bipolar disorders (BD)**. There is some evidence for dysfunctional VS activity

bipolar disorders (BD) Characterized by typically recurring cycles of manic episodes, euthymia, and major depressive episodes.

Figure 7.5 In contrast with healthy participants, individuals with bipolar disorders who are experiencing a euthymic state exhibit increased vlPFC activity during the anticipation of winning money but not of losing money. Note that 0 represents baseline activity in these data. (After Nusslock et al., 2012.)

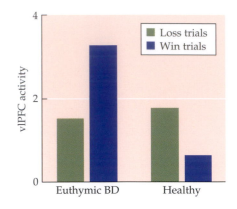

during monetary incentive delay tasks in BD when experiencing a manic phase. However, this dysfunction is not clearly one of relative hypoactivity in comparison with controls. Rather, there appears to be a lack of differential VS activity to positive versus negative outcomes (i.e., winning or not winning money). While in healthy participants VS activity is higher in response to positive outcomes relative to negative outcomes, in manic individuals VS activity is consistently high for both outcomes. A similar pattern of undifferentiated activity is seen in the midbrain ventral tegmental area. Thus, the "gate" and "key" of the corticostriatal circuit may not discriminate between clearly rewarding and nonrewarding outcomes in BD during a manic episode. A similar lack of discrimination exists at the behavioral level, where manic individuals show generally poor judgment and hyperactivity, often including increased sex drive and drug abuse. Interestingly, these response patterns in the VS and VTA may reflect disorder in prefrontal regions responsible for the regulation and planning of goal-directed behavior.

As was true for the corticolimbic circuit, abnormal activity of the vlPFC may be critical in the emergence of dysfunction in other circuit nodes. Results from one study indicate that during manic episodes the vlPFC does not appropriately track changes in anticipating reward. Specifically, in comparison with healthy participants, there is an exaggerated decrease in vlPFC activity during anticipation of smaller amounts of money and an exaggerated increase with larger amounts. The opposite pattern emerges during anticipation of relatively smaller or larger losses of money. Thus, activity in the vlPFC of manic individuals appears to overestimate the value of potential gains and underestimate the value of potential losses. Again, this pattern is consistent with behavior during manic episodes, when individuals with BD take greater risks and believe themselves to be more capable than they actually are. Importantly, vlPFC dysfunction during reward anticipation has also been observed during euthymic states, suggesting that disorder in top-down prefrontal regulation of the corticostriatal circuit may be a trait-like feature of BD (**Figure 7.5**).

Posttraumatic stress disorder

posttraumatic stress disorder (PTSD) Complex pattern of dysfunctional responses following exposure to a discrete, identifiable traumatic event or experience involving threat of death or serious bodily harm.

As reviewed in Unit I, a wealth of existing research implicates dysfunction of the corticolimbic circuit, particularly during fear extinction and recall, as contributing to the core symptoms of **posttraumatic stress disorder**, or **PTSD**. Recent research suggests that disorder of the corticostriatal circuit

BD	bipolar disorders	**vlPFC**	ventrolateral prefrontal cortex
VS	ventral striatum	**VTA**	ventral tegmental area

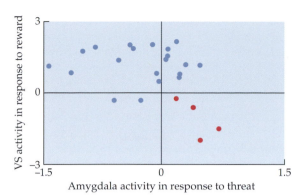

Figure 7.6 Medics in the Israeli Defense Forces who have both relatively high threat-related amygdala activity and low reward-related VS activity (bottom right quadrant) are the most vulnerable for developing PTSD-like symptoms after combat exposure. Note that 0 represents mean activity in these data. (After Admon et al., 2013.)

may exaggerate the effects of this core corticolimbic circuit dysfunction. In another prospective study of Israeli soldiers, investigators again identified relatively increased predeployment threat-related amygdala activity with increased levels of PTSD-like symptoms. However, unlike the earlier work described in Chapter 4, in this study relatively decreased reward-related VS activity postdeployment but not predeployment also predicted increased PTSD-like symptoms. Moreover, the combination of relatively low VS activity and high amygdala activity postdeployment characterized the soldiers at highest risk for developing PTSD-like symptoms (**Figure 7.6**). Thus, decreased reward-related VS activity following exposure to stressors compounds the risk for PTSD associated with increased threat-related amygdala activity. This pattern may reflect an inability to maintain positive affect during stressful times in particularly sensitive individuals. Recent work from my laboratory, described in the Research Spotlight on p. 131, further suggests that complex interactions between threat-related amygdala activity and reward-related VS activity may better explain psychopathology than does dysfunction of either hub alone.

Attention deficit hyperactivity disorder

Attention deficit hyperactivity disorder, or **ADHD**, is the first new form of psychopathology we encounter in our discussion of corticostriatal circuit dysfunction. While there is little evidence for corticolimbic circuit disorder in the emergence of symptoms common to ADHD, there is evidence for additional dysfunction of the corticohippocampal circuit, which we will consider in detail in Unit III.

ADHD is one of the most common behavioral disorders of childhood and may occasionally continue through adolescence and even into adulthood. The core symptoms of ADHD include inattention, impulsivity, and hyperactivity. To be formally diagnosed with the disorder, a child must have these symptoms for 6 months or longer, and to a degree that is greater than other children of the same age. While some children experience only symptoms of inattention or only symptoms of impulsivity and hyperactivity, the majority of children with ADHD experience inattention, hyperactivity, *and* impulsivity. ADHD is more often diagnosed in boys than in girls, although the nature of this sex difference is unclear, and may, in part, represent differing gender norms and expectations as much as biological factors.

Symptoms of inattention in ADHD include being easily distracted; daydreaming; trouble following instructions and missing details; forgetting

attention deficit hyperactivity disorder (ADHD) Characterized by persistent inattention, impulsivity, and/or hyperactivity that exceed what is typical in children of the same age.

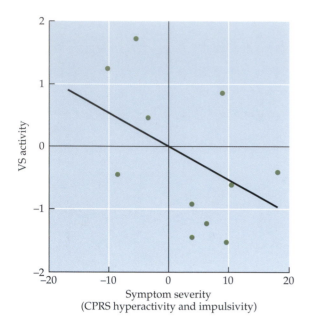

Figure 7.7 VS activity during reward anticipation in ADHD predicts higher levels of hyperactivity and impulsivity (but not inattention) as measured using the Conners' Parent Rating Scale (CPRS). Note that 0 represents mean activity and mean symptom severity in these data. (After Scheres et al., 2007.)

things; and frequently switching from one activity to another. The last symptom is further expressed as difficulty focusing on one thing and becoming bored with a task after only a few minutes. As you can imagine, teachers are often the first to notice these symptoms of inattention, and teacher report can be a key factor in ADHD diagnosis. Not surprisingly, symptoms of inattention in ADHD most clearly reflect disorder in prefrontal regions responsible for attentional focus, planning, and response selection; thus, we will revisit these symptoms in Unit III on the corticohippocampal circuit. For now, we turn to the symptoms of impulsivity and hyperactivity, which reflect disorder in the corticostriatal circuit.

Symptoms of hyperactivity in ADHD generally involve motor behaviors in children, such as fidgeting in their seats in school or at the dinner table, dashing around the schoolyard or house, and otherwise moving nonstop; these children find it very difficult to be still or complete quiet tasks such as reading, working on a puzzle, or drawing. Some symptoms of impulsivity manifest as cognitive forms of hyperactivity. These cognitive symptoms, which broadly represent the inability to regulate behaviors, emerge specifically in children with ADHD as being impatient when required to wait; interrupting the activities of others; expressing inappropriate or rude comments; and acting without regard for consequences. These symptoms of impulsivity are particularly salient in the context of corticostriatal circuit contributions to delayed gratification, reviewed in Chapter 6. Not surprisingly, the ability to delay gratification is significantly lacking in children with ADHD.

Hypoactivity of the VS during the anticipation of monetary reward has been reported in ADHD. In contrast, no difference in VS activity has been observed during reward outcome. Interestingly, the magnitude of VS activity during anticipation of reward is negatively correlated with the symptoms of hyperactivity and impulsivity specifically (**Figure 7.7**). Similar VS hypoactivity has been reported in individuals with ADHD during a delay discounting task where choices were made between smaller immediate amounts of money or larger delayed amounts (**Figure 7.8**). Individuals with ADHD exhibited decreased VS activity during anticipation of immediate or delayed rewards, which is consistent with data from MID tasks. In contrast, the dorsal striatum exhibited hyperactivity during anticipation of delayed rewards. Moreover, the magnitude of DS activity during anticipation of delayed but not immediate rewards was positively correlated with symptoms of hyperactivity and impulsivity specifically.

These patterns suggest that the symptoms of hyperactivity and impulsivity in ADHD may reflect a failure to activate the VS gate in anticipation of rewarding stimuli. This failure subsequently results in deficits in reward learning and generating adaptive goal-directed behaviors. Rather, in ADHD there is the expression of inappropriate behavioral responses that are not

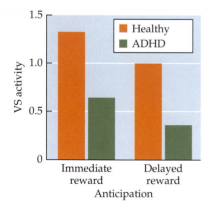

Figure 7.8 There is VS hypoactivity during anticipation of either immediate or delayed rewards in ADHD. Note that 0 represents baseline activity in these data. (After Plitchta et al., 2009.)

ADHD	attention deficit hyperactivity disorder	MID	monetary incentive delay
VS	ventral striatum	DS	dorsal striatum

tuned or sculpted to produce positive rewarding effects. One downstream consequence of this VS gate failure may be the observed hyperactivity of the DS during periods of time when behavioral responses are not appropriate (i.e., when one has to wait for a reward to arrive). As we have seen, the DS provides an interface through which the VS can activate goal-directed behaviors through cortical motor systems. In the absence of appropriate VS activity during the anticipation of reward, particularly when it is delayed, there may be inappropriate or "runaway" activity in the DS, and subsequently, behavioral hyperactivity and impulsivity.

Abnormal DA signaling during reward learning—expressed as the failure to shift activity and subsequent DA release in the VS from the initial experience of an unexpected reward to the cues that predict the reward—has been theorized as a molecular basis of ADHD (**Figure 7.9**). This more pervasive dysfunction in reward learning resulting from abnormal DA signaling may explain why VS hypoactivity predicts impulsivity in ADHD when, more generally, VS hyperactivity predicts impulsivity across the normative range in healthy individuals, as described in Chapter 6. Thus, disorder of the corticostriatal circuit associated with pathological levels of impulsivity and hyperactivity in ADHD may be fundamentally different from aspects of circuit function (e.g., VS hyperactivity) associated with broader variability in reward-related behaviors, including impulsivity.

Ventral Striatum Hyperactivity

In contrast to the relatively decreased VS activity described in the previous sections, relatively increased VS activity in response to typically rewarding stimuli such as food and money is often observed in psychopathology characterized by maladaptive motivations and actions. However, in many cases VS hyperactivity is observed in response to stimuli not generally found to be rewarding or pleasant (e.g., inflicting pain on others or observing images of emaciated bodies). Similarly, the goal-directed behaviors associated with the motivation for these stimuli are counterproductive to general well-being and health.

Antisocial personality disorder

As we saw in Unit I, **antisocial personality disorder (ASPD)** is characterized by a lack of regard for others and inability to follow moral, societal, or legal rules. Individuals with ASPD are generally hypersensitive to threat and exhibit reactive aggression, which is associated with amygdala hyperactivity to threatening stimuli such as angry facial expressions. In extreme cases such as psychopathy, there is also proactive or instrumental aggression, which along with callous and unemotional traits, is associated with amygdala hypoactivity, particularly to signals of distress such as fearful facial expressions.

While these aggression-related symptoms of ASPD are clearly associated with disorder of the corticolimbic circuit, recent research suggests that other

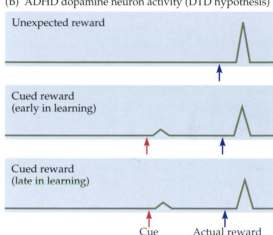

Figure 7.9 (A) Normally, dopamine neuron activity transfers from an unexpected reward to cues that come to predict the reward. (B) The dopamine transfer deficit (DTD) model of ADHD posits that hyperactivity and impulsivity may emerge when there is a failure of dopamine neuron activity to transfer from the actual reward to the cues that predict reward. (After Tripp & Wickens, 2009.)

antisocial personality disorder (ASPD) Characterized by disregard for the needs, safety, and well being of others as well as an inability to follow moral, societal, or legal rules.

core symptoms may be more closely associated with disorder of the cortico-striatal circuit. Specifically, corticostriatal circuit dysfunction appears to be linked with committing delinquent and antisocial acts typical in ASPD, such as assault, larceny, arson, and destruction of property.

In a seminal study published in 2010, Josh Buckholtz, then working in the laboratory of David Zald at Vanderbilt University, used a combination of fMRI and PET to implicate corticostriatal circuit dysfunction in the emergence of impulsive antisocial traits (**Figure 7.10**). Buckholtz and his colleagues found that DA release in the VS, measured with PET, predicted increased VS activity to monetary reward, measured with fMRI. This general relationship is consistent with basic corticostriatal circuit anatomy and function and thus is expected. However, Buckholtz and colleagues were able to demonstrate that both the magnitude of DA release and the activity of the VS predicted antisocial traits, specifically those related to committing impulsive and delinquent acts such as assault and larceny. Subsequent work has confirmed the positive association between reward-related VS activity and the expression of antisocial traits generally; however, the extension of these patterns to clinical populations with ASPD remains unclear as of now, although a recent study did report that VS activity to monetary reward predicted the severity of antisocial traits in a small sample of incarcerated men.

Other studies in individuals with ASPD have reported decreased activity of prefrontal regions during reward processing but no differences in VS activity. Regardless, the general pattern emerging from these studies, especially those examining dimensional traits related to antisocial behavior, is one wherein there is hyperactivity of the VS gate and DA key. Such "unlocking" of the corticostriatal circuit may be further exacerbated by decreased activity of prefrontal regions necessary for behavioral regulation. These patterns, unlike those found in ADHD, are consistent with the generally positive correlation between VS activity and impulsivity found in healthy individuals, suggesting that antisocial traits, particularly those that are impulsive in nature, may represent a more general lack of behavioral control. The additional deficits in corticolimbic circuit function (especially prefontal hypoactivity) observed

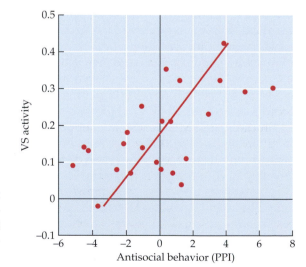

Figure 7.10 Impulsive antisocial behavior, particularly committing delinquent acts, as measured by the Psychopathic Personality Inventory (PPI) is positively correlated with VS activity during the anticipation of monetary reward. Note that 0 represents mean activity and mean antisocial behavior in these data. (After Buckholtz et al., 2010.)

ASPD	antisocial personality disorder
DA	dopamine
VS	ventral striatum
ADHD	attention deficit hyperactivity disorder

in ASPD may help explain the expression of this more general impulsivity as antisocial acts, specifically in these individuals.

It will be interesting to examine whether the observed hyperactivity of the VS gate and DA key, as well as hypoactivity of the prefrontal cortex to generally rewarding stimuli (e.g., money), also occur in response to antisocial or delinquent stimuli/scenarios specifically (e.g., hurting someone for personal gain). Such work will help us better understand whether antisocial behaviors are part of a broader pattern of general impulsivity or a unique expression of maladaptive response to activities and stimuli that most of us do not find pleasant or rewarding.

Eating disorders

Eating disorders (ED), which are most common among girls and women, are characterized by severe disturbances in eating behavior, spanning both under- and overeating, as well as significant distress and concern about body weight or image. There is high comorbidity between ED and other psychopathology, particularly mood and anxiety disorders. In Western industrialized nations, ED are accompanied by the highest rates of physical morbidity and mortality among all psychopathology. These devastating consequences largely reflect the distress and dysfunction that emerge in multiple organ systems (cardiovascular, endocrine, reproductive, and gastrointestinal) as individuals with ED become increasingly malnourished.

Two common forms of ED studied using neuroimaging are **anorexia nervosa (AN)** and **bulimia nervosa (BN)**. They key features of AN are distorted body image and excessive dieting that leads to severe weight loss, with a pathological fear of becoming fat. To induce weight loss and/or limit weight gain, individuals with AN typically engage in restricting their caloric intake or purging immediately after eating. Individuals with BN, like those with AN, also have a severe fear of gaining weight. However, individuals with BN maintain a normal weight through cycles of binge eating followed by purging, fasting, or excessive exercise.

Despite diagnosis-specific features, AN and BN are both characterized by striking abnormalities in motivation (e.g., striving for lower weight) and goal-directed behaviors (e.g., purging, restriction, binging), which have been mapped onto disorder of the corticostriatal circuit. Neuroimaging studies of AN have typically focused on "recovered" individuals who have normal weight and no current signs of disorder. While this strategy is adopted to avoid confounding the studies by symptoms of medical illness (e.g., disrupted glucose metabolism and blood flow) that might affect the BOLD signal, it also works to reveal patterns of dysfunction that may represent preexisting traits that increase risk for ED rather than neural consequences of the disease process.

Studies using MID tasks have reported a failure of individuals with AN to differentiate between losing and winning. Specifically, while VS activity increases in response to winning and decreases in response to losing in healthy women, there is consistently high VS activity to both winning and losing in women with AN. A similar lack of differential VS activity to winning and losing money has been reported in women who have recovered from BN. These findings suggest that a general inability to learn the value of relative gains and losses through differential VS gate activity may represent a trait-like risk factor in both AN and BN. A failure to shape goal-directed behaviors through

eating disorders (ED) Characterized by severe disturbances in eating behavior, spanning both under- and overeating, as well as significant distress and concern about body weight or image.

anorexia nervosa (AN) Eating disorder characterized by distorted body image and excessive dieting that leads to severe weight loss, with a pathological fear of becoming fat.

bulimia nervosa (BN) Eating disorder characterized by severe fear of gaining weight, but maintenance of normal weight through cycles of binge eating followed by purging, fasting, or excessive exercise.

ED eating disorders
AN anorexia nervosa
BN bulimia nervosa
MID monetary incentive delay

differential VS gate function may manifest as the maladaptive patterns of dysregulated eating and distorted body image in ED broadly.

Recent studies have moved beyond general reward-related circuit disorder to focus on corticostriatal contributions to specific symptoms of ED, most notably distorted body image in AN. In one fMRI study, women with acute AN were asked to view computer-generated pictures of nude women varying from severely underweight to overweight (**Figure 7.11A**). The women were asked to make two different appraisals. First, how would you feel if you had this body weight? Second, estimate the weight of the person. Consistent with the severe fear of weight gain, women with AN felt worst not only when imagining themselves with the overweight bodies, but also the normal weight bodies (**Figure 7.11B**). Their distorted body images were evident in their ratings of feeling best when imagining themselves with the underweight bodies. Healthy women, in contrast, felt best when imagining themselves with the

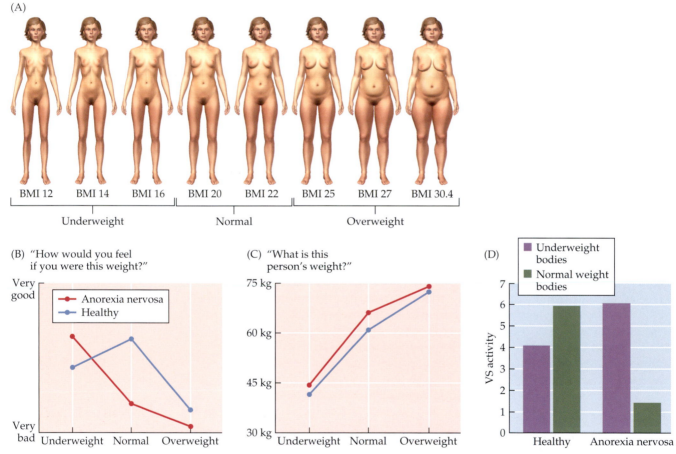

Figure 7.11 (A) Examples of visual stimuli depicting a female body with underweight, normal weight, and overweight features according to standardized body mass index (BMI). (B) Women with AN strongly preferred the underweight bodies, while healthy women strongly preferred the normal weight bodies. Both healthy women and women with AN "disliked" the overweight bodies. (C) Women with AN were just as accurate as healthy women in estimating body weight. (D) Women with AN exhibited significantly greater VS activity to underweight bodies than to normal weight bodies, while healthy women exhibited the opposite pattern. Note that 0 represents baseline activity in these data. (After Fladung et al., 2010.)

AN	anorexia nervosa	BMI	body mass index
BN	bulimia nervosa	ED	eating disorders
VS	ventral striatum		

normal weight bodies and worse with either the overweight or underweight bodies.

Interestingly, women with AN were as accurate as healthy women in estimating the weight of each body (**Figure 7.11C**). This suggests that the preference for thinner bodies and aversion to normal or heavier bodies is not simply a reflection of abnormal perception in AN, but rather abnormal motivation. Remarkably, differences in VS activity to the body images mapped onto these differences in subjective preference or motivation. Specifically, women with AN exhibited higher VS activity in response to the underweight bodies in comparison to normal weight bodies (**Figure 7.11D**). Healthy women showed the opposite pattern of VS activity, and neither group showed significant VS activity to the overweight bodies. These data suggest that abnormal VS

RESEARCH SPOTLIGHT

While not an officially recognized form of psychopathology, obesity is a significant health problem with emerging links to disordered neural circuit function. Obesity is generally defined by a body mass index (BMI) in excess of 30, with normal BMI ranging from 18 to 25. Emerging studies of obese individuals have revealed an interesting pattern of corticostriatal circuit dysfunction in response to highly palatable, calorie-enriched foods like milkshakes, cheeseburgers, and cakes.

Specifically, VS activity when consuming such foods is negatively correlated with obesity (**Figure 7.12A**). That is, as VS activity during the consumption of calorie-rich foods increases, obesity decreases. Thus, opening of the VS gate in response to primary reinforcers may protect against becoming obese by readily registering reward and pleasure during eating. In contrast, VS activity during the anticipation of these foods is positively correlated with subsequent weight gain, specifically BMI, extending into the range of obesity (**Figure 7.12B**). Taken together, these findings suggest that increased VS activity during the anticipation of highly palatable foods and decreased VS activity during consumption of these foods is associated with weight gain and obesity. In other words, having a corticostriatal circuit that is driven to seek calorie-rich foods (high VS activity during anticipation) but that does not recognize their arrival (low VS activity during consumption) sets the stage for overeating and subsequent weight gain.

Consistent with these observations, another study using a classical conditioning paradigm reported significantly decreased VS activity to visual cues predicting delivery of sugar water in obese individuals, indicative of deficient reward learning. In contrast, individuals with AN exhibited significantly increased VS activity to the visual cues, suggesting hypersensitive reward learning, which could contribute to or allow for the restricted eating in this condition (i.e., getting a larger reward signal than healthy individuals for the same amount of food).

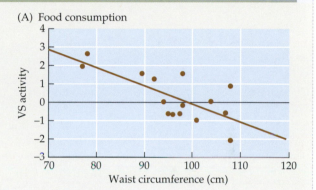

(A) Food consumption

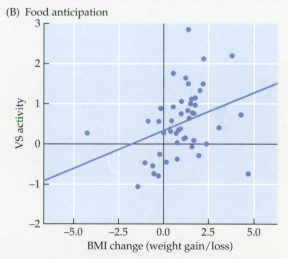

(B) Food anticipation

Figure 7.12 (A) Higher waist circumference is negatively correlated with VS activity during the consumption of sugar- and fat-rich foods (e.g., milkshake). (B) In contrast, VS activity during anticipation of sugar- and fat-rich foods (i.e., viewing food images) is positively correlated with subsequent weight gain as indexed by BMI. Note that 0 represents mean activity and mean change in BMI in these data. (A after Green et al., 2011; B after Demos et al., 2012.)

activity in response to pictures of underweight bodies may reflect abnormal reward-learning in AN, thereby generating motivation to be underweight as well as driving maladaptive goal-directed behaviors to satisfy this motivation (e.g., restriction, purging).

Substance use disorder

Substance use disorder (SUD), more commonly referred to as **addiction**, is characterized by persistent patterns of substance use leading to significant impairment and distress. While historically the **substance** in SUD referred specifically to drugs (e.g., alcohol, tobacco, cocaine, cannabis), the word now also encompasses the nondrug end points of pathological gambling, Internet use, and online or electronic gaming. For convenience and clarity, in considering corticostriatal circuit disorder in SUD we will consistently use the term *drug* to refer broadly to all substances, drug and nondrug. This terminology usefully captures and conveys the severity and maladaptive nature of gambling, Internet use, and gaming in their disordered forms. For individuals suffering from these forms of SUD, gambling, Internet use, and gaming become, in effect, drugs. In many ways, SUD best captures the expression of corticostriatal circuit disorder through its core features of pathological motivation (drug craving) and maladaptive goal-directed behavior (drug seeking).

Nora Volkow and colleagues have developed one prominent model of drug addiction, components of which map consistently onto corticostriatal circuit disorder (**Figure 7.13**). Their model emphasizes a cycle of impaired reward learning and loss of behavioral control. Necessarily, the cycle begins with use or exposure leading to intoxication. Initial exposure leads to episodes of bingeing, with escalation in the quantity consumed or compulsive use of the drug for longer periods than intended. Bingeing and compulsive use are indicative of reduced behavioral control. Periods between heavy or repeated drug use are characterized by withdrawal and craving. During withdrawal, addicted individuals typically lack motivation, experience anhedonia and negative emotion such as irritability and depression, and become more sensitive to stress. Eventually, addicted individuals develop a drug craving leading to drug-seeking behavior designed to satisfy the craving. Importantly, drug craving can be either explicit (i.e., conscious desire for the drug) or implicit (i.e., unconscious expression of conditioned responses to drug cues). When obtaining and consuming the drug satisfies the craving, (i.e., leads to intoxication), the cycle begins again.

substance use disorder (SUD; addiction) Characterized by persistent patterns of maladaptive substance use leading to significant impairment and distress.

substance As used in substance use disorder, refers to any rewarding stimulus or activity resulting in dysfunction of the corticostriatal circuit and the development of pathological motivation and action.

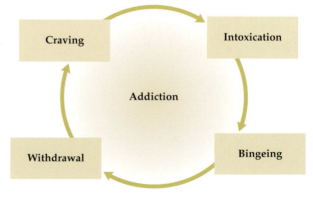

Figure 7.13 One model of addiction depicts a cycle of clinical symptoms including intoxication, bingeing, withdrawal, and craving. Corticostriatal circuit disorder is associated with drug craving and, subsequently, drug-seeking behavior as well as intoxication and bingeing. (After Goldstein & Volkow, 2011.)

VS   ventral striatum
AN   anorexia nervosa
SUD   substance use disorder

Of these four model components, corticostriatal circuit disorder is most clearly linked with drug craving and, subsequently, drug-seeking behavior. In addition, individual differences in corticostriatal circuit function, particularly VS gate and DA key activity, contribute to the experience of intoxication and the likelihood of escalation to bingeing and compulsive use. The associated lack of behavioral control, in contrast, largely reflects disorder in top-down prefrontal circuits and will be considered in Unit III on the corticohippocampal circuit.

A large number of studies have identified the response of the corticostriatal circuit to the administration of drugs. We briefly considered these studies in Chapter 6 while examining the role of the corticostriatal circuit, particularly the VS gate and DA key, in responding to primary reinforcers. Studies of corticostriatal circuit disorder in addiction have employed intravenous, oral, and respiratory modes of administering drugs ranging from cocaine to alcohol to nicotine. Regardless of the administration technique employed, these studies collectively reveal strong activity of both the VS gate and DA key during drug consumption (**Figure 7.14**). This pattern is consistent with activation of corticostriatal circuit nodes by primary reinforcers generally, as well as DA release caused by drugs specifically. Addiction develops, in part, because drugs can open the VS gate through direct release of the DA key. The magnitude of this activity further predicts the subjective experience of

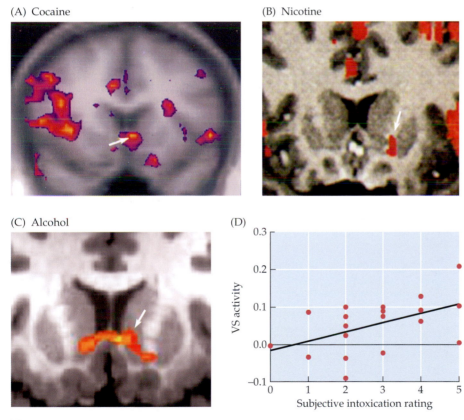

(A) Cocaine

(B) Nicotine

(C) Alcohol

(D)

Figure 7.14 Administration of cocaine (A), nicotine (B), and alcohol (C) all produce activity in the VS. (D) The magnitude of VS activity following drug administration typically predicts the subjective experience of intoxication, as represented by these data from an alcohol study. Note that 0 represents mean activity in these data. (A from Breiter et al., 1997; B from Stein et al., 1998; C,D from Gilman et al., 2012.)

intoxication or the drug "high," which likely reflects direct drug activation of "hedonic hot spots" in both the ventral striatum and ventral pallidum (see the Research Spotlight on p. 99).

The drug-induced activation of the VS gate and DA key, as well as hedonic hot spots, further functions to reinforce the behaviors that precede drug consumption. Because the magnitude of this direct activation by drugs may be larger for some individuals than that produced by other primary reinforcers such as food and sex, there is often very rapid reinforcement of associated behaviors. Some refer to this process as "hijacking" of an otherwise adaptive corticostriatal circuit for reward learning by drugs, resulting in reinforcement of maladaptive patterns of goal-directed behaviors, which emerge as the idiosyncratic habits or rituals of addicts in search of the next fix. While all individuals are vulnerable to these addictive properties of drugs, some are more vulnerable than others. Individual differences in the magnitude of drug-induced activation of the VS gate and DA key are important factors in the emergence of this vulnerability. However, other factors, both neural and environmental, are also important, as discussed in the Research Spotlight on p. 144.

The contribution of corticostriatal circuit disorder to addiction, of course, extends beyond this "hijacking" by drugs that act as primary reinforcers. Specifically, corticostriatal circuit involvement extends to the development of maladaptive conditioned responses to drug-related cues. This is consistent with the function of the circuit in mediating reward-related learning through the association of primary and secondary reinforcers as reviewed in Chapter 6. For example, studies exposing addicted individuals to conditioned stimuli, including images of glass paraphernalia used for smoking cannabis or even the taste of beer in the absence of actual alcohol, elicit strong activity of the VS gate and DA key. Even the smell of alcohol, specifically beer, in the absence of a drink elicits strong activity in the VS gate (**Figure 7.15**). The relative increase in VS activity in addicts occurs not only in response to cues associated with

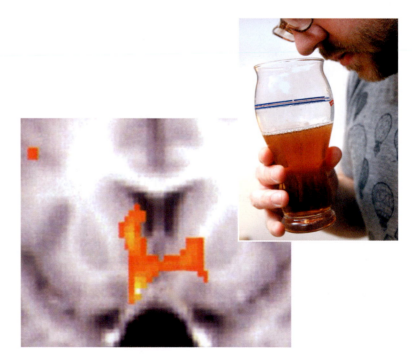

Figure 7.15 The aroma of beer functions as a secondary reinforcer for the primary reinforcer alcohol; even this aroma alone elicits activity in the VS. (fMRI from Kareken et al., 2004; photo © Tom Wallace/Corbis.)

| VS | ventral striatum |
| DA | dopamine |

(A)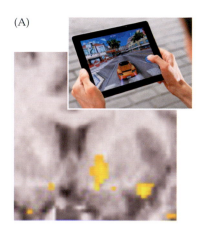

(B)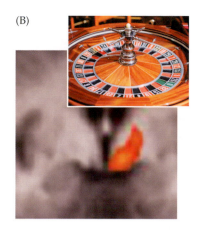

Figure 7.16 Visual cues related to gaming (A) or gambling (B) elicit VS activity in individuals who have developed pathological patterns of use that impairs daily functioning. (A, fMRI from Ko et al., 2009, photo © Bloomua/Shutterstock; B, fMRI from Frosini et al., 2010, photo © Zveaghintev/Shutterstock.)

traditional drugs of abuse but also in response to cues related to Internet use and online gaming as well as pathological gambling (**Figure 7.16**).

In effect, both classical conditioning and operant conditioning, in which DA release and subsequent opening of the VS gate are shifted from the drug to cues predicting the drug, are intimately involved in the development of addiction. The magnitude of cue-induced activity, particularly in the VS gate, predicts the severity of craving in addicts. Moreover, individuals at increased risk for addiction typically show exaggerated VS gate and DA key activity to conditioned drug stimuli in comparison to those at decreased risk.

Corticostriatal circuit disorder also contributes to the development of drug tolerance and the emergence of drug withdrawal in addicts. Both of these processes reflect alterations in the functioning of the DA key in the VS gate. Drug tolerance represents the need for increasing quantities and/or concentrations of a drug over repeated use to achieve the same level of "high" or intoxication. Studies using PET to directly measure DA signaling in the VS of addicts suggest that tolerance reflects the downregulation or decreased signaling of DA in the striatum (**Figure 7.17**). This downregulation is, in fact, a natural homeostatic response to the repeated drug-induced triggering of DA release. The DA system attempts to reestablish balance in signaling by decreasing the numbers of receptors through which DA modulates activity of the striatum, particularly in the VS. After all, the system is flooded with DA following drug consumption, so why maintain more receptors than necessary? However, this creates a DA system that becomes less sensitive to the original doses (and effects) of the drug because there are now fewer dopamine receptors to act on. Hence, a tolerance develops for prior dose levels, and the addicted individual

(A) Healthy Addicted

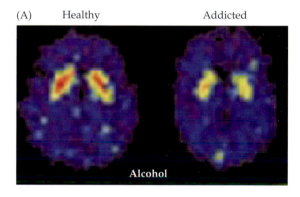

(B)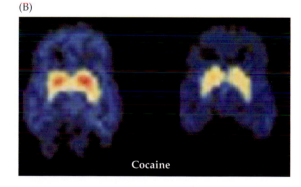

(C)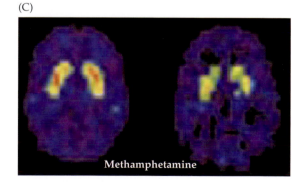

Figure 7.17 Prolonged use of drugs such as alcohol (A), cocaine (B), and methamphetamine (C) is associated with diminished DA function in the striatum related to the emergence of drug withdrawal and drug tolerance. (From Goldstein & Volkow, 2002.)

RESEARCH SPOTLIGHT

Understanding why some individuals are more likely than others to develop addiction is a major thrust of ongoing research. Relative risk can emerge at different stages of the addiction cycle (e.g., there can be risk of transition from regular use to bingeing, or risk of increased tolerance). However, identifying factors that predict individual tendencies to begin substance use may be most important, because prevention is better than treatment.

A common approach to understanding vulnerability is to compare individuals with and without a family history of addiction. A wealth of epidemiologic data indicates that a positive family history significantly increases the odds of individual risk. It remains unclear, however, how this risk manifests at the level of neural circuit function. Available studies suggest that individuals at high risk for addiction may exhibit relatively increased VS gate and DA key activity to drugs.

Interestingly, studies of high-risk individuals reveal differences not only in the activity of the corticostriatal circuit to reward, but also that of the amygdala and corticolimbic circuit to threat. Some data suggest that high-risk individuals (i.e., those with a positive family history of addiction) have relatively blunted amygdala activity to threat. This has been interpreted as a possible deficit in recognizing the harmful consequences of persistent drinking. Work from my lab has explored the interactions of reward-related VS activity and threat-related amygdala activity in the emergence of problem drinking in response to stress in college students. We found that stress-related problem drinking is particularly pronounced in individuals with relatively high reward-related VS activity and relatively low threat-related amygdala activity (**Figure 7.18**). This pattern may reflect an increased drive to pursue rewards (high VS activity) to offset stressful experiences, *coupled with* a reduced ability to detect the potentially harmful consequences of drinking (low amygdala activity). In an expanded sample of the same study, we found that stress is also associated with problem drinking in those with relatively low VS activity and high amygdala activity. Stress does not, however, correlate with problem drinking in individuals whose VS and amygdala function are in a state of equilibrium (i.e., both low or both high).

Collectively, our findings support the existence of two distinct neural profiles associated with stress-related problem drinking: one associated with an increased drive to pursue rewards and reduced threat sensitivity, possibly reflecting drinking for stimulation and positive emotion enhancement (i.e., drinking for enjoyment); and another associated with decreased reward drive and increased sensitivity to threat, possibly reflecting drinking to reduce negative emotion (i.e., drinking to cope). Our findings also suggest the existence of two distinct protective patterns of neural functioning: one where threat and reward responsiveness are both high, and another where they are both low. The notion that a functional balance between these circuit hubs is critical for adaptive response to stress is further supported by observations that relatively heightened functional connectivity between the BLA and VS is associated with *reduced* stress-related problem drinking.

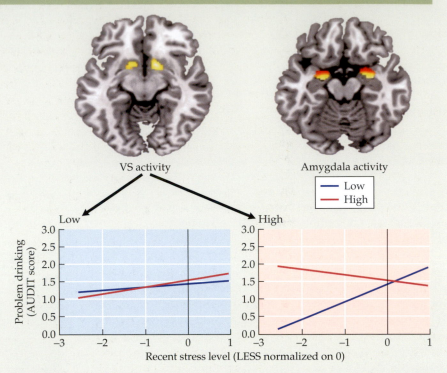

Figure 7.18 Problem drinking as measured by the Alcohol Use Disorder Identification Test (AUDIT) is reported by college students in relation to the subjective experience of stress in the past year as measured by the LESS only when they have a combination of relatively high reward-related VS activity and relatively low threat-related amygdala reactivity. (After Nikolova & Hariri, 2012.)

DA dopamine
VS ventral striatum
BLA basolateral complex of the amygdala

seeks greater quantities or concentrations of the drug to elicit the release of the DA key and activate the VS gate as well as the hedonic hot spots in the VS and ventral pallidum. Tolerance can become more pronounced with chronic drug use and may eventually lead to a state where an addicted individual cannot experience a drug high or consumes levels of a drug that are lethal.

Altered DA signaling and the resulting dysregulation of the corticostriatal circuit following chronic or heavy drug use also contributes to the phenomenon of withdrawal, a period without or with insufficient (following tolerance) drug consumption during which the addicted individual may experience mood disturbances, especially anhedonia. The downregulation of DA signaling in the striatum following heavy or chronic drug use results in decreased sensitivity of the VS gate and hedonic hot spots to otherwise rewarding stimuli (e.g., food, sex) and interactions (e.g., talking with friends). In turn, an addicted individual is unable to experience positive emotion in response to normal daily activities and experiences, leading to anhedonia. Furthermore, decreased VS gate activity leads to a weakening of reward learning and a decline in goal-directed behaviors, which further contribute to disturbances in mood.

Decreased DA signaling in the striatum further contributes to withdrawal by indirectly impairing the function of prefrontal regions supporting emotion regulation. This prefrontal dysfunction, which will be considered in more detail in Unit III on the corticohippocampal circuit, leads to irritability and increased sensitivity to stress. Unfortunately, the symptoms of withdrawal are typically only relieved through drug consumption, the quantity of which must increase due to tolerance, thereby triggering release of striatal DA large enough to open the VS gate to restore goal-directed behaviors and the experience of pleasure. Although DA signaling and corticostriatal circuit functioning can recover following extended periods of drug abstinence, the available data suggest that this recovery may never be complete (i.e., return to levels of functioning in healthy, never-addicted individuals). This persistent corticostriatal circuit disorder is one reason recovered addicts are vulnerable to relapse.

Summary

Disorder of the corticostriatal circuit typically emerges as abnormal motivation and maladaptive actions in pursuit of a goal. Relative ventral striatum hyperactivity to both primary and secondary reinforcers is typically associated with lack of behavioral control and poor decision making, particularly with regard to appetitive or rewarding stimuli. Hyperactivity in the VS may also occur in response to otherwise unrewarding stimuli (e.g., extremely low body weight in eating disorders), and such maladaptive opening of the VS gate may be related to abnormal signaling of the dopamine key. Hyperactivity of both the DA key and VS gate also contribute to impulsive antisocial or delinquent behaviors reflecting a failure to consider the consequences of one's actions, as often seen in antisocial personality disorder. Relative hypoactivity of the VS gate, while less common, is also observed in some psychopathology. For example, VS hypoactivity to rewarding stimuli is associated with the core symptom of anhedonia in major depressive disorder. In attention deficit hyperactivity disorder, VS hypoactivity associated with behavioral impulsivity and hyperactivity may reflect broader deficits in the normal shift in dopamine signaling from primary to secondary reinforcers during reward learning. VS hypoactivity to otherwise rewarding stimuli can also emerge as a consequence of psychopathology, particularly addiction, through disruption of DA signaling. Finally, VS gate dysfunction can further manifest as indiscriminate responses to rewarding and nonrewarding outcomes as well as a failure in reward learning, as has been observed in bipolar disorders.

Literature Cited & Further Reading

Abler, B., Greenhouse, I., Ongur, D., Walter, H., & Heckers, S. (2008). Abnormal reward system activation in mania. *Neuropsychopharmacology*, 33: 2217–2227.

Admon, R., Lubin, G., Rosenblatt, J. D., Stern, O., Kahn, I., Assaf, M., & Hendler, T. (2013). Imbalanced neural responsivity to risk and reward indicates stress vulnerability in humans. *Cerebral Cortex*, 23: 28–35.

Bermpohl, F., and 12 others. (2010). Altered representation of expected value in the orbitofrontal cortex in mania. *Human Brain Mapping*, 31: 958–969.

Bjork, J. M., Chen, G., & Hommer, D. W. (2012). Psychopathic tendencies and mesolimbic recruitment by cues for instrumental and passively obtained rewards. *Biological Psychology*, 89: 408–415.

Breiter, H. C., & 12 others (1997). Acute effects of cocaine on human brain activity and emotion. *Neuron*, 19: 591–611.

Buckholtz, J. W., & 13 others. (2010). Mesolimbic dopamine reward system hypersensitivity in individuals with psychopathic traits. *Nature Neuroscience*, 13: 419–421.

Carré, J. M., Hyde, L. W., Neumann, C. S., Viding, E., & Hariri, A. R. (2012). The neural signatures of distinct psychopathic traits. *Social Neuroscience*, 8: 122–135.

Crowley, T. J., Dalwani, M. S., Mikulich-Gilbertson, S. K., Du, Y. P., Lejuez, C. W., Raymond, K. M., & Banich, M. T. (2010). Risky decisions and their consequences: Neural processing by boys with antisocial substance disorder. *PLoS One*, 2010 Sep 22; 5(9):e12835.

Demos, K. E., Heatherton, T. F., & Kelley, W. M. (2012). Individual differences in nucleus accumbens activity to food and sexual images predict weight gain and sexual behavior. *Journal of Neuroscience*, 32: 5549–5552.

Epstein, J., & 9 others. (2006). Lack of ventral striatal response to positive stimuli in depressed versus normal subjects. *American Journal of Psychiatry*, 163: 1784–1790.

Filbey, F. M., Schacht, J. P., Myers, U. S., Chavez, R. S., & Hutchison, K. E. (2009). Marijuana craving in the brain. *Proceedings of the National Academy of Sciences USA*, 106: 13016–13021.

Fladung, A. K., & 8 others. (2010). A neural signature of anorexia nervosa in the ventral striatal reward system. *American Journal of Psychiatry*, 167: 206–212.

Frank, G. K. W., Reynolds, J. R., Shott, M. E., Jappe, L., Yang, T. T., Tregallas, J. R., & O'Reilly, R. C. (2012). Anorexia nervosa and obesity are associated with opposite brain reward response. *Neuropsychopharmacology*, 37: 2031–2046.

Frosini, D., & 8 others. (2010). Parkinson's disease and pathological gambling: Results from a functional MRI study. *Movement Disorders*, 25: 2449–2453.

Gilman, J. M., Ramchandani, V. A., Crouss, T., & Hommer, D. W. (2012). Subjective and neural responses to intravenous alcohol in young adults with light and heavy drinking patterns. *Neuropsychopharmacology* 37: 467–477.

Glahn, D. C., Lovallo, W. R., & Fox, P. T. (2007). Reduced amygdala activation in young adults at high risk of alcoholism: Studies from the Oklahoma Family Health Patterns Project. *Biological Psychiatry*, 61: 1306–1309.

Goldstein, R. Z., & Volkow, N. D. (2002). Drug addiction and its underlying neurobiological basis: Neuroimaging evidence for the involvement of the frontal cortex. *American Journal of Psychiatry*, 159: 1642–1652.

Goldstein R. Z., & Volkow N. D. (2011). Dysfunction of the prefrontal cortex in addiction. *Nature Reviews Neuroscience*, 12: 652–667.

Green, E., Jacobson, A., Haase, L., & Murphy, C. (2011). Reduced nucleus accumbens and caudate nucleus activation to a pleasant taste is associated with obesity in older adults. *Brain Research*, 1386: 109–117.

Kareken, D. A., & 10 others. (2004). Alcohol-related olfactory cues activate the nucleus accumbens and ventral tegmental area in high-risk drinkers: Preliminary findings. *Alcoholism: Clinical and Experimental Research*, 28: 550–557.

Knutson, B., Bhanji, J. P., Cooney, R. E., Atlas, L. Y., & Gotlib, I. H. (2008). Neural responses to monetary incentives in major depression. *Biological Psychiatry*, 63: 686–692.

Ko, C.-H., Liu, G.-C., Hsiao, S., Yen, J.-Y., Yang, M.-J., Lin, W.-C., Yen, C.-F., & Chen, C.-S. (2009). Brain activities associated with gaming urge of online gaming addiction. *Journal of Psychiatric Research*, 43: 739–747.

Nikolova, Y. S., & Hariri, A. R. (2012). Neural responses to threat and reward interact to predict stress-related problem drinking: A novel protective role of the amygdala. *Biology of Mood &Anxiety Disorders*, 2: 19.

Nikolova, Y. S., Bogdan, R., Brigidi, B. D., & Hariri, A. R. (2012). Ventral striatum reactivity to reward and recent life stress interact to predict positive affect. *Biological Psychiatry*, 72: 157–163.

Nusslock, R., Almeida, J. R. C., Forbes, E. E., Versace, A., Frank, E., LaBarbara, E. J., Klein, C. R., & Phillips, M. L. (2012). Waiting to win: Elevated striatal and orbitofrontal cortical activity during reward anticipation in euthymic bipolar disorder adults. *Bipolar Disorders*, 14: 249–260.

Oberlin, B. G., Dzemidzic, M., Tran, S. M., Soeurt, C. M., Albrecht, D. S., Yoder, K. K., & Kareken, D. A. (2013). Beer flavor provokes striatal dopamine release in male drinkers: Mediation by family history of alcoholism. *Neuropsychopharmacology*, 38: 1617–1624.

Pizzagalli, D. A., & 9 others. (2009). Reduced caudate and nucleus accumbens response to rewards in unmedicated individuals with major depressive disorder. *American Journal of Psychiatry*, 166: 702–710.

Plichta, M. M., Vasic, N., Wolf, R. C., Lesch, K.-P., Brummer, D., Jacob, C., Fallgatter, A. J., & Grön, G. (2009). Neural hyporesponsiveness and hyperresponsiveness during immediate and delayed reward processing in adult attention-deficit/hyperactivity disorder. *Biological Psychiatry*, 65: 7–14.

Pujara, M., Motzkin, J. C., Newman, J. P., Kiehl, K. A., & Koenigs, M. (2013). Neural correlates of reward and loss sensitivity in psychopathy. *Social Cognitive & Affective Neuroscience*, 9: 794–801.

Scheres, A., Milham, M. P., Knutson, B., & Castellanos, F. X. (2007).Ventral striatal hyporesponsiveness during reward anticipation in attention deficit/hyperactivity disorder. *Biological Psychiatry*, 61: 720–724.

Schlaepfer, T. E., & 9 others. (2008). Deep brain stimulation to reward circuitry alleviates anhedonia in refractory major depression. *Neuropsychopharmacology*, 33: 368–377.

Steele, J. D., Kumar, P., & Ebmeier, K. P. (2007). Blunted response to feedback information in depressive illness. *Brain*, 130: 2367–2369.

Stein, E. A., & 9 others. (1998). Nicotine-induced limbic cortical activation in the human brain: A functional MRI study. *American Journal of Psychiatry*, 155: 1009–1015.

Stoy, M., & 13 others. (2011). Hyporeactivity of ventral striatum towards incentive stimuli in unmedicated depressed patients normalizes after treatment with escitalopram. *Journal of Psychopharmacology*, 26: 677–688.

Tripp, G., & Wickens, J. R. (2009). Neurobiology of ADHD. *Neuropharmacology*, 57: 579–589.

Völlm, B., & 8 others. (2010). Neuronal correlates and serotonergic modulation of behavioural inhibition and reward in healthy and antisocial individuals. *Journal of Psychiatric Research*, 44: 123–131.

Wagner, A., & 10 others. (2010). Altered striatal response to reward in bulimia nervosa after recovery. *International Journal of Eating Disorders*, 43: 289–294.

Wagner, A., & 12 others. (2007). Altered reward processing in women recovered from anorexia nervosa. *American Journal of Psychiatry*, 164: 1842–1849.

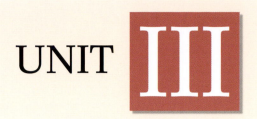

UNIT **III**

The Corticohippocampal Circuit for Memory and Executive Control

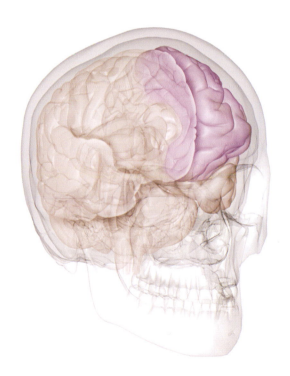

8

The Corticohippocampal Circuit
Anatomy

Our last unit focuses on the corticohippocampal circuit. Unlike the circuits described in Units I and II, each of which supports distinct yet equally critical life-sustaining behaviors, this final circuit is best characterized by its more general regulation and nuanced control of these and all other behaviors through *memory* and *executive control*.

The corticohippocampal circuit (**Figure 8.1**) is comprised of the following interconnected structures:

1. Dorsolateral prefrontal cortex
2. Hippocampal formation
3. Sensory association areas
4. Midbrain

The dorsolateral prefrontal cortex (dlPFC) is the hub of the corticohippocampal circuit. As the hub, the dlPFC not only organizes the flow of information through the other corticohippocampal circuit nodes but also regulates the activity and output of both the corticolimbic and corticostriatal circuits.

In Chapter 9 we will consider how information processing within the corticohippocampal circuit supports memory and executive control in the context of regulating our behavior. In Chapter 10, we conclude by reviewing how disorder within the corticohippocampal circuit manifests as specific symptoms of psychopathology, including memory loss in amnesic syndromes, and disordered thinking and lack of control in schizophrenia and obsessive-compulsive disorder. For now, we turn to the general anatomy and basic connections of key corticohippocampal circuit nodes.

The Dorsolateral Prefrontal Cortex

In contrast to the clearly defined structural shape and anatomical divisions of the amygdala and ventral striatum hubs of the corticolimbic and corticostriatal circuits, respectively, there is little that distinguishes the dlPFC hub of the corticohippocampal circuit at the level of gross anatomy. Broadly, *prefrontal cortex* refers to cortical regions of the frontal lobe that are anterior to the motor and premotor cortices (**Figure 8.2**). In addition to the dlPFC circuit hub, subdivisions of the PFC have been established based on their relative locations. They include the ventromedial PFC (vmPFC), dorsomedial PFC (dmPFC),

Figure 8.1 The four key nodes of the corticohippocampal circuit and their basic connections. The dorsolateral prefrontal cortex is the central hub of the circuit through which activity and information processing in the other nodes is orchestrated. Notice that, in contrast to the corticolimbic and corticostriatal circuits (see Figures 2.1 and 5.1), all pathways of the corticohippocampal circuit are bidirectional, reflecting the continuous flow of information necessary for maintaining the core circuit functions of memory and executive control.

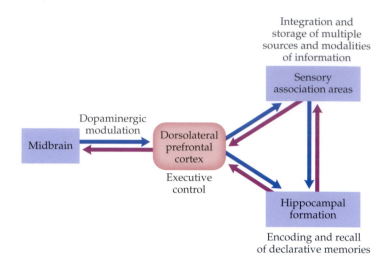

and ventrolateral PFC (vlPFC). The ventral surfaces of the vmPFC and vlPFC may also be referred to as the orbitofrontal cortex in recognition of their location above the ocular orbits of the skull. We have already considered the importance of the vmPFC, dmPFC, and vlPFC within the corticolimbic circuit and have described the contribution of the dlPFC within the corticostriatal

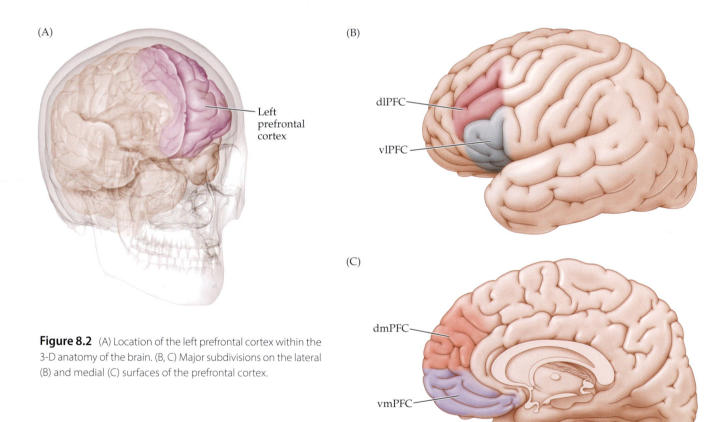

Figure 8.2 (A) Location of the left prefrontal cortex within the 3-D anatomy of the brain. (B, C) Major subdivisions on the lateral (B) and medial (C) surfaces of the prefrontal cortex.

vlPFC	ventrolateral prefrontal cortex	**vmPFC**	ventromedial prefrontal cortex
dlPFC	dorsolateral prefrontal cortex	**dmPFC**	dorsomedial prefrontal cortex

circuit. In this chapter we will focus on which unique features of the dlPFC position it as the hub of the corticohippocampal circuit. In Chapters 9 and 10, we will pay particular attention to the critical importance of the dlPFC in mediating executive control.

Cytoarchitectonics and Brodmann areas

In addition to having spatially based anatomical subdivisions, the PFC is further subdivided on the basis of local composition, arrangement, and connections of neurons, collectively referred to as cytoarchitectonics (literally, "cell architecture"). The cytoarchitectonics of the PFC forms the basis of a commonly employed classification scheme developed by the German neurologist Korbinian Brodmann in the early 1900s. Using painstaking and meticulous dissection, Brodmann described unique patterns of cellular anatomy across regions of the cortex, including the PFC. During this process, he consecutively numbered each unique region he encountered, leading to what is now known as Brodmann areas, or BA. Unfortunately, Brodmann did not conduct his dissections in any obvious anatomical order (e.g., anterior to posterior, or dorsal to ventral), so his overall numbering scheme is a haphazard one that belies decoding (**Figure 8.3**).

There is approximate correspondence between the gross anatomical and cytoarchitectonic subdivisions of the PFC, with BA46 and lateral aspects of BA9 corresponding to the dlPFC hub; BA44, BA45, and BA47 corresponding to the vlPFC; and BA12 and BA32 as well as medial aspects of BA9, BA10, and BA11 corresponding to subregions of the vmPFC and dmPFC. Of note, BA24 captures the anterior cingulate cortex (including its dorsal subregion, or dACC), which plays a key role in executive control in the form of conflict monitoring. However, it is often the cellular anatomy captured by Brodmann areas, not necessarily the spatially based superficial anatomy, that is of critical importance in supporting the role of the PFC broadly in generating executive control, and the role of the dlPFC specifically as the corticohippocampal circuit hub.

The majority of the neurons in the PFC (approximately 80%) are excitatory glutamatergic pyramidal neurons; the remaining 20% or so are inhibitory GABA interneurons. Despite this bias in absolute numbers, it is the minority population of inhibitory interneurons that ultimately determines the executive control function of the dlPFC. As we saw earlier, our refined and controlled behaviors generally emerge as a function of discrete, stimulus-dependent patterns of selective inhibition, or by "sculpting in negativity" (see Chapter 2). In Chapter 9, we will see how input-dependent inhibition of pyramidal neurons by interneurons in the dlPFC is critical for executive control. In this chapter, we will consider how the arrangement of the PFC's two primary neuronal populations

cytoarchitectonics Detailed cellular anatomy and arrangement of neurons; literally "cell architecture."

Brodmann areas (BA) Common notation for identifying cytoarchitectonically and functionally distinct subregions of the cortex, based on the work of Korbinian Brodmann.

pyramidal neurons Named for the shape of their cell bodies, these are large, glutamatergic neurons common to the cortex. (Glutamate is the primary excitatory neurotransmitter in the brain.)

interneurons Small, inhibitory GABA neurons positioned to regulate the activity of neighboring pyramidal neurons in the cortex. (GABA is gamma-aminobutyric acid, the primary inhibitory neurotransmitter in the brain.)

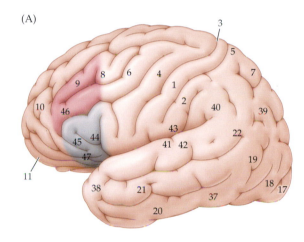

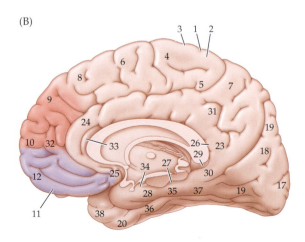

Figure 8.3 Lateral (A) and medial (B) views of the human brain depicting the major cytoarchitectonic divisions identified by Brodmann (Brodmann areas). Shaded regions overlap with the major anatomical subdivisions of the prefrontal cortex depicted in Figure 8.2.

PFC   prefrontal cortex
dACC   dorsal anterior cingulate cortex

Figure 8.4 This stylized reconstruction illustrates the typical columnar and laminar (layered) organization of sensory cortex, in this case from an area of the rat brain that processes sensory information from the whiskers. (From Meyer et al., 2013; prepared by Marcel Oberlaender et al.)

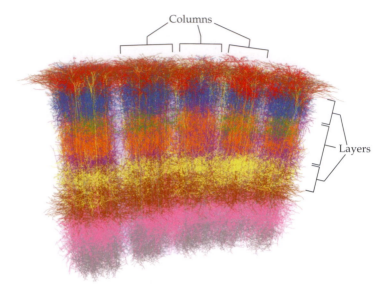

into horizontal layers and vertical columns (**Figure 8.4**), helps set the stage for executive control.

Horizontal layers

All subregions of the PFC (and most other cortical areas) are broadly organized into six horizontal layers (**Figure 8.5**). In fact, Brodmann based his cytoarchitectonic labels on the specific distribution of excitatory pyramidal neurons and inhibitory interneurons and their connections within these layers. Generally, the two innermost layers (V and VI) contain pyramidal neurons whose axons

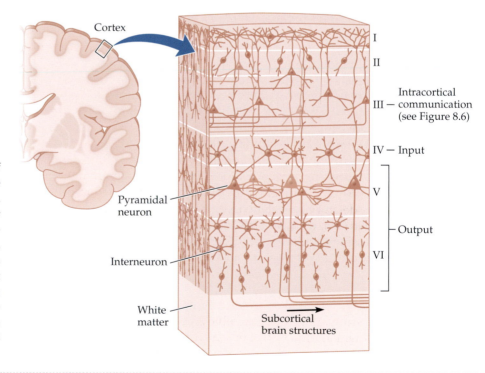

Figure 8.5 Laminar organization of human cortex within columns and the general flow (arrows) of input and output. Layers I through III represent the majority of intracortical connections. Layer IV represents the majority of inputs to the cortex, coming largely from thalamic relays. Layers V and VI represent the majority of output projections to subcortical structures such as the amygdala, ventral striatum, and hippocampus as well as the thalamus and, via the spinal cord, the peripheral nervous system.

PFC   prefrontal cortex

project to all subcortical targets, including the hippocampus, amygdala, ventral striatum, thalamus, and brainstem. Thus, these layers facilitate the output of the PFC and, through this output, its regulation of other brain regions. In contrast, all input to the PFC, largely via thalamic relays, arrives in layer IV, which contains populations of both pyramidal neurons and interneurons. Communication between different subdivisions of the PFC, as well as between the PFC and other cortical regions, is largely conducted within connections of layers I, II, and III. The **neuronal ensembles** of layer III are particularly critical in supporting the communication between the dlPFC and other subregions of the PFC that is necessary for executive control (**Figure 8.6**). Collectively, it is the staggering density and variety of afferent and efferent connections maintained throughout the horizontal layers of the dlPFC that help form the anatomical foundation for executive control.

Vertical columns

The nature of corticohippocampal circuit function, particularly executive control, is further reflected in the second form of anatomical order in the cortex: vertical columns. There are approximately 500,000 columns in the human cortex, and each column is made up of approximately 70,000 neurons. In sensory cortices, each column receives a unique set of inputs (e.g., different aspects of visual information from the retinal cells of the eyes) and, through local filtering of the information and feedforward processing, contributes to the representation of these inputs as a specific sensory experience (e.g., sight). The columns within the PFC, in contrast, largely receive input from sensory association areas (e.g., the dorsal "where" stream and ventral "what" stream), which function to develop the overall representation of sensory inputs from primary sensory cortices. Thus, the PFC, especially dlPFC, is positioned to execute higher-order processes in service of integrating our multimodal sensory experiences, as is characteristic of memories, rather than to piece together individual stimulus inputs. Likewise, the selection of appropriate responses and execution of adaptive behaviors reflect the dynamic processing of converging inputs to these columns.

This convergence of inputs reaches its zenith in the dlPFC, which maintains afferent and efferent connections with all subregions of the PFC (see Figure 8.6) as well as sensory association areas and the HF. Fine-tuning of column activity through selective inhibition of pyramidal output neurons results in the top-down executive control of downstream target regions. We will consider in greater detail how executive control and memory are supported by dlPFC function in Chapter 9, and in Chapter 10 we will see how abnormal information processing within the dlPFC emerges as specific symptoms of cognitive dysfunction and disordered thinking.

The Hippocampal Formation

As we saw in our study of the corticolimbic and corticostriatal circuits, the HF provides important information about the context of our experiences (i.e., where, when, what, and whom). As a node within the corticolimbic circuit,

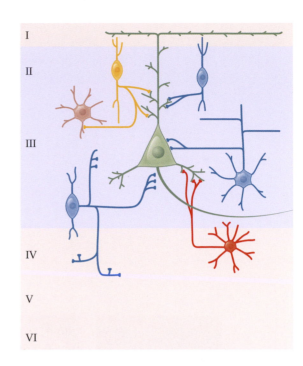

Figure 8.6 Typical arrangement of inhibitory interneurons (blue, red, and yellow) and their inputs to an excitatory pyramidal neuron (green) within layer III of the dlPFC.

neuronal ensembles A complex of pyramidal neurons and interneurons in the cortex that form the foundation of information processing during executive control.

dlPFC   dorsolateral prefrontal cortex
HF   hippocampal formation

RESEARCH SPOTLIGHT

Much is made of the large size of the human brain in comparison to the brains of other animals. However, the most remarkable difference is visible only at the microscopic level. Detailed anatomical studies of cortical columns across mammalian species reveal that it's not the number of neurons that distinguishes humans from other animals, but the number of connections these neurons make with each other. Cortical columns in humans are significantly thicker than those in rats and mice, as would be expected from the overall size differences in the brains of these species. Despite the size differences favoring humans, the columns in both rats and mice have more neurons than those in humans. However, the neurons of humans have many more connections, or synapses, on average.

This relative richness in synaptic density allows the cortical columns of the human brain and the broader regions they comprise to process and integrate more information and, in turn, to effect more nuanced and flexible responses. The greater synaptic density of neurons in the human cortex, most importantly the PFC, further allows for a dizzying array of combinations in information processing and, as a result, some uniquely human behaviors such as art, creativity, and invention. The abilities afforded by this anatomy, however, are not without drawbacks. The complexity of the human brain, particularly the PFC, requires a protracted period of development before reaching maturity (**Figure 8.7**). This leaves the PFC highly vulnerable to insult and injury, which may be expressed as disordered thought and impoverished executive control.

(A)   1 month   6 years

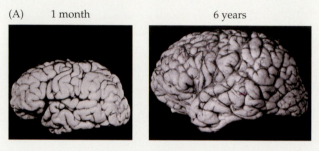

(B)   1 month   6 years

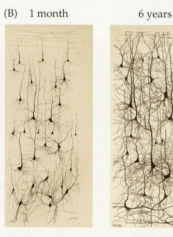

Figure 8.7 (A) Between 1 month and 6 years of age the human brain enlarges approximately fourfold. (B) A significant proportion of this brain growth reflects not an increase in the number of neurons, but rather an exponential increase in the connections between existing neurons, especially those of the cortex. (From DeFelipe et al., 2002.)

the HF further functions to regulate the activity of the hypothalamic-pituitary-adrenal axis in response to stressful situations or experiences. Here we focus on the detailed intrinsic anatomy of the HF that allows us to first create (i.e., encode) and subsequently access (i.e., recall) long-term declarative memories.

In our description of corticolimbic circuit anatomy, we briefly described the HF as including several interconnected and contiguous regions of the medial temporal lobes. The hippocampus, the core of the HF, is located immediately posterior to the amygdala (**Figure 8.8**; also see Figure 2.12). The HF includes the parahippocampal cortex, entorhinal cortex, perirhinal cortex, subiculum, and dentate gyrus. These regions function as an interface or relay for communication between the hippocampus and other brain regions, including the amygdala, ventral striatum, sensory association areas, and PFC.

The HF, and the hippocampus specifically, is one of the most remarkable brain structures from the perspective of gross anatomy. As with the amygdala, early anatomists named this brain structure for its general shape and appearance. The word *hippocampus* is Greek for "seahorse," which this brain region resembles. Like the seahorse, the brain's hippocampus can be viewed as having a head, body, and tail, which curves gently along the ventral surface

HF   hippocampal formation
PFC   prefrontal cortex

Figure 8.8 General location of the hippocampus within the medial temporal lobe posterior to the amygdala. The gross anatomy is reminiscent of a seahorse, from which the word *hippocampus* is derived.

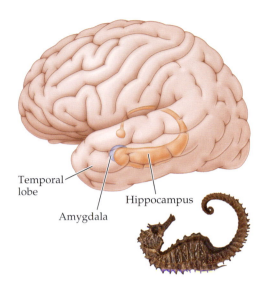

Temporal lobe

Amygdala

Hippocampus

of the medial temporal lobe (see Figure 8.8). In Chapter 9, we will see that long-term declarative memory is supported by waves of activity that travel along this long axis of the hippocampus and HF.

The internal anatomy of the HF is almost as striking as its external anatomy (**Figure 8.9**). When viewed along the coronal plane, the HF can be seen as a unique layering of gray and white matter into two intersecting semicircles, which are comprised of the hippocampus, dentate gyrus, subiculum, entorhinal cortex, perirhinal cortex, and parahippocampal cortex. Because of its cross-sectional appearance, the gray matter of the hippocampus is referred to as the **cornu ammonis (CA)**, which is Latin for "horns of Amun" (Amun being an ancient Egyptian god whose temple was guarded by rams with curved horns). At the cellular or cytoarchitectonic level, the cornu ammonis is divided into contiguous subregions known as CA1, CA2, CA3, and CA4. A characteristic flow of information along the HF subregions revealed in the coronal plane, like that along the long axis of the entire HF, supports the formation of long-term memories. We will further consider this information processing flow in Chapter 9.

cornu ammonis (CA) Subregions of the hippocampus named for their curved appearance in the coronal section; literally "horns of Ammon."

(A)

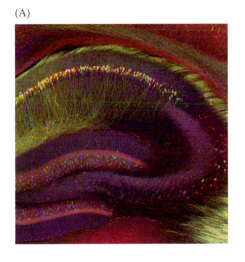

(B)

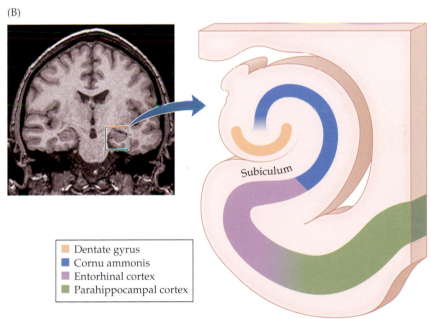

Subiculum

- Dentate gyrus
- Cornu ammonis
- Entorhinal cortex
- Parahippocampal cortex

Figure 8.9 (A) The hippocampal formation of a transgenic mouse (coronal view). To create this "brainbow," the mouse's genome was modified to express different fluorescent proteins (cyan, yellow, and red) in different subsets of neurons, resulting in a clear visualization of the curved structure of the HF. (B) Coronal section of the human hippocampal formation depicting the general layout of the dentate gyrus and cornu ammonis as well as the subiculum, entorhinal cortex, and parahippocampal cortex. (A, photograph by Tamily Weissman, Lichtman Lab, Harvard University Medical School.)

RESEARCH SPOTLIGHT

Of the varied and vast contributions of noninvasive human neuroimaging to our understanding of order and disorder inside the brain, perhaps none eclipse those revealing the rather spectacular waves of brain development over time. Here the work of Jay Giedd at the National Institute of Mental Health and Paul Thompson at the University of Southern California is exemplary. Working with structural neuroimaging data collected in normally developing individuals every 2 years between the ages of 4 and 25, these investigators and their colleagues have documented unique profiles for the maturation of the HF and PFC (**Figure 8.10**). Consistent with data from animal models, the human HF, specifically the hippocampus, reaches its mature adult form relatively early in development, as no changes in total gray matter volume are observed between ages 4 and 25. However, there are small increases and decreases in gray matter within specific subregions of the hippocampus (e.g., in its head, body, and tail).

The functional importance of these subregional changes in hippocampal gray matter is currently unknown. In contrast, cortical regions exhibit significant waves of change in gray matter volume throughout the developmental window from 4 to 25 years. Remarkably, primary sensory cortices mature before the sensory association areas to which they forward information. The PFC, and the dlPFC in particular, receive information from sensory association areas and are the last cortical regions to mature. Thus, there is a wave of development from more posterior to more anterior aspects of the cortex over time. The relatively protracted maturation of the dlPFC reflects the time needed to establish and refine the tremendous complexity of connections that ultimately allow this circuit hub to effect executive control. This long window of development until maturity, unfortunately, also leaves the PFC most vulnerable to potential damage from stress and trauma.

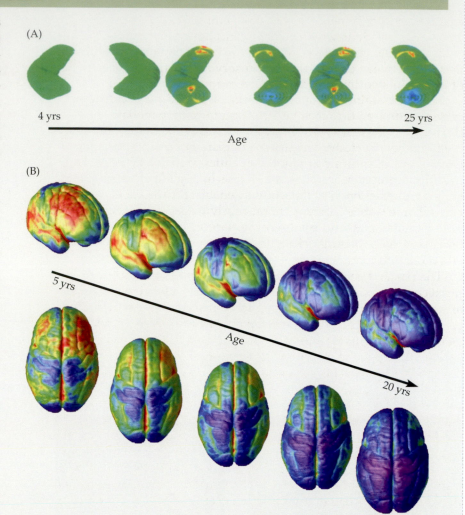

(A)

4 yrs   25 yrs

Age

(B)

5 yrs

Age

20 yrs

Figure 8.10   (A) Analyses of repeated MRI scans reveals that the general structure of the human hippocampus is relatively unchanged (green areas) between the ages of 4 and 25, but there are some small but significant changes in some subregions (blue, red, yellow). (B) In contrast to the hippocampus, which matures relatively early in life, the cortex exhibits dramatic changes in structure across the first three decades. This is particularly true for the prefrontal cortex, which continues to develop well into our 20s. Purple represents a relatively mature state. (From Gogtay et al., 2004, 2006.)

PFC   prefrontal cortex
dlPFC   dorsolateral prefrontal cortex

Sensory Association Areas

While the HF plays a fundamental role in the encoding and recall of long-term memories, it does so through its rich reciprocal connections with multiple cortical regions. Of particular importance for these mnemonic processes are interconnections between the HF and the sensory association areas of the brain's cortex, which function to integrate multiple sources of incoming sensory information. Unlike the cortical regions dedicated to processing specific information modalities (e.g., the primary somatosensory, visual, auditory, and motor cortices), sensory association areas are capable of processing and integrating multiple modalities of information. In other words, sensory association areas help generate our perceptual experiences of the world by enabling associations between many different and simultaneously occurring inputs. This capacity reflects the position of sensory association areas downstream of cortical regions dedicated to specific inputs and modalities.

The parietal cortex and the ventral aspects of the temporal cortex are two prime examples of sensory association areas that figure prominently in memory and executive control. The parietal cortex helps create our concrete sense of where we are in relation to other objects in space, as well as the more abstract ability to relate information in a virtual space (e.g., when working on a complex algebraic formula). The ventral temporal cortex, in contrast, provides details about what specific objects occupy our space. These parallel but related pathways are thus commonly referred to as the dorsal "where" stream and ventral "what" stream, respectively (**Figure 8.11**). In the context of long-term declarative memory, the forwarding of integrated inputs from sensory association areas into the HF creates vivid details for the what, where, when, and whom of our memories. For executive control, interactions between the dlPFC hub and other sensory association areas, particularly the parietal cortex, allow for the goal-directed manipulation of complex information (e.g., using a map to travel from one location to another).

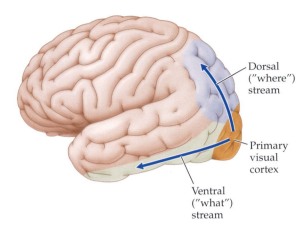

Dorsal ("where") stream

Primary visual cortex

Ventral ("what") stream

Figure 8.11 Two sensory association areas—the dorsal parietal cortex (blue) and ventral temporal cortex (green)—help us become aware of what objects exist around us (the ventral "what" stream) and where, specifically, these objects are located in space (the dorsal "where" stream).

dorsal "where" stream Sensory association areas encompassing the parietal lobes contributing to our perception of where objects exist in space around us.

ventral "what" stream Sensory association areas encompassing the temporal lobes contributing to our perception of what objects exists around us.

The Midbrain

Within the corticohippocampal circuit, dopamine signaling generated by cells in the midbrain is critically involved in the active modulation of dlPFC hub activity. In this capacity, an optimal level of dopamine signaling from the midbrain ventral tegmental area specifically is critical for the activity- and input-dependent tuning of the dlPFC necessary for generating adaptive and flexible executive control. We will further describe this "tuning" function of dopamine in the context of executive control of our behavior in Chapter 9. We will revisit this important modulatory role of midbrain dopamine when we discuss schizophrenia in Chapter 10.

HF   hippocampal formation
VTA   ventral tegmental area

Summary

Information processing through the interconnected nodes of the corticohippocampal circuit forms the basis of two critical behavioral processes: memory and executive control. The structures of the hippocampal formation, most notably the hippocampus, mediate long-term declarative memory through their dynamic interactions with sensory association areas as well as the prefrontal cortex. Executive control also reflects dynamic interactions but throughout the extensive afferent and efferent connections within and between cortical columns of the prefrontal cortex (most notably the dorsolateral prefrontal cortex circuit hub) as well as sensory association areas. In support of executive control, dopaminergic cells of the midbrain ventral tegmental area function to modulate the activity and effectiveness of the circuit hub. The complexity of these corticohippocampal circuit nodes and their interconnections simultaneously reflect the unparalleled capacity of the human brain for sophisticated cognition and manipulation of both our external and internal worlds, as well as our unique vulnerability to disorders of thought such as those characteristic of schizophrenia.

Literature Cited & Further Reading

Badre, D. (2008). Cognitive control, hierarchy, and the rostro-caudal organization of the frontal lobes. *Trends in Cognitive Science*, 12: 193–200.

Brodmann, K. (1909). *Vergleichende Lokalisationslehre der Grosshirnrinde in ihren Prinzipien dargestellt auf Grund des Zellenbaues*. Barth, Leipzig.

DeFelipe, J., & 12 others. (2002) Neocortical circuits: Evolutionary aspects and specificity versus non-specificity of synaptic connections. *Journal of Neurocytology*, 31: 387–416.

DeFelipe, J. (2011). The evolution of the brain, the human nature of cortical circuits, and intellectual creativity. *Frontiers in Neuroanatomy*, 5 doi: 10.3389/fnana.2011.00029.

Dolcos, F., LaBar, K. S., & Cabeza, R. (2004). Interaction between the amygdala and the medial temporal lobe memory system predicts better memory for emotional events. *Neuron*, 42: 855–863.

Gogtay, N., & 11 others. (2004). Dynamic mapping of human cortical development during childhood through early adulthood. *Proceedings of the National Academy of Science USA*, 101: 8174–8179.

Gogtay, N., & 10 others. (2006). Dynamic mapping of normal human hippocampal development. *Hippocampus*, 16: 664–672.

Lewis, D. A., Hashimoto, T., & Volk, D. W. (2005). Cortical inhibitory neurons and schizophrenia. *Nature Reviews Neuroscience*, 6: 312–324.

MacLean, P. D. (1949). Psychosomatic disease and the visceral brain; recent developments bearing on the Papez theory of emotion. *Psychosomatic Medicine*, 11: 338–353.

Meyer, K., & 14 others. (2014). Direct conversion of patient fibroblasts demonstrates non-cell autonomous toxicity of astrocytes to motor neurons in familial and sporadic ALS. *Proceedings of the National Academy of Science USA*, 111: 829–832.

Miller, E. K. (2000). The prefrontal cortex and cognitive control. *Nature Reviews Neuroscience*, 1: 59–65.

Small, S. A., Schobel, S. A., Buxton, R. B., Witter, M. P., & Barnes, C. A. (2011). A pathophysiological framework of hippocampal dysfunction in ageing and disease. *Nature Reviews Neuroscience*, 12: 585–601.

9

The Corticohippocampal Circuit
Order

In this chapter, we will consider in detail how specific patterns of information processing through the corticohippocampal circuit generate and support the circuit's principal functions of memory and executive control. As noted in Chapter 8, the corticohippocampal circuit processes information broadly rather than selectively. There are no distinct triggers of circuit function like those found for the corticolimbic and corticostriatal circuits. Thus, the processes of memory and executive control described below are relevant and applicable to virtually all content, stimuli, and situations.

In many ways, memory and executive control are processes that operate above those concerned with specific stimuli (e.g., processing of threat through the corticolimbic circuit or reward through the corticostriatal circuit). With this in mind, we first consider how the hippocampal formation and interconnected sensory association areas form the foundation for memory. We then consider how the dorsolateral prefrontal cortex hub of the circuit contributes to memory and, moreover, directly supports executive control, which involves a second major form of memory: working, or short-term, memory.

Memory

As introduced in Chapter 8, *memory* within the corticohippocampal circuit refers to **declarative memory**, or the ability to consciously and explicitly recall information, which is broadly divided into **semantic memory** and **episodic memory**. Semantic memory refers to our factual or encyclopedic knowledge of the world (e.g., there are seven continents) and basic concepts (e.g., apples and oranges are fruits, and whales are actually mammals). A distinguishing feature of semantic memory, which is shared among many individuals, is the absence of details regarding the specific time and place where the information was acquired. In contrast, there *is* a specific time stamp for episodic memory, which typically reflects unique personal, or autobiographical, experiences or episodes of our lives. Examples of episodic memory include major life events such as births, anniversaries, deaths; first kiss (and first heartbreak); and first college acceptance letter. As these examples suggest, episodic memories are those most likely to be colored by the concurrent experience of emotions and, fittingly, can be heavily influenced by the corticolimbic and corticostriatal circuits (e.g., flashbulb memories). A useful way to distinguish these subforms

declarative memory The conscious and often goal-directed encoding and recall of information.

semantic memory Encoding and recall of general facts (i.e., encyclopedic knowledge).

episodic memory Encoding and recall of specific facts related to our unique experiences (i.e., autobiographical knowledge).

of declarative memory is to consider semantic memory as our shared knowledge of the multiplication table, and episodic memory as the specific time, place, and person from whom we learned this information (my mother, on the car ride to school, every day when I was in third grade—in case you were wondering).

Regardless of subform, declarative memory allows our acquired knowledge as well as personal experiences to shape our current behaviors and guide decisions about our future. This critical function is facilitated through the activity of the corticohippocampal circuit, particularly dynamic interactions between the prefrontal cortex and hippocampal formation. For now, we turn to consider how the orderly processing of information through the hippocampal formation represents the neural basis of declarative memory.

Memory and the hippocampal formation

Neuroimaging studies, particularly those employing fMRI, have repeatedly demonstrated widespread activity throughout the HF during both memory encoding and recall. Often, the strength of activity in the HF during encoding predicts the accuracy of subsequent memory during recall. These studies typically ask participants to first learn new information and then recall this information later during the experiment. This information can come in the form of words, pictures, faces, and even abstract fractal images. A common strategy is to ask participants to learn and subsequently recall the names that accompany new faces (**Figure 9.1**)—nicely capturing a process we all experience routinely. Participants are usually distracted by other tasks (e.g., counting or sorting information) between the encoding and recall stages of the experiment. The use of such distraction is critical, as it prevents participants from maintaining the new information in short-term, or working, memory, which is dependent not on the HF but rather on the dorsolateral PFC, as we will see later in the chapter.

Although the HF is critical for both the encoding and recall of declarative memories, it has become increasingly clear with continued research that the HF is *not* where memories are stored or consolidated. The storage of declarative memory likely occurs across distributed sensory association areas that each process specific aspects of information that collectively comprise a memory. For example, our visual memory of the facial features of a friend are likely stored in visual association cortices such as the posterior fusiform gyrus, while memory of a friend's voice is likely stored in auditory association areas along the superior temporal gyrus. The systematic strengthening of synaptic pathways or neuronal connections linking such modality-specific components associated with a person, experience, or stimulus between sensory association areas and the HF is believed to represent the fundamental basis of declarative memory.

At the cellular level, this phenomenon is called **long-term potentiation (LTP)**. Typically, LTP emerges through repetition, rehearsal, or practice. For example, we may not remember the name of a new person after an initial meeting, but after several encounters, we begin to remember not only his name but, as our relationship deepens, other characteristics ranging from the pragmatic, like his occupation and education, to the more personal, like his aspirations and fears. While these modality-specific components exist or are stored across distributed regions of the brain, they are linked together accurately and consistently over time through the HF to generate our expression and experience of memory. We

long-term potentiation (LTP) Cellular and molecular changes resulting in strengthening of connections and communication between neurons that support learning and memory.

HF   hippocampal formation
PFC   prefrontal cortex
LTP   long-term potentiation

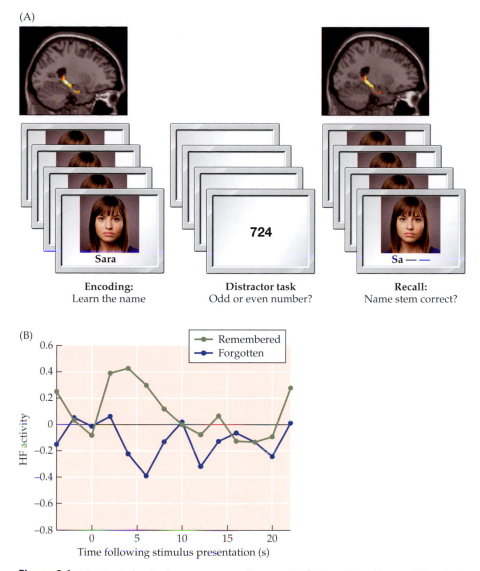

Figure 9.1 (A) A typical episodic memory paradigm used in fMRI studies asking participants to learn names of new faces. During encoding, participants are asked to learn the names of new faces. During recall, participants are asked to remember if a name stem is correctly paired with a face. In between blocks of encoding and recall, participants are required to perform distractor tasks designed to prevent them from rehearsing or maintaining the face-name pairs in working memory. There is robust activity throughout the HF during both the encoding (left panel) and recall (right panel) of face-name pairs. (B) During encoding (i.e., time following stimulus presentation), face-name pairs that are remembered correctly (green) are associated with increased HF activity, while those that are forgotten (blue) are associated with decreased HF activity. (B after Dickerson & Eichenbaum, 2010.)

next consider in detail how the coordinated flow of modality-specific information into and out of the HF supports declarative memory (**Figure 9.2**).

First, information from primary sensory cortices that is processed within sensory association areas is fed forward into the HF in a topographically distinct pattern. Information regarding the locations of items or objects in space is relayed from the dorsal "where" stream to the parahippocampal

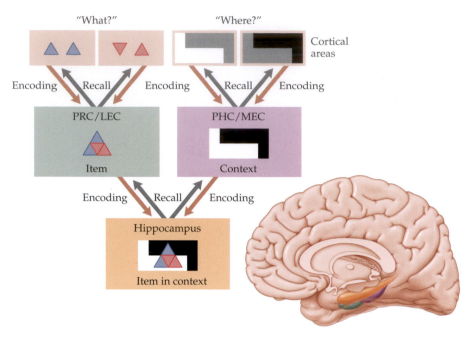

Figure 9.2 A proposed functional organization of declarative memory within the corticohippocampal circuit. Details about item features ("what") from sensory association areas along the *ventral* visual stream are relayed through the perirhinal cortex (PRC) and lateral entorhinal cortex (LEC), whereas details about item context ("where") from sensory association areas along the *dorsal* visual stream are relayed through the parahippocampal cortex (PHC) and medial entorhinal cortex (MEC). These streams converge in the hippocampus, which represents items in the context in which they are experienced. Reverse projections through the PHC-MEC support recall of "where," and those through the PRC-LEC support recall of "what." (After Dickerson & Eichenbaum, 2010.)

cortex (PHC), and from the PHC to the medial entorhinal cortex (MEC), and from the MEC into the hippocampus. At the same time, object or item information is relayed from the ventral "what" stream to the perirhinal cortex (PRC), and from the PRC to the lateral entorhinal cortex (LEC), and from the LEC to the hippocampus.

Then, having converged through these distinct topographic pathways onto the hippocampus, information regarding both "where" and "what" is serially processed within another anatomical loop (**Figure 9.3**). Beginning with the superficial layers of the entorhinal cortex, information is relayed to the dentate gyrus (DG); from the DG to CA3 and then CA1 of the hippocampus; from CA1 to the subiculum; and from the subiculum to the deep layers of the entorhinal cortex. From there, information processing flows back out to

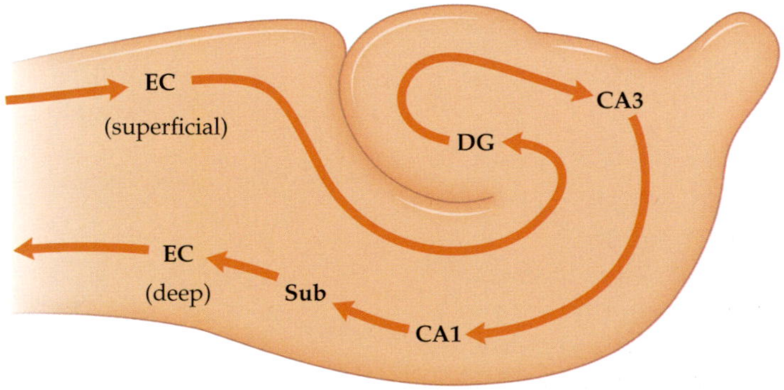

Figure 9.3 Information flow within the HF supporting declarative memory. Note that information both enters and leaves the hippocampus through layers of the entorhinal cortex. EC = entorhinal cortex. Sub = subiculum; DG = dentate gyrus; CA = cornu ammonis.

PHC	parahippocampal cortex	PRC	perirhinal cortex
MEC	medial entorhinal cortex	LEC	lateral entorhinal cortex

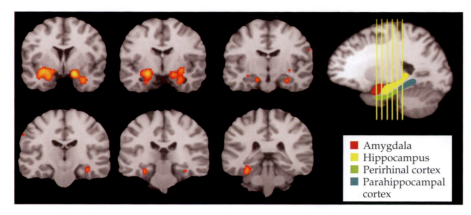

Figure 9.4 During encoding of emotionally charged stimuli such as fearful or angry facial expressions, there is activity both in the amygdala and throughout the HF. Locations of the coronal planes are shown by the yellow lines in the sagittal image on the right, with the most anterior plane corresponding to the top left image and the most posterior plane to the bottom right image. (From Murty et al., 2010.)

the sensory association areas of origin. Through this flow of information, the HF broadly and the hippocampus specifically function to bind "what" and "where" in real time to create a complete memory of a person, experience, or stimulus. In other words, the HF serves as the anatomical nexus through which memories are first formed *and* later remembered. A useful albeit dated analogy is that the HF functions less like a library where information is stored and more like a card catalog through which we can access specific information inside the library.

Not surprisingly, within pathways between the DG and the CA3 and CA1 subregions, LTP in response to the convergence of "where" and "what" information is particularly critical for the binding of memories during encoding. In addition, the concurrent experience of a strong emotion such as fear in response to a threat (**Figure 9.4**) or happiness in response to a reward, through the amygdala and VS, respectively, can further strengthen LTP along these pathways, leading to emotional "flashbulb" memories. Reactivation of these potentiated hippocampal pathways—which can occur even when we encounter a single-component element of a memory, like a person's voice—are likewise critical for recall or remembering.

Finally, consistent with the anatomical location of the PHC and PRC, memory for objects and items is typically reflected by primary activity in the anterior hippocampus, and for spatial location in the posterior hippocampus. Of course, actual memory is rarely so piecemeal but typically is of a complete experience or episode (i.e., the binding of items in context) and thus is reflected in activity along the entire HF.

Memory and the prefrontal cortex

While our declarative memories of people, places, and experiences are valuable simply for the pleasure and joy they can create by their remembrance, such memories may be even more valuable in the context of guiding our behavior and informing our decision making. This is particularly true of semantic memories and the worldly knowledge they communicate. After all,

DG	dentate gyrus	VS	ventral striatum
CA	cornu ammonis	LTP	long-term potentiation
HF	hippocampal formation		

RESEARCH SPOTLIGHT

Until quite recently, it was nearly impossible to study the flow of information throughout the human HF during memory encoding and recall. The intricate cross-sectional anatomy of the HF perplexes as much as it awes and inspires. Specifically, the tightly rolled anatomy of the HF makes it extremely difficult to map memory-related activity measured with fMRI onto specific subregions such as the hippocampus, dentate gyrus, and subiculum. The general methods for analyzing fMRI data simply don't allow for such precision. In fact, much of our understanding of information flow through the HF is based on non-human animal studies, with their detailed mapping of neuronal connections and direct electrophysiological recording of activity within and between HF subregions.

However, in 2003 a remarkable fMRI study by Michael Zeineh and Susan Bookheimer at UCLA provided the first glimpse into this information flow in the human HF (**Figure 9.5**). The key to their breakthrough was the application of then novel processing algorithms to virtually "unroll" the HF along the entirety of its longitudinal axis. These algorithms were originally developed in part to "flatten" the cortical surface, thereby making activity in deep sulci visible like that in gyri. This was particularly important for investigators seeking to map the representation of our complex, three-dimensional worlds onto the visual cortex.

Applying these analytic techniques to fMRI data collected while participants learned the names associated with new faces, Zeineh and colleagues were able to map encoding- and retrieval-related activity within component subregions of the HF that were virtually flattened onto a continuous surface. Encoding of novel face-name pairs was primarily associated with activity in the anterior hippocampus,

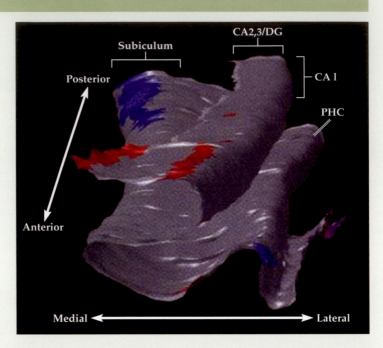

Figure 9.5 Activity during encoding and retrieval within component subregions of the HF that have been "flattened" onto a continuous surface. Encoding of novel face-name pairs was primarily associated with activity (red) in the anterior hippocampus, dentate gyrus, and subiculum. In contrast, recall of previously learned face-name pairs was primarily associated with activity (blue) in the posterior subiculum and parahippocampal cortex. DG = dentate gyrus; CA = cornu ammonis; PHC = parahippocampal cortex. (From Zeineh et al., 2003.)

dentate gyrus, and subiculum. In contrast, retrieval of previously learned face-name pairs was primarily associated with activity in the posterior subiculum and parahippocampal cortex. These results not only corroborate basic patterns derived from nonhuman animal studies, but also shed light on previously unknown contributions of specific HF subregions to components of human memory.

how can we be expected to make the best decisions about our present and future if these decisions aren't guided by our past knowledge as well as our personal experiences, be they good, bad, or otherwise? It is at this interface of information exchange between our declarative memory and goal-directed decision making that we first encounter the importance of the dlPFC hub of the corticohippocampal circuit.

As described in Chapter 8, the dlPFC has extensive connections with the HF and other sensory association areas, including the dorsal "where" and ventral "what" streams of sensory processing located in the parietal and temporal cortices, respectively. Through these connections, the dlPFC hub can work to

HF	hippocampal formation	**DG**	dentate gyrus
CA	cornu ammonis	**PHC**	parahippocampal cortex

Figure 9.6 Pattern of prefrontal activity reported across 37 fMRI studies of declarative memory. Each green dot represents an activation peak in an analysis that reported increased activation during encoding of items that were subsequently remembered, as compared with items that were subsequently forgotten. Similar activity throughout the PFC is observed during recall of previously encoded information. (From Blumenfeld & Ranganath, 2007.)

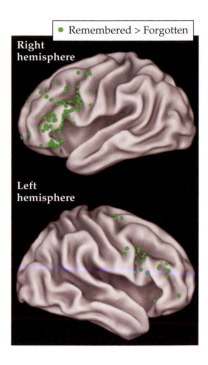

● Remembered > Forgotten

Right hemisphere

Left hemisphere

organize and prioritize information processing that allows for the creation of specific declarative memories. During encoding, the dlPFC generally functions to focus HF processing on goal-relevant information so that we can remember the important things while ignoring the bevy of distractions always around us. For example, hopefully right now your dlPFC is functioning to focus your attention and subsequent information processing on the text you are reading while it is simultaneously preventing you from being distracted by the music coming from next door or your roommate beckoning you to a party down the hall. (We will consider how the dlPFC accomplishes this monumental task in the following section on executive control.) In parallel to the attention-focusing activity of the dlPFC, the vlPFC, particularly subregions in the left hemisphere supporting language, help you to mentally rehearse the information you want to remember. This is particularly important when you review your notes after (again hopefully) having keenly attended to your professor's instruction during a lecture.

Collectively, this activity of the dlPFC and vlPFC functions to select what specific features of information are selectively processed within the HF and, ultimately, encoded into declarative memory (**Figure 9.6**). Likewise, activity in the dlPFC hub contributes to our ability to selectively remember or access specific information after it is stored in our declarative memory. This is accomplished when the dlPFC drives activity of distinct memory traces through the HF (as will almost certainly be necessary when you are tested on your grasp of this material). An equally important role of the dlPFC during recall specifically is to actively inhibit the engagement of a multitude of other memory traces through alternate HF pathways. This inhibitory effect of the dlPFC during goal-directed recall is critical because memory traces can also be activated through incidental exposure to cues.

For example, when taking your exam on the corticohippocampal circuit, you will want to selectively recall lecture material on this unit and not become confused or distracted by material from the prior two units. However, memory traces for all three units could be activated simply because all the lectures have been held in the same auditorium and you may have been sitting in the same seat and next to the same classmates during all the lectures. You have also learned about brain regions that contribute to all three foundational circuits, but need to selectively access memory for their specific contributions to the corticohippocampal circuit.

The dlPFC is ultimately responsible for your ability to selectively access the corticohippocampal circuit lectures and suppress the lectures for the other two circuits. By simultaneously activating goal-relevant and inhibiting goal-irrelevant memory traces embedded within the bidirectional pathways of the HF and sensory association areas, the dlPFC allows for such highly selective and flexible access to our declarative memories. Of course, there is memory (both encoding and recall) independent of such top-down direction from the dlPFC hub. Such memories are represented, for example, by contextually

dlPFC   dorsolateral prefrontal cortex
vlPFC   ventrolateral prefrontal cortex

appropriate fear or extinction following fear learning. Such basic forms of memory, while also supported by the connections between the HF and sensory association areas, are relatively crude—and typically subconscious—mechanisms for shaping behavior. In contrast, declarative memories emerging from conscious thought and deliberation depend on dynamic interactions between the dlPFC and HF.

Executive Control

executive control The capacity to generate and orchestrate complex plans and goal-directed behaviors through attention, working memory, and response selection as well as declarative memory.

Outside of its specific contribution to first creating and then accessing declarative memories, the dlPFC hub is quintessential for generating the second major function of the corticohippocampal circuit: executive control. Broadly, executive control refers to our conscious ability to direct and redirect behavioral and physical resources in the service of achieving specific goals based on not only our current circumstances but also our past experiences. Looked at in this way, executive control can be considered a top-down process in contrast to the bottom-up responses of the other circuits. In fact, we have encountered executive control in our earlier consideration of the corticolimbic and corticostriatal circuits.

Recall the famous "marshmallow test," where kids are given one marshmallow to eat right away, but are also told that if they wait only a few minutes before eating it, they will receive a second marshmallow. In Chapter 6, we considered the more impulsive decision to not wait and eat one marshmallow immediately, a bias reflected in increased activity of the VS gate of the corticostriatal circuit. In contrast, the decision to wait for the second marshmallow reflects the operation of executive control, in this case manifesting as the decision to inhibit the desire to eat the first marshmallow.

Of course, executive control is informed, even guided, by our past experiences. In the marshmallow test, the memory of whether a previous promise was kept or broken shapes the decision to eat one marshmallow right away or trust the investigator and wait for two marshmallows. In fact, successful executive control often requires that we explicitly access memories that are relevant for our current decision making through dlPFC activation of the HF.

More abstractly, executive control is reflected in our decisions to invest in the future through retirement plans and investments, to forgo parties in favor of studying for exams, and to pass on a second helping of dessert and swim an extra lap in the pool to keep our weight down and our heart healthy. Likewise, executive control can overcome biases associated with fear or negative emotions. For example, we can consciously decide to hike along a trail where we have previously encountered a snake. In this case, executive control is consciously inhibiting the expression of fear that would keep us away from the trail, thereby allowing us to resume an otherwise pleasurable activity. Importantly, this explicit control of fear is different from fear extinction, which is an unconscious or implicit process reflecting a parallel learning trace in the medial PFC. We will learn shortly that executive control, as exemplified by the conscious ability to either delay gratification or overcome fear, is supported by information processing in the dlPFC hub.

Components of executive control

Regardless of its specific application or expression, there are three broad component processes that together allow for the emergent property of executive

| HF | hippocampal formation | VS | ventral striatum |
| dlPFC | dorsolateral prefrontal cortex | PFC | prefrontal cortex |

control. They are (1) attention, (2) working memory, and (3) response selection. The first component, attention, refers to selectively concentrating on one aspect of an experience, the environment, or even a discrete stimulus while ignoring others. By such selective concentration, attention allows us to allocate processing resources to specific features that are relevant for achieving our goals. Attention is like the mind's spotlight, which can be shone on different objects or even parts of objects to increase the clarity of our perception and deepen our processing of information in the service of achieving a specific goal.

The second component of executive control, working memory, refers to the ability to briefly maintain information in mind and subsequently manipulate that information in the service of achieving our goals. This form of memory is sometimes referred to as short-term memory. In effect, working memory is like a mental notepad where we can jot down information to help us complete tasks in real time. In contrast to declarative memory, the information represented in working memory is not typically consolidated or stored, and thus is not available to us over long intervals of time. Furthermore, working memory has a much more limited capacity, and we can maintain and manipulate only so much information in real time. Ideally, our working memory is cleared or reset after achieving a specific goal. However, this reset also occurs if we are distracted by other information or if we shift goals, after which we either can't or don't maintain the prior information through mental rehearsal.

The third component of executive control, response selection, refers to the conscious ability to direct and redirect our behavioral responses, ranging from simple motor actions to complex, long-term plans, according to changing needs or task demands. One specific type of response selection, response inhibition, plays a prominent role in the top-down regulatory effects of executive control. Response inhibition is the explicit ability to withhold behavioral responses when they are inconsistent with our goals or with task demands.

We can use a scenario familiar to many students to illustrate these three component processes of executive control. Imagine you are studying in the library with a group of friends. Many varied distractions abound (e.g., conversations between other students, openings of books, keystrokes on nearby computers, texting from smartphones). However, you focus on your class notes to prepare for an upcoming exam. This is an example of the first component process of attention. This selective attention to your notes also contributes to the long-term encoding of the information through the HF. After many hours, you decide to take a study break and head over to the student union for a double espresso to carry you through the rest of the night. Being a good friend, you ask your study partners if they want something as well. The second component process of working memory allows you to maintain the list of drinks for your friends as you make your way to the coffee bar and then give the barista your order. Once you place the order and deliver the drinks to your friends, you forget this information, clearing working memory for new information (maybe there's a doughnut run in your future). The third component process of response selection comes into play because the main walkway you've used for 3 years to travel from the library to the union is under construction and you need to inhibit your habitual response to head toward that walkway and head instead toward an alternate, unfamiliar path on the other side of the quad. As with the example from the marshmallow test above, throughout this scenario specific declarative memories (e.g., for

attention Selectively concentrating on one aspect of an experience or stimulus while ignoring others to help achieve a specific goal.

working memory The ability to briefly maintain information in mind and subsequently manipulate that information in the service of achieving our goals.

response selection The ability to direct and redirect our behavioral responses according to changing needs or task demands.

routes, locations of campus buildings, and the fact that there is construction underway) are being accessed via top-down dlPFC activation of the HF that inform and guide the expression and application of executive control.

While it's impossible to use the above scenario in an fMRI study, a number of commonly used experimental paradigms for engaging executive control have been adapted for use with neuroimaging. These paradigms allow us to identify corticohippocampal circuit activity supporting executive control broadly, as well as each of the three component processes described above. Because these paradigms almost universally require participants to provide specific responses to specific cues, they inherently involve allocation of resources to task demands through selective attention. Similarly, most of these paradigms require working memory, if for no other reason than to maintain task instructions to properly manipulate information during the scans. Finally, many of these paradigms include an explicit response selection component wherein participants are required to select appropriate and inhibit inappropriate responses or to switch between different responses, depending on task demands.

The Wisconsin Card Sorting Test (WCST; **Figure 9.7A**) is often used to measure executive control, both inside and outside the scanner. During the WCST, a participant is asked to sort a deck of cards into four piles representing the color, shape, or number of symbols printed on the cards. Initially, the participant must randomly select one of the three properties and receive feedback about whether that selection was correct or incorrect. If the selection was correct, the participant must continue to sort cards based on this property. The WCST then becomes a function of working memory as the participant

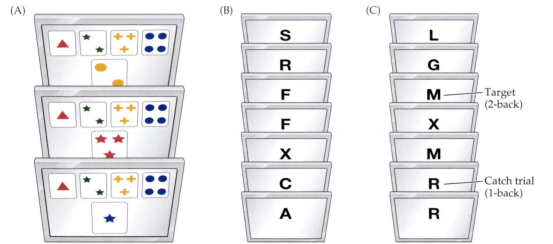
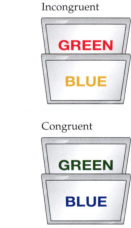

Figure 9.7 Commonly used paradigms to examine corticohippocampal circuit activity supporting executive control. (A) The Wisconsin Card Sorting Test. Each card in the deck has 1, 2, 3, or 4 triangles, circles, stars, or crosses that are all red, green, yellow, or blue. The participant is told to sort the cards into four different piles but is not told on what basis the sorting is to be accomplished. After each card is placed in a pile, the participant is told whether or not it was correctly placed. For example, at first the participant must learn to sort by color, but once this sorting principle is learned, the correct principle changes without warning, from color to either form or number. (B) The Conners' Continuous Performance Test: press key for all letters except X. (C) Letter "*n*-back" task: with 2-back, look for matches two steps into the past and avoid catch trials (e.g., matches only 1 step back). (D) Color Stroop: name the ink color. This is harder when the color word and the ink color are incongruent.

dlPFC dorsolateral prefrontal cortex
HF hippocampal formation
WCST Wisconsin Card Sorting Test

keeps in mind that cards should be sorted according to, for example, color and then manipulates the cards drawn from the deck by placing them in the correct color piles. Attention is also in operation, as the participant must focus on the color of the symbols rather than their shape or frequency. This phase of the WCST is typically called "maintenance." If the initial selection was incorrect, the participant must move through the other stimulus properties (shape and number) until the correct property is identified. After several correct responses (typically five), the contingency is changed and the participant receives feedback that the current stimulus property is no longer correct. At this time, the participant must select one of the other two stimulus properties until once again receiving feedback that it is correct. This phase of the WCST is called the "switch" and requires the addition of response selection (stopping selection based on color) to the attention (focusing on the different symbols and feedback) and working memory (keeping track of which properties have already been tried) already engaged by maintenance. In this way, the WCST engages all three component processes of executive control in a relatively seamless and integrated manner.

In contrast to the WCST, other paradigms are designed to measure distinct components of executive control. For example, the Conners' Continuous Performance Test (**Figure 9.7B**) specifically measures attention and response selection. This task requires participants to keep track of letters presented on a screen and press a button for every letter except X. In this way, the task measures sustained attention (monitoring the letters) and response selection (not pressing the space bar when X appears). Not surprisingly, this task and similar continuous performance tasks are commonly used to examine inattention and impulsivity in attention deficit hyperactivity disorder.

The "*n*-back" task is a common probe of working memory that requires participants to indicate when a current stimulus (e.g., letter, number, picture, face) matches the one from *n* steps earlier in a sequence (**Figure 9.7C**). Importantly, the load factor *n* can be adjusted to make the task more (e.g., 2-back or 3-back) or less (1-back) difficult. This allows investigators to challenge the working memory capacity of participants to the point where the task is effortful but not impossible. In turn, they can use fMRI to track corticohippocampal circuit activity supporting such effortful working memory performance. We will revisit the critical importance of manipulating working memory load and the resulting effects on performance and circuit activation when reviewing schizophrenia in Chapter 10.

Finally, a multitude of tasks evoke response selection. Of these, the color Stroop test (**Figure 9.7D**) may be the most commonly used. In this paradigm, participants are presented with words for primary colors printed in different-colored inks (e.g., the word *green* printed in red ink instead of green ink). The participants are asked to identify the ink color while ignoring the word itself, and they are slower and less accurate when the color of the ink doesn't match the name of the color (i.e., ink and word are incongruent). The decrement in accuracy and reaction time arises because the automatic process of reading, where the mind automatically determines the semantic meaning of the word (it reads the word *green* and thinks of the color green), must be inhibited, and instead the ink color of the word (red) must be identified. This is a classic example of response selection wherein a prepotent, incorrect response (reading) must be suppressed in favor of a more effortful, correct response (color identification). Of course, there also is a significant need for selective

Figure 9.8 (A) Meta-analysis of 31 fMRI and PET studies reveals activity in a distributed set of corticohippocampal circuit nodes, including the dlPFC, vlPFC and parietal cortex, when maintaining information in working memory. (B) In contrast to the more distributed pattern of activity during the maintenance of information in working memory, switching behavioral responses or strategies following negative feedback is associated with highly focused activity in the dACC. (From Wager et al., 2004.)

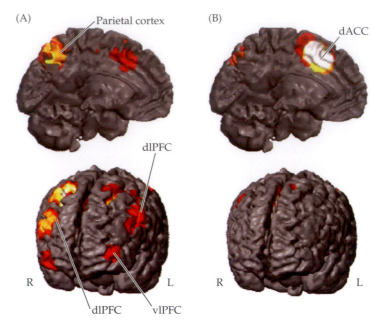

attention to the different qualities of the stimulus with the color as well as other versions of the Stroop test.

Across all these many and varied paradigms, a wealth of neuroimaging studies have consistently revealed that distributed activity in the corticohippocampal circuit supports executive control (**Figure 9.8**). At the center of this circuit activity is the dlPFC hub. In the next section we will consider in detail how the unique anatomy of the dlPFC, described in Chapter 8, allows for flexible processing of information in support of executive control. For now, we briefly consider additional brain regions implicated in meta-analyses of executive control studies.

Activity in the bilateral posterior parietal cortex and in the dACC is often observed during executive control. Activity in the former region along with that in the dlPFC primarily occurs during working memory and related processes (e.g., the maintenance phase of the WCST). In contrast, activity in the dACC occurs most prominently during response selection (e.g., the switch phase of the WCST). The dACC exhibits activity across other component processes of executive control, reflecting its contribution to the general monitoring of behavior. This pattern of activity is consistent with the important function of the dACC for detecting conflict (or error) and relaying this information to the dlPFC for the formation of a new plan (or correction). This dACC activity further contributes to the capacity for selective attention through the dlPFC by signaling whether a specific stimulus property is relevant to current task demands (there is low conflict; attend to stimulus) or irrelevant (high conflict; ignore).

Executive control central: The dlPFC

While the posterior parietal cortices and dACC both play important roles in generating executive control, the dlPFC represents the critical hub through which activity in these brain regions (and all others) is orchestrated in the service of effecting executive control and generating complex, adaptive responses. The dlPFC, if you will, is the conductor of a large and intricate orchestra, the

dlPFC   dorsolateral prefrontal cortex
dACC   dorsal anterior cingulate cortex
WCST   Wisconsin Card Sorting Test

RESEARCH SPOTLIGHT

The featured importance and hub status of the dlPFC in executive control has been powerfully illustrated through the application of a relatively new research tool in neuroscience and psychology known as transcranial magnetic stimulation, or TMS (**Figure 9.9**). With TMS, investigators can deliver a brief and focused magnetic pulse to specific regions of the cortex to generate electrical currents that temporarily disrupt local function. Early applications of TMS focused on demonstrating the importance of primary sensory and motor cortices to basic functions such as vision and movement. As the technique became more common, investigators began using TMS to study cognitive functions supported by the PFC. These cognitive applications include examining the differential contributions of prefrontal subregions to component processes of executive control.

One study applied TMS to three prefrontal regions—the dlPFC, dmPFC, and vlPFC—during working memory tasks for either faces or the locations of objects (**Figure 9.10**). Disruption of the dmPFC produced specific deficits in working memory for object location but not for faces. In contrast, disruption of the vlPFC produced specific deficits in working memory for faces but not for object location. These crossover effects of subregional TMS reflect the modality-specific processing of object location information through the dmPFC as a continuation of the dorsal "where" stream, and of face information through the vlPFC as a continuation of the ventral "what" stream. TMS directed at the dlPFC, however disrupted working memory for *both* faces and object location. This

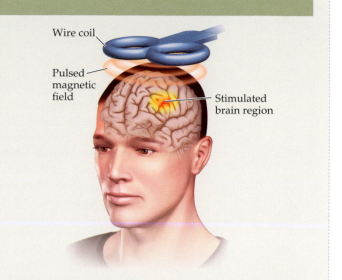

Figure 9.9 General experimental apparatus and setup for TMS studies of prefrontal function.

is consistent with the central role of the dlPFC in working memory (i.e., maintenance and manipulation of information) regardless of modality and further, reflects the convergence of input from other modality-specific prefrontal subregions into the dlPFC. This hub function of the dlPFC extends to executive control broadly including the component processes of attention and response selection, which again are not limited to any specific modality.

Figure 9.10 Effects of TMS within PFC subregions on working memory for faces and location of objects. Disruption (orange bars) of the dmPFC produced specific deficits in working memory for location but not for faces. Disruption of the vlPFC produced specific deficits in working memory for faces but not location. In contrast, TMS directed at the dlPFC disrupted working memory for *both* faces and location. Of note, the transient nature of TMS is evident by the recovery of function in all three regions evident at 5 minutes post-TMS, and full recovery after 10 minutes. (After Robertson et al., 2003.)

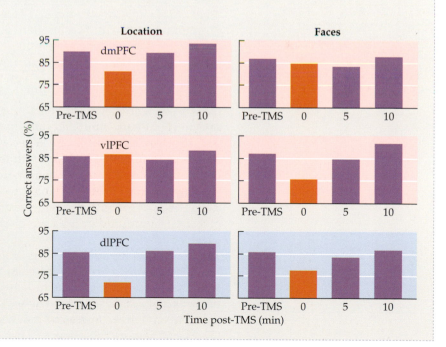

vlPFC ventrolateral prefrontal cortex
dmPFC dorsomedial prefrontal cortex
TMS transcranial magnetic stimulation

members of which represent the rest of the brain. Two anatomical features described in Chapter 8 afford the dlPFC this privileged position within the neural architecture of the brain: extensive interconnections with other brain regions, and a complex of excitatory pyramidal neurons and inhibitory interneurons that allow task-dependent, goal-directed selective information processing.

First, the ability of the dlPFC to broadly effect executive control reflects its extensive afferent and efferent connections with other cortical as well as subcortical brain regions. Of particular importance is the convergence (through layers I–III) of information from all other prefrontal regions and sensory association areas, such as the dorsal and ventral visual streams. These intracortical connections allow the dlPFC to simultaneously monitor and influence essentially all our experiences and behaviors. In turn, subcortical afferents (via layer IV) allow our experiences to modulate information processing in the dlPFC. Most notably, these subcortical afferents mediate cholinergic potentiation of dlPFC activity through either the corticolimbic (via the NBM) or corticostriatal (via the VP) circuit.

Efferents (via layers V and VI) allow the dlPFC to regulate activity of subcortical structures such as the VS and HF to generate goal-directed behaviors and access declarative memory, respectively. The dlPFC can also exert inhibitory control over the amygdala. However, as we learned in Units I and II, the influence of the dlPFC on the VS and amygdala is mediated indirectly through the vmPFC. Regardless, through these extensive cortical and subcortical connections, the dlPFC is uniquely positioned to monitor our experiences, including bottom-up affective drives, and exert control over these experiences in the service of generating maximally adaptive responses in both the present and future.

The second anatomical feature of the dlPFC, the pyramidal neuron-interneuron complex, supports the task- and goal-dependent filtering and organization of information to prioritize, process, and sculpt behavior. As described in Chapter 8, the majority of neurons in the cortex, including the dlPFC, are glutamatergic pyramidal neurons. These excitatory neurons, particularly in layer III, provide the foundation for intracortical information processing. In other words, they are the targets of afferents as well as the source of efferents through which the dlPFC simultaneously monitors experiences and controls behaviors. Subcortical afferents likewise synapse onto these glutamatergic pyramidal neurons to modulate their activity. Pyramidal neurons exist within an extensive lattice of inhibitory gamma aminobutyric acid (GABA) neurons across all six layers of cortex. Although in the minority, these inhibitory "interneurons," as they were called in Chapter 8, are critical for establishing selectivity of both input and output, ultimately allowing for the expression of executive control (**Figure 9.11**).

At any moment in time, a multitude of sensory information arrives in the dlPFC. Each stimulus, or even a single feature of a stimulus, can be mapped onto a subset of glutamatergic neurons organized along columns within the dlPFC. However, an appropriate action often depends on selective processing of a specific stimulus or feature. For example, in the color Stroop test, we are expected to identify the ink color rather than the color word by inhibiting our automatic reading response. This is achieved within the dlPFC when the pyramidal neurons processing ink color inhibit those processing the color word through the GABA interneurons between them. That is, activity in pyramidal neurons processing ink color drives a subset of interneurons that inhibit other pyramidal neurons processing the color word or any other irrelevant features (e.g., font, location on the screen). This, in turn, increases the task-relevant signal

dlPFC	dorsolateral prefrontal cortex	**HF**	hippocampal formation
NBM	nucleus basalis of Meynert	**vmPFC**	ventromedial prefrontal cortex
VS	ventral striatum	**GABA**	gamma aminobutyric acid

from these neurons and decreases task-irrelevant signals from other neurons, thereby allowing the task-relevant ink color-processing pyramidal neurons in the dlPFC to bias output, which in this case is to identify the ink color and not read out the word. In effect, this is the neural basis of attention.

With the color Stroop test, the identification of which input is signal that should be amplified and which is noise that should be silenced reflects the explicit task instructions. These instructions are maintained in a subset of dlPFC neurons, which allow for the information to be manipulated more easily and accurately vis-à-vis the increase in signal and decrease in noise. The dlPFC thus maintains that the task is to identify the ink color and not read the word, and it allows you to manipulate the stimuli as appropriate. In this way, processing of information within the dlPFC supports the component process of working memory as well as attention. Likewise, the dlPFC pyramidal neurons that are selectively processing task-relevant information and those that are representing the task instructions send efferent signals to neurons in other sensory areas to produce appropriate behaviors including, when necessary, response selection (e.g., identifying ink color and suppressing automatic reading).

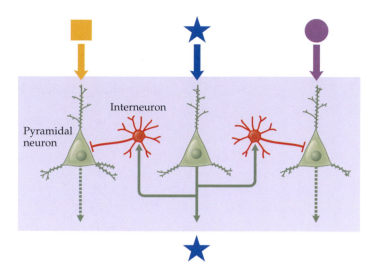

Figure 9.11 Selective processing of a specific stimulus or feature (blue star) is achieved within layers I–III of the dlPFC when the pyramidal neurons (green) processing the selected feature inhibit those processing other features (yellow square, purple circle) through the GABA interneurons (red) between them.

In the real world, both short-term and long-term goals can be represented by selective information processing within the dlPFC, which subsequently amplifies relevant signals and silences irrelevant noise, allowing us to exert control over our behaviors. When you are a student, doing well on your next exam is an example of a short-term goal (a related long-term goal may be to have a high enough GPA to get into a top graduate program). This short-term goal is represented in the dlPFC and biases information processing in favor of goal-relevant stimuli like your lecture notes, while simultaneously suppressing the processing of goal-irrelevant stimuli like Tweets about a huge party later that night. The dlPFC further functions to select and generate goal-directed behaviors, such as studying and not going to the party.

Strong affective drive from either the corticolimbic (e.g., threat) or corticostriatal (e.g., reward) circuit can further shape which stimuli or stimulus features become signals that influence our behaviors. The influence of either circuit is mediated through the common pathway of cholinergic drive via the NBM or VP to potentiate processing of concurrent information in the dlPFC (e.g., the banding pattern on a snake to help determine if it is poisonous or the sequence of cards dealt before a winning hand in poker). In these and other ways, executive control and its component processes of attention, working memory, and response selection are maintained by the dlPFC through a dynamic process of input-dependent selective inhibition or "sculpting in negativity."

A final contribution to dlPFC activity supporting executive control originates in dopamine signaling from the midbrain ventral tegmental area. Specifically, pyramidal neurons in the dlPFC project to dopamine neurons in the VTA, which in turn project back onto these same pyramidal neurons. Thus, when dlPFC neurons are engaged during executive control, their activity drives the release of dopamine from the VTA back onto their local synaptic connections

| VP | ventral pallidum |
| VTA | ventral tegmental area |

RESEARCH SPOTLIGHT

Work in my lab has demonstrated that the ability of the amygdala to drive activity in the PFC in response to threat-related angry and fearful facial expressions depends on cholinergic activity in the NBM. Specifically, we observed that increased activity in the NBM was associated with increased functional connectivity between the BLA and prefrontal cortex, particularly the vmPFC, consistent with the direct anatomical projections between these regions (**Figure 9.12**). This data provides evidence in humans consistent with the documented importance of NBM cholinergic signaling in driving activity of PFC neurons in animals. As discussed above, such cholinergic drive can selectively tune information processing to relevant stimuli in our environment. With our data, this tuning is toward signals of potential threat that elicit amygdala activity. We observed a similar effect of NBM cholinergic activity on the functional connectivity between the amygdala and HF, which likely reflects increased encoding of the face stimuli, which could further guide future responses if these stimuli are encountered again.

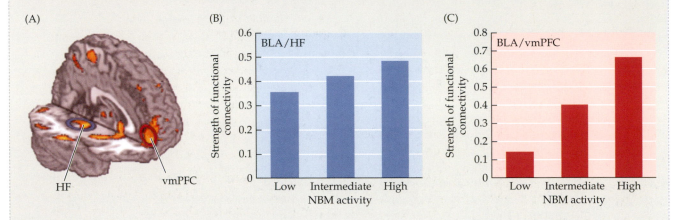

Figure 9.12 (A) The HF and vmPFC exhibit increased functional connectivity with the BLA as a function of cholinergic activity in the NBM. (B,C) Bar graphs depicting this moderated strength of functional connectivity in the right hemisphere between BLA and HF (B) and between BLA and vmPFC (C). Note that 0 represents baseline activity in these data. (After Gorka et al., 2014.)

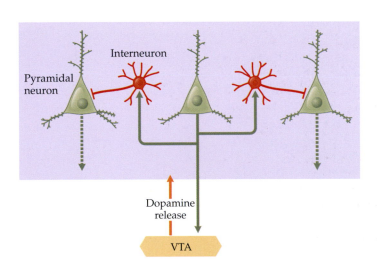

Figure 9.13 By driving dopamine release from the VTA back onto itself, a feature-specific pyramidal neuron can maintain an optimal signal-to-noise ratio during processing of task- or goal-relevant information.

(**Figure 9.13**). This dopamine signaling functions to maintain activity of dlPFC neurons processing task- or goal-relevant information while suppressing activity of dlPFC neurons processing task- or goal-irrelevant information. This pattern of activity-dependent dopamine release increases the signal-to-noise ratio in dlPFC neurons, thereby allowing for more efficient, selective, and prolonged information processing. Such tonic (i.e., steady) dopamine signaling supporting the maintenance of dlPFC activity contrasts with the phasic (i.e., periodic) dopamine signaling that regulates VS "gate" activity in the corticostriatal circuit supporting reward learning.

NBM	nucleus basalis of Meynert	**dlPFC**	dorsolateral prefrontal cortex
BLA	basolateral complex of the amygdala	**VTA**	ventral tegmental area
vmPFC	ventromedial prefrontal cortex	**VS**	ventral striatum
HF	hippocampal formation		

Summary

Through the distributed processing of information, the corticohippocampal circuit supports the related functions of memory and executive control. The hippocampal formation represents the circuit foundation for both semantic and episodic forms of declarative memory. More specifically, declarative memory emerges through strengthening of synaptic connections (via long-term potentiation) within the hippocampal formation that function to link specific features of a stimulus or experience that are represented in distributed sensory association areas. In this way, memories for both general knowledge and unique experiences are first formed and subsequently remembered through activity of the hippocampal formation. The memories, however, are stored as independent features in the distinct sensory association areas. Conscious access to our declarative memories is critical in guiding our behavior in the present and future. The dorsolateral prefrontal cortex circuit hub is responsible for orchestrating the creation of specific declarative memories as well as controlling explicit, goal-directed access to these memories. Such goal-directed access to declarative memories contributes to the broader circuit function of executive control.

The network of extensive connections with all other cortical association areas as well as key subcortical structures (e.g., hippocampal formation and ventral striatum) is one feature that allows the dlPFC circuit hub to generate and maintain executive control. A second feature contributing to the hub function of the dlPFC is the complex of excitatory glutamatergic pyramidal neurons and inhibitory GABA interneurons, particularly within layers I–III, of the cortex, that allow for task and goal-dependent selection of competing information. This process generates an increase in processing of goal-relevant signals within specific dlPFC pyramidal neurons, and a concurrent decrease in processing of goal-irrelevant signals in other pyramidal neurons.

The differentiation of goal-relevant and goal-irrelevant information (i.e., signal and noise) can be enhanced through cholinergic potentiation in response to affective drives and bottom-up signaling from both corticolimbic and corticostriatal circuits. Moreover, activity-dependent tonic dopamine release onto dlPFC neurons can help maintain goal-relevant information processing by further enhancing the signal-to-noise ratio. These fundamental features of the dlPFC allow for executive control and its component processes of attention, working memory, and response selection, which support not only top-down control of our basic behavioral drives but also how we ultimately navigate our complex environments and social interactions to maximize success in all our endeavors.

Literature Cited & Further Reading

Blumenfeld, R. S., & Ranganath, C. (2007). Prefrontal cortex and long-term memory encoding: An integrative review of findings from neuropsychology and neuroimaging. *The Neuroscientist*, 13: 281–291.

Dickerson, B. C., & Eichenbaum, H. (2010). The episodic memory system: Neurocircuitry and disorders. *Neuropsychopharmacology*, 35: 86–104.

Dolcos, F., LaBar, K. S., & Cabeza, R. (2004). Interaction between the amygdala and the medial temporal lobe memory system predicts better memory for emotional events. *Neuron*, 42: 855–863.

Duncan, J. (2001). An adaptive coding model of neural function in prefrontal cortex. *Nature Reviews Neuroscience*, 11: 820–829.

Gorka, A. X., Knodt, A. R., & Hariri, A. R. (2014). Basal forebrain moderates the magnitude of task-dependent amygdala functional connectivity. *Social Cognitive & Affective Neuroscience*, 2014: doi:10.1093/scan/nsu080.

Mansouri, F. A., Tanak, K., & Buckley, M. J. (2009). Conflict-induced behavioural adjustment: A clue to the executive functions of the prefrontal cortex. *Nature Reviews Neuroscience*, 10: 141–152.

Mecklinger, A. (2010). The control of long-term memory: Brain systems and cognitive processes. *Neuroscience & Biobehavioral Reviews*, 34: 1055–1065.

Mecklinger, A., Zimmer, H., & Klimesch, W. (2010). Binding processes: Neurodynamics and functional role in memory and action. *Neuroscience & Biobehavioral Reviews*, 34: 979–980.

Murty, V. P., Ritchey, M., Adcock, R. A., & LaBar, K. S. (2010). fMRI studies of successful emotional memory encoding: A quantitative meta-analysis. *Neuropsychologia*, 48: 3459–3469.

Niendam, T. A., Laird, A. R., Ray, K. L., Dean, Y. M., Glahn, D. C., & Carter, C. S. (2013). Meta-analytic evidence for a superordinate cognitive control network subserving diverse executive functions. *Cognitive Affective & Behavioral Neuroscience*, 12: 241–268.

Owen, A. M., McMillan, K. M., Laird, A. R., & Bullmore, E. (2005). *N*-back working memory paradigm: A meta-analysis of normative functional neuroimaging studies. *Human Brain Mapping*, 25: 46–59.

Robertson, E. M., Théoret, H., & Pascual-Leone, A. (2003). Studies in cognition: The problems solved and created by transcranial magnetic stimulation. *The Journal of Cognitive Neuroscience*, 15: 948–960.

Simons, J. A., & Spiers, H. J. (2003). Prefrontal and medial temporal lobe interactions in long-term memory. *Nature Reviews Neuroscience*, 4: 637–648.

Wager, T. D., Jonides, J., & Reading, S. (2004). Neuroimaging studies of shifting attention: A meta-analysis. *NeuroImage*, 22: 1679–1693.

Zeineh, M. M., Engel, S. A., Thompson, P. M., & Bookheimer, S. Y. (2003). Dynamics of the hippocampus during encoding and retrieval of face-name pairs. *Science*, 299: 577–580.

10 *The Corticohippocampal Circuit* Disorder

In this final chapter, we review how disorder of the corticohippocampal circuit manifests as dysfunction in memory and executive control. We will first review evidence that disorder of the hippocampal formation (HF) is a central feature of memory and memory-related disorders such as Alzheimer's disease. We then focus on disorder of the dorsolateral prefrontal cortex (dlPFC) as a central feature of dysfunction in executive control, best exemplified by thought disorders such as schizophrenia. We also consider the contribution of dlPFC dysfunction to mood, anxiety, and substance use disorder, particularly in the context of the inability to regulate bottom-up drive from the amygdala and ventral striatum.

Unlike disorders of the corticolimbic and corticostriatal circuits, disorder of the corticohippocampal circuit is not readily characterized by either increased or decreased activity of the HF or the dlPFC hub. Rather, corticohippocampal disorder emerges as more complex patterns of dysfunction reflected as increased *and* decreased activity depending on multiple factors, and is thus better described as "inefficient" processing of information, particularly in the dlPFC hub. We first consider evidence for such inefficient information processing within the HF in mild cognitive impairment, a precursor of Alzheimer's disease. Then we will consider evidence for inefficient information processing within the dlPFC hub, particularly in schizophrenia.

Disorder of the Hippocampal Formation and Long-Term Memory

This is not our first encounter with HF dysfunction in the context of psychopathology. In the context of the corticolimbic circuit, we noted in Chapter 4 that individuals suffering from posttraumatic stress disorder (PTSD) have relatively decreased HF activity during recall of fear extinction. We further considered evidence that the magnitude of HF activity during fear extinction learning predicts the subsequent ability of those with PTSD to adaptively learn and express extinction. These patterns reflect the important role of the HF for encoding the context of our specific experiences and, through modulation of fear or extinction neurons in the amygdala, guide the expression of contextually appropriate behaviors (e.g., fear in a dangerous context, extinction in a safe context).

implicit recall   Memory that helps guide behavior without conscious thought (e.g., fear learning).

explicit recall   Memory that helps guide behavior through conscious thought (e.g., declarative memory).

retrograde amnesia   The inability to recall long-term declarative memories; literally, "backward in time."

anterograde amnesia   The inability to create new long-term declaration memories; literally, "forward in time."

Similar contributions of the HF to contextual memory for rewarding experiences were described in Unit II for the corticostriatal circuit. Within the corticostriatal circuit, contextual memory for rewarding experiences helps unlock the VS gate, thereby triggering goal-directed behaviors only in appropriate contexts (e.g., ordering a hamburger at McDonald's and not the doctor's office). However, such contextual memory for aversive or appetitive experiences typically occurs automatically (**implicit recall**) and does not involve or require conscious access to the memory (**explicit recall**).

We now specifically consider abnormal HF activity associated with dysfunction of declarative memory for factual knowledge (semantic memory) and for personal experiences (episodic memory) rather than implicit contextual memory occurring within the corticolimbic and corticostriatal circuits. We begin with amnesic syndromes, which refer to primary deficits in declarative memory, associated with significant structural damage to the HF. We next consider how more moderate but progressive dysfunction of the HF contributes to the gradual emergence of deficits in declarative memory like that seen in mild cognitive impairment. Finally, we briefly consider the importance of the HF and its connections with the amygdala in the emergence of a very rare group of disorders called delusional misidentification syndromes.

Amnesic syndromes

Damage to the HF typically arises from oxygen deprivation. This deprivation can be due to heart attack, carbon monoxide poisoning, or near-drowning. HF damage emerges functionally as a loss of memory, or amnesia, which occurs in two common forms: **retrograde amnesia** and **anterograde amnesia**. *Retrograde* literally means "backward in time," while *anterograde* means "forward in time." An individual with retrograde amnesia cannot remember past events or information. In contrast, anterograde amnesia is the inability to form new long-term memories. While individuals with profound damage to the HF almost always exhibit both retrograde and anterograde amnesia—reflecting the critical role of the HF in both creating and recalling memories—these forms of amnesia are also observed independently.

Although the exact anatomical and functional nature of retrograde and anterograde amnesia remains unclear, it is possible that the independent expression of the two forms reflects specific patterns of damage or dysfunction. For example, the presence of anterograde but not retrograde amnesia may reflect more distributed damage in sensory association areas but relative sparing of the HF, such as might follow traumatic brain injuries. The damage in sensory association areas may preclude the consolidation (i.e., storage) of component features of new memories, but the HF may be able to retrieve older memories that were consolidated before damage occurred. In contrast, the presence of retrograde but not anterograde amnesia may reflect highly localized damage to specific pathways in the HF, such as might occur from prolonged oxygen deprivation, which mediate access to the features or elements of past experiences represented in distributed sensory association areas. These sensory association areas, however, may be unaffected and available for the consolidation of new memories through pathways that remain intact in the HF.

Mild cognitive impairment and Alzheimer's disease

Severe amnesic syndromes like that of H.M. are exceptionally rare. Gradual loss of memory, however, is more common and, in some contexts, even

| HF | hippocampal formation |
| VS | ventral striatum |

RESEARCH SPOTLIGHT

Much of our initial understanding not only of the critical importance of the HF in long-term memory but also of the very existence of different forms of memory can be traced back to the brain of one man (**Figure 10.1**). Henry Molaison, or H.M. as he was known throughout the scientific community until his death in 2008, is arguably the most studied research subject in history. He developed epilepsy as a child, possibly the result of head trauma suffered during a bicycle accident. By his late twenties, H.M.'s epileptic seizures could no longer be controlled with medication and became completely debilitating. Having no other medical options, H.M. and his family consented to allow a neurosurgeon, William Scoville, to perform a radical and experimental procedure: removal of his medial temporal lobe in both hemispheres. These regions were targeted because of prior work, some in animals, that revealed them to be common foci of the kind of spontaneous electrical activity associated with epileptic seizures. Remarkably, the operation, known as a bilateral temporal lobectomy, was a success and provided H.M. immediate relief from his seizures. However, the operation produced an equally immediate and unexpected effect: profound anterograde amnesia. After the operation, H.M. was unable to form new semantic or episodic long-term memories. It thus became clear that the hippocampus and adjacent structures of the HF were critical for forming long-term memories. Until this observation in H.M., the generally accepted model was that memory was an emergent property, reflecting activity throughout the entire brain.

There is in fact some truth to this model, as the consolidation of memory occurs in distributed sensory association areas. However, the HF represents a necessary structure for creating and subsequently retrieving long-term memories. Interestingly, while

H.M. also had retrograde amnesia, this memory deficit was more modest than his anterograde amnesia. His retrograde amnesia was also temporally graded—that is, he had some preoperative memories, but these became fewer and fewer and eventually nonexistent as the timeline neared his operation. This temporally graded retrograde amnesia may reflect the fact that a small section of H.M.'s left posterior HF was intact. This is consistent with the fMRI study of Zeineh and colleagues, described in Chapter 9, which demonstrated that memory retrieval may be preferentially supported by the posterior hippocampus and subiculum. Thus, memories of H.M.'s preoperative life, which were consolidated in distributed sensory areas, may have been partially accessible via this intact portion of the HF.

In addition to illuminating the critical importance of the HF for long-term memory, pioneering studies of H.M. by Brenda Milner, Suzanne Corkin, and others revealed that there are distinct and largely independent forms of memory. For example, H.M. had normal working memory, which we now understand reflected his intact dlPFC. H.M. also had normal procedural or implicit memory such as that used in learning a complex sequence of movements to achieve a task. Familiar examples of procedural memory include learning to swim, ride a bicycle, or play a musical instrument. We now know that such "muscle memory" is supported not by the HF, but by long-term potentiation of circuits in the dorsal striatum and associated motor cortices as a function of practice or repetition. Like the dlPFC, these circuits were intact in H.M.

Today it is hard to imagine that up until the detailed research done with H.M., the distinct forms of memory (long-term, working, and procedural) all were believed to reflect the same underlying processes and brain functions.

(A)   (B)   (C)

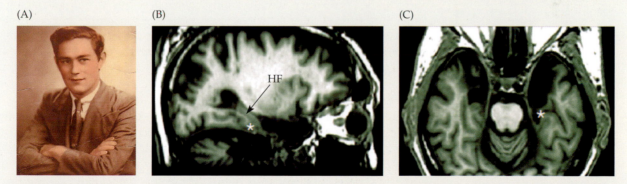

Figure 10.1 (A) Photograph of the famous amnesic patient H.M. around age 20, a few years before he underwent surgery. Sagittal (B) and axial (C) structural MRIs of H.M.'s brain at the age of 62 show the extent of surgical resection, which included the amygdala and most but not all of the hippocampal formation. A small section of the left posterior HF was not removed (asterisks). (From Corkin, 2002.)

Alzheimer's disease (AD) Neurological disorder characterized by initial impairments in declarative memory and progression to dementia.

dementia Characterized by deterioration of cognitive and emotional functions.

mild cognitive impairment (MCI) Characterized by impairments in declarative memory; an early precursor in individuals with Alzheimer's disease.

normal. Most of us will experience some decline in memory as we get older, so be kind to your professors. This normal age-related decline in memory is associated with the inevitable loss of gray matter in the HF and associated sensory association areas. Unfortunately, some individuals develop a more significant and progressive loss of memory as a component of **Alzheimer's disease (AD)**. While AD is the most common disorder of memory, it encompasses other significant deficits. Most notably, there is a general deterioration of cognitive and emotional functions known as **dementia**, which is diagnostic of AD and rooted in the progressive effects of the disease throughout the brain, especially the PFC. However, the majority of individuals who go on to develop AD first experience **mild cognitive impairment (MCI)** and isolated memory loss before the emergence of dementia. In fact, some older individuals exhibit MCI but never progress to AD. Studies of individuals with MCI, particularly milder forms associated primarily with impairments in declarative memory, have revealed distinct patterns of HF dysfunction.

Surprisingly, studies of declarative memory in individuals with MCI have generally observed relatively *increased* activity of the HF during encoding and retrieval of novel information (e.g., face-name pairs). This pattern is surprising because, as we learned in Chapter 9, increased HF activity, particularly during encoding, predicts better memory in healthy individuals. Why then would there be relatively increased activity in individuals with MCI, who have generally poorer memory? This pattern of HF hyperactivity is believed to reflect a compensatory response to another related pattern: a relative loss of neurons as reflected by decrease in the volume of gray matter in the HF.

In individuals with MCI, HF hyperactivity during memory encoding is inversely correlated to the amount of gray matter volume loss. This decrease in gray matter volume is observable on structural MRI (**Figure 10.2A**) and is itself directly predictive of deficits in memory. The compensatory nature of relatively increased activity of the HF is further reflected in memory performance, which is no worse in individuals with MCI than in healthy individuals. This relatively increased HF activity simply allows individuals with MCI to maintain average levels of memory performance in the face of neuron loss (**Figure 10.2B**). In other words, those HF neurons that remain functional in MCI must work harder to achieve the same level of memory observed in healthy individuals. While the pathophysiological basis of this structural damage is poorly understood, it is clear that gray matter loss is generally progressive, with almost complete loss of the HF in individuals with advanced AD. At this point there is no possibility of compensatory hyperactivity and memory loss is nearly total.

Delusional misidentification syndromes

In the classic 1950s science fiction film *Invasion of the Body Snatchers*, a small-town doctor returns from vacation to find several of his patients suffering from paranoid delusions that their friends and relatives have been replaced by imposters who not only look and act exactly like their friends and relatives, but also know the intimate details of each person's life. In the movie, we eventually learn that these doppelgängers are alien creatures that intend to take over the Earth by replacing humans with alien duplicates (who emerge from giant seed pods).

Such a sensational plot may seem possible only through the lens of Hollywood. In fact, however, this plot was based on a very small number of

HF	hippocampal formation
AD	Alzheimer's disease
PFC	prefrontal cortex
MCI	mild cognitive impairment

(A)

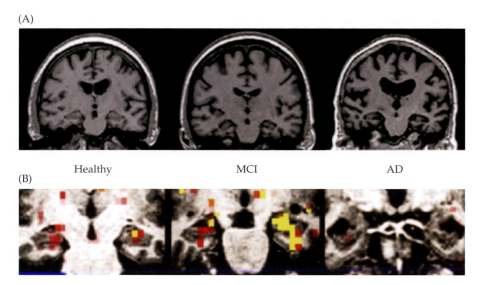

Healthy   MCI   AD

(B)

Figure 10.2 (A) Structural MRIs depicting the typical loss of gray matter in the HF of a healthy 75-year-old person in comparison with individuals of the same age suffering from either MCI or AD. Note that in AD there is significant loss of gray matter in the cortex, including the PFC, which contributes to the dementia that characterizes the disease. (B) Compensatory HF hyperactivity associated with gray matter loss in MCI compared with healthy participants while encoding novel face-name pairs. No such compensatory hyperactivity is present in AD, as no HF gray matter remains. (A from Schuff et al., 2009; B from Dickerson & Sperling, 2008.)

individuals who suffer from such bizarre paranoid delusions in real life. These individuals exhibit behaviors that fall under the umbrella category of **delusional misidentification syndromes**. One specific form, **Capgras syndrome**, is particularly reminiscent of the movie plot because these individuals believe that an imposter has replaced a familiar person (e.g., a sibling or spouse). The imposters look and behave exactly like the people they replaced and even know all the details and memories of the "real" people. However, the imposters fail to generate any of the familiar feelings or emotions associated with the real people.

The neurologist and neuroscientist Vilayanur Ramachandran at the University of California San Diego has vividly discussed this peculiar dissociation between the physical and emotional recognition of a familiar individual. He and his colleagues have argued that Capgras syndrome emerges following disconnection of pathways between the amygdala and regions of the ventral visual stream supporting face recognition. This is consistent with the respective roles of the amygdala and ventral visual stream for generating emotional signatures and explicit recognition. This hypothesis is further consistent with the observation of Capgras syndrome subsequent to a traumatic brain injury, which could disrupt these structural pathways. In addition, the often modality-specific nature of the delusion further implicates this pathway. Most patients with Capgras syndrome, including a young man studied by Ramachandran and colleagues, exhibit the delusion only through the visual domain. That is, when these patients see a familiar person, they believe that person must be an imposter because the sight of them does not generate any familiar feelings. But when such patients only *listen* to the person's voice, they regain the sense of familiarity and recognize the person as authentic.

delusional misidentification syndromes A rare group of disorders characterized by delusions regarding the identity of familiar individuals.

Capgras syndrome One form of delusional misidentification syndrome; characterized by the belief that an imposter has replaced a once-familiar individual.

Anterior

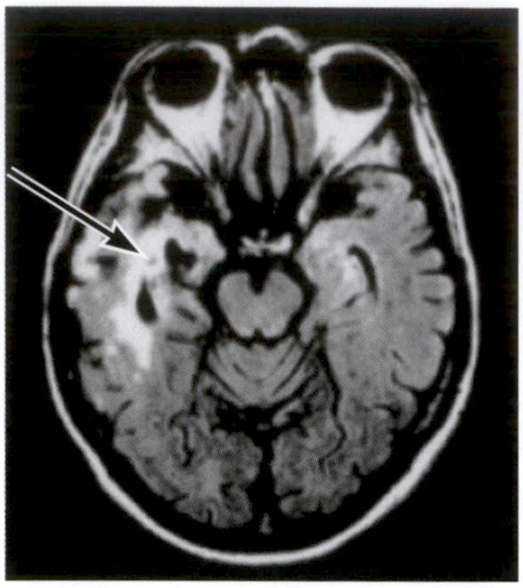

Posterior

Figure 10.3 Example of structural damage (arrow) to the left medial temporal lobe, encompassing the hippocampal formation and amygdala in a patient who suffers from a delusional misidentification syndrome similar to Capgras syndrome. (From Hudson & Grace, 2000.)

Although compelling, there is a critical gap in the above model of Capgras syndrome. Specifically, this model of primary disconnection between the amygdala and ventral visual stream fails to account for the memory component of the syndrome. Individuals with Capgras syndrome fail to remember prior emotional experiences associated with familiar individuals; they don't exhibit primary deficits in experiencing emotions or responding to emotional stimuli. Thus, the key dysfunction is a *failure to assign or remember prior emotional experiences* with specific physical features of a familiar individual. In fact, Arnold Pick, who in 1903 first described delusional misidentification syndromes, maintained that they represented a disorder of memory.

Deficits in memory, of course, implicate dysfunction of the HF. In Capgras syndrome there appears to be a failure of the HF broadly and hippocampus specifically to bind "person in context" by accessing the distributed components of memory that create our recognition of familiar individuals (e.g., by binding emotional experiences through the amygdala with facial features through the ventral visual stream). Dysfunction of discrete memory circuits within the HF rather than general disconnection between sensory processing streams and the amygdala could further explain the remarkable specificity of delusions experienced in Capgras syndrome, where a mother could be viewed as an imposter while the father was perceived as authentic.

Further support for a central role of the HF in Capgras syndrome and related delusional disorders is provided by a small number of neuroimaging studies identifying damage to the HF and adjacent regions of the medial temporal lobes including the amygdala (**Figure 10.3**). Moreover, delusional misidentification syndromes have been observed in patients suffering from epileptic seizures localized to the medial temporal lobes as well as in patients with cardiovascular disease affecting cerebral blood flow and oxygenation. The latter association is interesting because the hippocampus is more sensitive to oxygen deprivation than most other brain structures. Both acute transient events, such as a traumatic brain injury or heart attack, and chronic diseases such as epilepsy can damage the HF. While it remains unclear whether such damage causes delusional misidentification syndromes, these rare disorders nevertheless further illustrate the remarkable and delicate importance of the HF and interconnected structures in creating the memories that add color to our experiences and guide our behaviors.

Disorder of the Prefrontal Cortex and Executive Control

An inability to exert executive control can manifest as dysfunction of nearly every behavioral domain. This diffuse and pervasive pattern reflects the importance of executive control in the top-down, conscious regulation of implicit or reflexive responses such as those generated by the corticolimbic circuit to threat. Executive control via the dlPFC is similarly important for generating and, when necessary, correcting or adjusting goal-directed plans such as those executed through the corticostriatal circuit in search of rewards. Executive control and its component processes of attention, working memory, and response selection are further critical for our more general ability to think and plan. More specifically, executive control allows us to track and sort streams of information arising from either within or without in the service of identifying useful patterns that can guide our behavior in the present and future. It is the disintegration of this more general ability as a consequence of dysfunctional executive control that characterizes disorder of the dlPFC hub. Before we

HF hippocampal formation
dlPFC dorsolateral prefrontal cortex

Figure 10.4 Meta-analysis of 38 fMRI studies involving viewing of emotional facial expressions reveals consistent evidence for relative hypoactivity of the dlPFC in MDD in comparison with healthy participants. (From Hamilton et al., 2012.)

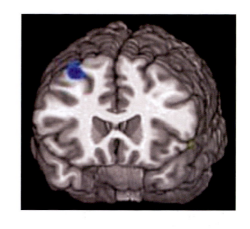

turn to this primary form of dlPFC disorder and dysfunctional executive control, largely as manifested in schizophrenia, we will consider how an inability to recruit the dlPFC in the context of regulating emotional responses and appetitive drives contributes to mood and anxiety disorders as well as addiction.

Mood and anxiety disorders

In addition to the persistent hyperactivity of corticolimbic circuit nodes that is common across mood and anxiety disorders, as reviewed in Chapter 4, there is converging evidence for general hypoactivity of the dlPFC (**Figure 10.4**). Dysfunction of the dlPFC in mood and anxiety disorders becomes most evident when patients are asked to explicitly regulate their emotional responses to different triggers (e.g., threatening facial expressions, aversive pictures, sad movie clips, or autobiographical passages). In fMRI experiments, emotion regulation is often achieved through the process of reappraisal wherein one considers alternate contexts, motivations, or outcomes in relation to a given stimulus or scenario. For example, one may be shown an emotionally provocative image (e.g., someone being threatened with a gun) and asked to reappraise the stimulus as not being real (e.g., it is only a scene acted out for a movie) or to project a positive outcome (e.g., the victim is not injured and the perpetrator is punished). In this way, emotion regulation strategies such as reappraisal require engagement of all component processes of executive control: attention (e.g., shifting your eye gaze away from negative features or characteristics), working memory (e.g., maintaining stimulus features but manipulating them into a different context), and response selection (e.g., inhibiting your spontaneous negative emotions).

When healthy individuals enlist such explicit emotion regulation strategies, there is increased activity in the dlPFC as well as the vlPFC, mPFC, and dACC. Often, there is also a concurrent decrease in amygdala activity. These changes are in comparison to activity when emotional responses are not explicitly regulated (i.e., allowed to be experienced spontaneously during passive viewing). At the subjective level, reappraisal is associated with a decrease in negative emotions such as anger, fear, or sadness, and the magnitude of this decrease in experiencing negative emotions is predicted by the ability to engage prefrontal regions, particularly the dlPFC, and subsequently to inhibit the amygdala.

In depressed individuals, there is relatively decreased activity of the dlPFC during emotion regulation, which is associated with diminished ability to downregulate amygdala activity (**Figure 10.5**). Furthermore,

Figure 10.5 (A) Activity in the dlPFC increases when healthy participants but not individuals with MDD are asked to regulate their negative emotional responses through reappraisal. (B) This increase in dlPFC activity predicts greater decrease in amygdala activity in healthy participants compared with depressed individuals. (C) In MDD, the ability to downregulate amygdala activity predicts less severe depression symptoms, as measured by the Hamilton Depression Rating Scale (HDRS). Note that 0 represents mean activity in these data. (After Erk et al., 2010.)

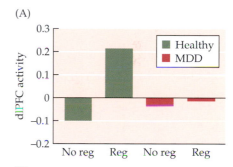

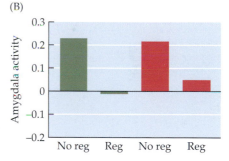

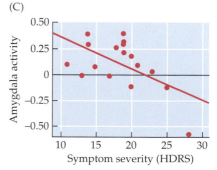

mPFC	medial prefrontal cortex	
vlPFC	ventrolateral prefrontal cortex	
dACC	dorsal anterior cingulate cortex	
MDD	dorsal anterior cingulate cortex	

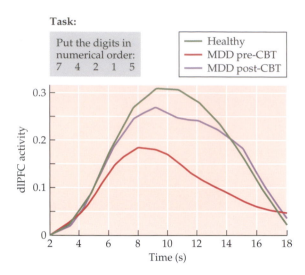

Task:

Put the digits in numerical order:
7 4 2 1 5

— Healthy
— MDD pre-CBT
— MDD post-CBT

Figure 10.6 In Chapter 4, we reviewed a study reporting that CBT was associated with decreased amygdala activity in response to self-referential negative words in MDD. Here we consider that this decrease in amygdala activity was associated with increased dlPFC activity post-CBT during a task requiring executive control. This pattern is consistent with the importance of the dlPFC in effecting top-down regulation of the amygdala, and it suggests that one mechanism through which CBT can relieve depression is by strengthening the ability of the dlPFC to effect this top-down control. Note that 0 represents baseline activity in these data. (After DeRubeis et al., 2008.)

the severity of depression symptoms is inversely related to the extent that patients are able to downregulate amygdala activity. In other words, when individuals with MDD are able to downregulate their amygdala activity, they report fewer or less intense symptoms. Finally, there is growing evidence that cognitive behavioral therapy (CBT) in depression may act to improve symptoms by increasing the capacity of the dlPFC to process information and, subsequently, effect better regulation of the amygdala (**Figure 10.6**). Increased activity of the dlPFC during emotion regulation also contributes to symptom improvement in response to drug therapies, which unlike CBT do not directly act on higher-order cognitive processes. Direct electrical stimulation of the dlPFC likewise improves symptoms in depression.

Given the high comorbidity between depression and anxiety, it comes as little surprise that similar deficits in engaging the dlPFC and inhibiting the amygdala during regulation of negative emotion are observed across anxiety disorders. Moreover, there is evidence in anxiety disorders that there is also decreased activity of the dmPFC during emotion regulation. This is consistent with the direct role of the dmPFC in mediating top-down inhibition of the amygdala. As there are no direct anatomical connections between the dlPFC and amygdala, the executive control mediated by the dlPFC must be relayed via the dmPFC to ultimately regulate amygdala activity. In addition, the magnitude of activity in both the dlPFC and dmPFC are inversely correlated with severity of anxiety symptoms (**Figure 10.7**). Those individuals who are better able to activate the dlPFC and dmPFC during emotion regulation experience fewer and less severe anxiety symptoms. Although not clearly observed in negative emotion regulation studies in depression, similar deficits in dmPFC function are almost certainly occurring.

Dysfunction of the dlPFC in mood and anxiety disorders is not limited to deficits in the ability to decrease negative emotional responses. Consistent with the general importance of the dlPFC for coordinating information processing of all stimuli as well as regulating responses from both the corticolimbic and corticostriatal circuits, activity in this region also supports the ability to maintain positive emotional

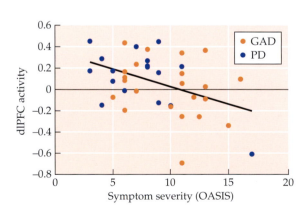

● GAD
● PD

Figure 10.7 Decreased activity in dlPFC during negative emotion regulation in either generalized anxiety disorder or panic disorder is associated with symptom severity and impairment as measured by the Overall Anxiety Severity and Impairment Scale (OASIS). Note that 0 represents mean activity in these data. (After Ball et al., 2013.)

MDD	major depressive disorder
CBT	cognitive behavioral therapy
dlPFC	dorsolateral prefrontal cortex
dmPFC	dorsomedial prefrontal cortex

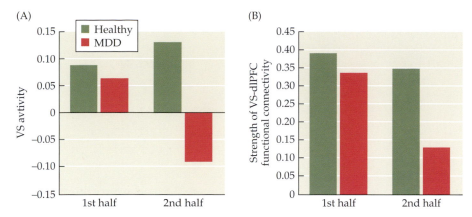

Figure 10.8 (A) In comparison with healthy participants, VS activity decreases in individuals with MDD from the first to the second half of a scan session during which they are asked to maintain a positive emotional response. (B) This inability to maintain VS activity is associated with relatively decreased functional connectivity between the VS and dlPFC from the first to second half of the scan. Note that 0 represents mean activity in A and baseline functional connectivity in B. (After Heller et al., 2009.)

states or mood over time. In other words, activity in the dlPFC helps us keep a good thing going. This reflects the importance of the dlPFC for focusing our attention on positive aspects of our experiences and maintaining these experiences in our working memory. As we learned in Unit II, individuals with depression often struggle to experience pleasure or enjoy activities that are normally pleasurable and enjoyable. Such anhedonia is a core deficit in depression that maps onto decreased ventral striatum activity in response to reward. Recent work indicates that anhedonia is further reflected in deficits in engaging the dlPFC and subsequently maintaining activity of the VS gate in response to positive or rewarding stimuli (**Figure 10.8**). Specifically, in comparison to healthy participants, functional connectivity between the dlPFC and VS decreases over time in individuals with depression. The inability to maintain VS gate activity further predicts the severity of anhedonic symptoms. Thus, dlPFC dysfunction manifests not only as a deficit in down-regulating amygdala activity associated with negative emotion, but also as a deficit in maintaining VS activity in response to positive emotion. In this way, dlPFC dysfunction contributes to both core deficits of depression— depressed mood and anhedonia—through selective deficits in its interactions with the amygdala and VS, respectively.

Bipolar disorders

Although not explicitly associated with dysfunction in emotion regulation as characterized in the previous section, a clear disturbance of the PFC exists in bipolar disorders (BD), as reviewed in Chapters 4 and 7. In BD, however, the available evidence implicates the vlPFC more than the dlPFC. Specifically, studies have consistently found relative vlPFC hypoactivity across depressed, manic, and euthymic states. In contrast, the functional connectivity or coupling between the vlPFC and amygdala is state-dependent, with increased connectivity during depressive episodes and decreased connectivity during manic episodes. During reward processing in manic patients, dysfunctional activity in the vlPFC is associated with overestimating the value of potential gains and underestimating the value of potential losses. There is, however,

VS	ventral striatum	PFC	prefrontal cortex
BD	bipolar disorders	vlPFC	ventrolateral prefrontal cortex

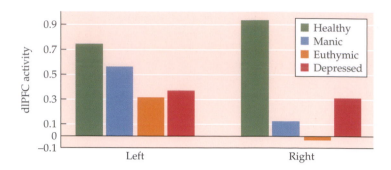

Figure 10.9 There is a persistent, trait-like decrease in dlPFC activity during working memory across depressed, manic, and euthymic states in individuals with bipolar disorders. Note that 0 repesents baseline activity in these data. (After Townsend et al., 2010.)

emerging evidence for persistent dlPFC hypoactivity during working memory tasks across states in BD (**Figure 10.9**). Thus, dysfunction of the vlPFC, which supports reappraisal of our experiences, likely converges with dysfunction of the dlPFC and the associated deficits in executive control, contributing to the emergence of abnormal cycling between mood states that characterizes BD.

Substance use disorder

Interactions between the dlPFC and VS gate also play an important role in substance use disorder or addiction. In one study, smokers were asked to regulate their craving for a cigarette when viewing cues like an open pack of cigarettes or an ashtray, by contemplating the later negative health consequences of smoking. Considering these future negative effects of smoking rather than the immediate benefits significantly reduced the magnitude of craving, a reduction associated with an increase in dlPFC activity and a decrease in VS activity (**Figure 10.10**). Moreover, the level of increase in dlPFC activity predicted how much smokers were able to reduce their craving through the reduction in VS activity. Thus, the capacity to engage the dlPFC while contemplating the later negative consequences of drug use—a common strategy in the treatment of addiction—is important for curbing drug craving, an effect that is mediated by reductions in activity of the VS gate.

In contrast, using transcranial magnetic stimulation (TMS) to reduce activity in the dlPFC when a cigarette is immediately available actually lowers craving. Consistent with the reduction in craving, TMS targeting the dlPFC is associated with reduced activity of the VS gate. This pattern reflects the

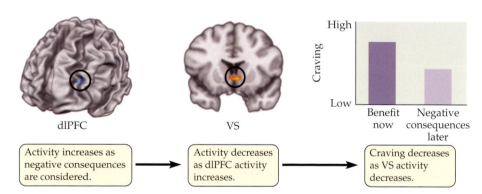

dlPFC	VS
Activity increases as negative consequences are considered.	Activity decreases as dlPFC activity increases.

Craving decreases as VS activity decreases.

Figure 10.10 Increased dlPFC activity when imagining the later negative consequences of smoking predicts a decrease in VS activity to visual cues of cigarettes, and this decrease in VS activity predicts reductions in subjective craving for cigarettes. (After Kober et al., 2010.)

dlPFC	dorsolateral prefrontal cortex	**VS**	ventral striatum
BD	bipolar disorders	**TMS**	transcranial magnetic stimulation
vlPFC	ventrolateral prefrontal cortex		

importance of the dlPFC for generating goal-directed plans (e.g., smoking a cigarette) that are executed through the VS gate as a component of the corticostriatal circuit for motivation and action. It further suggests that relative hyperactivity of the dlPFC (and associated increases in VS activity) in response to cues indicating immediate availability of drugs is a component of addiction.

As evidenced by the above, dysfunction of the dlPFC in addiction emerges as complex behavioral effects. During explicit regulation of drug craving, *increased* dlPFC activity is associated with decreased VS activity and reduced craving. When presented with the opportunity to satisfy a craving immediately, however, *decreased* dlPFC activity is associated with decreased VS activity and reduced craving. This divergent pattern reveals the multifaceted role of the dlPFC in regulating behavior broadly and for generating goal-directed plans specifically. Similarly complex effects of dlPFC dysfunction were described above for mood and anxiety disorders, particularly depression, where decreased activity is associated with deficits in both reducing negative emotion (by failing to inhibit the amygdala) and maintaining positive emotion (by failing to drive the VS). Unfortunately, as we learned in Chapter 7, drugs of abuse disrupt dopamine signaling, which is critically important for the maintenance of prefrontal function and executive control. Thus, in addiction more than in other disorders, latent problems with executive control, often expressed as high impulsivity, associated with risk are further unmasked and deepened as a consequence of drug-induced deficits in the ability of dopamine to effectively modulate information processing through prefrontal circuits.

Attention deficit hyperactivity disorder

As described in Chapter 7, the primary symptoms of hyperactivity and impulsivity common to ADHD map onto dysfunction of the corticostriatal circuit. However, the primary symptom of inattention not surprisingly maps onto dysfunction of the corticohippocampal circuit, specifically the dlPFC and interconnected cortical regions. A pervasive pattern of relative hypoactivity in ADHD emerges in the dlPFC, dACC, and parietal cortex across studies requiring sustained attention, such as the Conners' Continuous Performance Test (**Figure 10.11**). Additional deficits also have been observed in the dorsal striatum and basal ganglia, likely reflecting downstream effects of the failure to engage the dlPFC and subsequently drive activity in circuits supporting motor output, as would be necessary for maintaining task performance on the CPT.

Thought Disorders

The contributions of dlPFC dysfunction in mood and anxiety disorders as well as addiction emerge as the inability to effectively regulate emotional responses and appetitive drives. In other words, dlPFC dysfunction exacerbates abnormalities of corticolimbic and corticostriatal circuit function in these disorders. As we learned in Units I and II, dysfunction of hubs and interconnected nodes

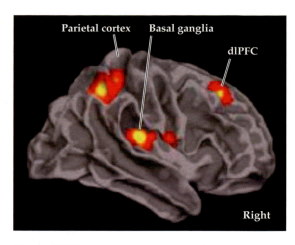

Figure 10.11 In comparison with healthy participants, individuals with ADHD exhibit consistent hypoactivity of the dlPFC as well as parietal cortex and basal ganglia during tasks requiring attention (e.g., Conners' Continuous Performance Test, or CPT). (From Hart et al., 2013.)

CPT   Conners' Continuous Performance Test
ADHD   attention deficit hyperactivity disorder
dACC   dorsal anterior cingulate cortex

thought disorders Characterized by deficits in following or generating a logical sequence of thoughts or ideas, profound difficulty in focusing and shifting attention, and inability to adapt behavioral responses to changing demands.

obsessive-compulsive disorder (OCD) Characterized by persistent, uncontrollable intrusive thoughts or impulses (i.e., obsessions) that typically elicit a pattern of equally uncontrollable ritualized or ceremonial behaviors (i.e., compulsions).

exists even in the absence of explicit regulation requiring engagement of the dlPFC. In contrast, thought disorders represent a primary dysfunction of the dlPFC hub and deficits in executive control. Thus, abnormalities in corticolimbic and corticostriatal circuit function observed in thought disorders are likely to be secondary effects of this primary dysfunction and are not explicitly considered below.

Broadly, **thought disorders** are characterized by deficits in following or generating a logical sequence of thoughts or ideas, profound difficulty in focusing and shifting attention, and inability to adapt behavioral responses to changing demands. These deficits often manifest as patterns of disorganized, bizarre, or illogical speech, writing, or behavior. The characteristic features and deficits of thought disorders map in a remarkably consistent way onto dysfunction of the component processes of executive control, namely attention, working memory, and response selection, and the underlying dysfunction of the dlPFC and other interconnected prefrontal and cortical areas. In the following sections, we consider evidence for such dysfunction in executive control and dlPFC activity in two common forms of thought disorders: obsessive-compulsive disorder and schizophrenia.

Obsessive-compulsive disorder

Obsessive-compulsive disorder (OCD) is characterized by persistent, uncontrollable intrusive thoughts or impulses—obsessions—that significantly impair normal functioning. In most cases, such obsessions elicit a pattern of equally uncontrollable ritualized or ceremonial behaviors—compulsions—designed to minimize or eliminate the obsessions. The nature of both obsessions and compulsions is extremely varied, ranging from contamination fears to violent impulses and from excessive hand washing to eliminating all contact with other people. Because obsessions and compulsions create great upheaval and chaos in normal living, individuals with OCD often experience significant levels of anxiety. In fact, OCD was formerly categorized (in *DSM*-IV) as an anxiety disorder. However, consistent with its distinction as an independent disorder in *DSM*-5, the available evidence from most fMRI studies, as well as some unique cognitive deficits, align OCD more closely with thought disorders than anxiety disorders.

First, OCD is often associated with cognitive deficits not observed in anxiety disorders. Specifically, individuals with OCD exhibit deficits in response inhibition and cognitive flexibility. For example, individuals with OCD are more likely to have difficulty switching response strategies on tasks like the Wisconsin Card Sorting Test or inhibiting prepotent responses on tasks like the color Stroop. In contrast, individuals with generalized anxiety disorder, specific phobia, panic disorder, social anxiety disorder, or PTSD typically show no such deficits. These specific deficits in cognitive flexibility and response inhibition in OCD are remarkably consistent with the hallmark obsessions and compulsions (e.g., being unable to stop hand washing because of the belief the the hands remain unclean).

Consistent with these cognitive deficits, the majority of fMRI studies in OCD reveal dysfunction in the dlPFC and associated prefrontal regions, including the vlPFC, vmPFC, and dACC (**Figure 10.12**). Generally, there is relative hypoactivity of these regions in OCD during executive control tasks such as the WCST and *n*-back tasks (see Figure 9.7). There is additional hypoactivity in the dorsal striatum during such executive control tasks. In contrast, there is evidence for hyperactivity of the dACC associated with error detection and conflict monitoring on tasks like the color Stroop. Hypoactivity of the dlPFC

dlPFC	dorsolateral prefrontal cortex	**PTSD**	posttraumatic stress disorder
OCD	obsessive-compulsive disorder	**vlPFC**	ventrolateral prefrontal cortex
WCST	Wisconsin Card Sorting Test	**vmPFC**	ventromedial prefrontal cortex

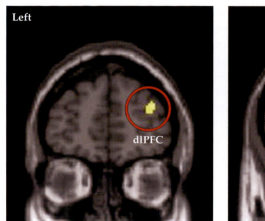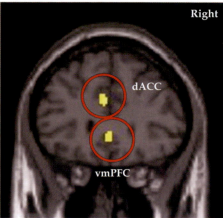

Figure 10.12 During task-switching requiring executive control, healthy participants show significantly greater activation in prefrontal regions (including the dlPFC, vmPFC, and dACC) in comparison with individuals with OCD. Not surprisingly, individuals with OCD make many more errors on such tasks. (From Gu et al., 2007.)

may manifest as an inability to shift attention away from intrusive thoughts or impulses (e.g., my hands are dirty because I touched a doorknob). Hyperactivity of the dACC may exaggerate perceived inadequacy in behavioral responses (e.g., washing my hands once did not get them clean), which may be further compounded by hypoactivity of the vmPFC and resulting deficits in integrating feedback (e.g., my hands feel clean). Finally, hypoactivity of the dorsal striatum may emerge as impairments in the ability to translate cognitive processes (e.g., I need to stop washing my hands) into actual changes in behavior.

It is further likely that dlPFC dysfunction, specifically hyperactivity, is central to the generation of obsessions as well as the inability of individuals with OCD to easily shift attention away from their obsessions or modify their behaviors. Anxiety in OCD generally emerges as a result of anticipating an episode of obsessive-compulsive behaviors rather than in response to discrete stimuli or external triggers. As we have learned, the core function of the amygdala and corticolimbic circuit for recognition and reaction is to respond to such triggers. In fact, there is little evidence of amygdala or extended corticolimbic circuit dysfunction in OCD, as is clearly observed in anxiety disorders. Although a few studies have reported increased amygdala activity in response to triggers of obsessive or intrusive thoughts, such as images of a dirty toilet for someone with a contamination obsession, such patterns are likely to reflect not primary dysfunction but rather impairments in top-down regulatory processes in prefrontal regions, including the dlPFC. Specifically, hyperactivity of the dlPFC associated with anticipating an episode of obsessive-compulsive behaviors may result in maladaptive top-down engagement of the amygdala, which in turn drives physiological arousal (e.g., increased heart rate, rapid breathing). Such maladaptive triggering of the amygdala and downstream arousal by dlPFC hyperactivity could then deepen obsessions and increase compensatory compulsions.

Interestingly, one of the most effective treatment approaches in OCD is a form of extinction or exposure therapy wherein patients experience their obsessive thoughts without opportunity to perform their compulsions (i.e., exposure and response prevention, or ERP). In this way, the cycle of

dACC   dorsal anterior cingulate cortex
ERP   exposure and response prevention

obsessive-compulsive behavior is broken and, over time, the intrusive thoughts are extinguished. Unlike exposure therapy in anxiety disorders, which generally promotes amygdala habituation to specific triggers (e.g., spiders in specific phobia), ERP encourages individuals with OCD to develop and strengthen executive control processes, including attention (e.g., shifting away from obsessions) and response selection (e.g., not engaging in compulsions). Not surprisingly, the brain regions commonly exhibiting dysfunction in OCD, particularly the dlPFC, are those that support these executive control processes.

Schizophrenia

The most common thought disorder, schizophrenia, literally refers to a "split mind." In schizophrenia there is near-complete disintegration of the ability to integrate higher mental processes—including cognition, emotion, and motivation—in the service of generating adaptive behavioral responses. As a result of this disintegration, schizophrenia can manifest as a number of varied symptoms and abnormal behaviors. For example, schizophrenia can be expressed as illogical, disorganized, even bizarre patterns of thought or speech. Powerful delusions and hallucinations, often of a persecutory nature, are not uncommon and can lead to violent outbursts; these are often referred to as positive symptoms. In contrast, the disorder can also be expressed as so-called negative symptoms, including loss of emotional responsiveness and motivation, even to the point of catatonia. These positive and negative symptoms are the most remarkable and familiar of schizophrenia. They are largely incidental, however, to its core deficit: the loss of executive control.

A growing body of evidence indicates that schizophrenia primarily reflects a failure of executive control processes to effectively regulate emotional responses and coordinate information processing. Subtle deficits in executive control are present before the onset of schizophrenia, which generally occurs suddenly in early adulthood in the form of positive symptoms (i.e., psychotic break). Deficits in executive control, including attention, working memory, and response inhibition, thus represent a risk factor for schizophrenia. These deficits also persist after onset and, unlike positive and negative symptoms, are generally unresponsive to antipsychotic drugs (the most common treatment option). Moreover, the severity of executive control deficits predicts treatment response, with individuals having better executive control generally showing greater improvement in both positive and negative symptoms. Thus, drug therapy in schizophrenia appears to simply augment what underlying capacity for executive control is left in an individual, thereby allowing for better orchestration and regulation of behavioral responses.

As suggested by the core deficit in executive control, dysfunction of the corticohippocampal circuit, particularly the dlPFC hub, is of central importance in schizophrenia. While abnormalities in corticolimbic and corticostriatal circuit function are commonly reported in schizophrenia, these, like positive and negative symptoms, are probably not primary deficits, but are secondary to dlPFC and broader corticohippocampal circuit dysfunction. Additionally, abnormal patterns of corticohippocampal circuit activity, particularly during executive control tasks, appear in individuals at risk for the disorder (e.g., unaffected siblings of individuals with schizophrenia; see the Research Spotlight on p. 194), persist after onset, and are less responsive to antipsychotic treatment.

schizophrenia Characterized by near-complete disintegration of the ability to integrate higher mental processes (including cognition, emotion, and motivation) in the service of generating adaptive behavioral responses; literally, "split mind."

positive symptoms In schizophrenia, exemplified by powerful delusions and hallucinations that may lead to violent behavior.

negative symptoms In schizophrenia, exemplified by the loss of emotional responsiveness and motivation, possibly to the extreme of catatonia.

catatonia State characterized by a near-complete lack of movement and interaction with or response to others or the environment.

psychotic break The first, often sudden and unexpected, episode of positive symptoms in an individual with schizophrenia, often requiring emergency hospitalization.

ERP	exposure and response prevention
OCD	obsessive-compulsive disorder
dlPFC	dorsolateral prefrontal cortex

Early studies of dlPFC dysfunction during executive control tasks reported relative hypoactivity in schizophrenia. This suggested that the commonly observed executive control deficits and associated positive and negative symptoms of schizophrenia reflect an inability to engage the dlPFC and associated circuits. This hypoactivity also was accompanied by poor task performance. Given the pronounced deficits in executive control described above, most individuals with schizophrenia cannot maintain levels of performance equivalent to those of healthy participants on typical executive control tasks such as the WCST. Thus, the dlPFC hypoactivity observed in schizophrenia likely reflects individuals giving up on tasks they find too difficult to keep up with. To address this confounding factor, investigators have employed tasks that afford opportunity to carefully control for performance differences between affected individuals and healthy participants.

Of particular importance in these efforts has been the *n*-back working memory task, which investigators can use to measure dlPFC activity across variable levels of task difficulty or load (i.e., 1-back, 2-back, 3-back). In this way, a participant with schizophrenia can be pushed to a point where the task is challenging (typically 2-back), but not to a point where they quit (typically 3-back). If they are not pushed far enough (e.g., 1-back), however, the task is not challenging enough to reveal what may be subtle deficits in dlPFC function.

Restricting analyses of *n*-back fMRI to those data where performance has been carefully matched between individuals with schizophrenia and healthy participants—and particularly using studies with larger numbers of participants, which generate a broader range of performance in affected individuals—has revealed two distinct patters of dlPFC dysfunction. In low-performing individuals with schizophrenia, there is relative hypoactivity. In high-performing individuals with schizophrenia, in contrast, there is relative hyperactivity of the dlPFC as well as associated neocortical association areas supporting executive control (e.g., vlPFC, parietal cortex). Interestingly, the relative extent to which individuals with schizophrenia are able to recruit the dlPFC in support of working memory, especially at higher loads (e.g., 2-back), may help them maintain some level of ordered thought and executive control (**Figure 10.13**).

The above patterns of dysfunctional dlPFC activity during executive control processes are interpreted as evidence of "inefficient" information processing in schizophrenia. That is, the dlPFC of an individual with schizophrenia who maintains relatively high performance must work harder than that of a healthy individual, while affected individuals with relatively low performance fail to sustain the necessary dlPFC activity (**Figure 10.14**). Such inefficient information processing, as evidenced primarily by relative hyperactivity, reflects

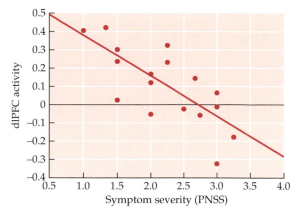

Figure 10.13 In schizophrenia, the magnitude of dlPFC activity during a working memory task, particularly at higher loads, is inversely correlated with the severity of symptoms related to disorganized thinking as measured using the Positive and Negative Syndrome Scale (PNSS). Note that 0 represents mean activity in these data. (After Perlstein et al., 2001.)

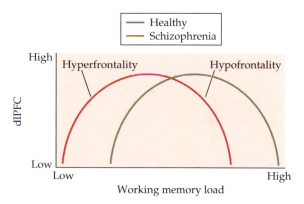

Figure 10.14 In comparison with healthy participants, individuals with schizophrenia exhibit relatively increased dlPFC activity (hyperfrontality) at low levels of working-memory load (when their performance is generally equal to that of healthy participants). However, they exhibit relatively decreased dlPFC activity (hypofrontality) at high levels of working memory load (when the task becomes too difficult and their performance falls below that of healthy participants). For this reason, the dlPFC of individuals with schizophrenia is said to be on a different "tuning curve" than that of healthy individuals, and they have a lower working memory capacity. (After Callicott et al., 2003.)

vlPFC ventrolateral prefrontal cortex
WCST Wisconsin Card Sorting Test

RESEARCH SPOTLIGHT

The "prefrontal inefficiency" model of schizophrenia has been advanced by a number of researchers and ongoing studies, most notably a sibling study conducted by Daniel Weinberger and colleagues first at the National Institute of Mental Health and now at the Lieber Institute for Brain Development. Through collection of clinical, behavioral, genetic, and neuroimaging data from large numbers of patients with schizophrenia and their unaffected siblings as well as healthy volunteers, Weinberger and his colleagues have made many seminal discoveries into the neurobiology of this disorder. One particularly important aspect of their ongoing work is to study patients during "drug-free" states when they are not taking antipsychotic or other psychotropic medication. Conducting studies during "drug-free" states under continuous medical supervision in a hospital setting allows for the expression of core deficits and symptoms, which are suppressed by medication, and the mapping of their underlying neural correlates. Using this powerful design, Weinberger and colleagues have repeatedly demonstrated that dysfunction of the dlPFC, particularly during tasks of executive control, is a core neural substrate of schizophrenia (**Figure 10.15**).

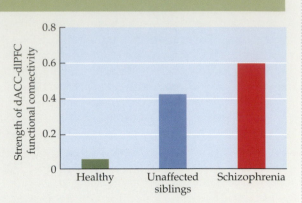

Figure 10.15 There is increased functional connectivity between the dACC and dlPFC during response inhibition in both individuals with schizophrenia and their unaffected siblings in comparison with healthy participants. As task performance did not differ between groups, the finding of increased connectivity is consistent with "inefficient" information processing in the dlPFC. Moreover, the observation of similar increases in affected individuals and their unaffected siblings suggests this pattern of dysfunction may represent a premorbid risk factor for the development of schizophrenia. (After Sambataro et al., 2013.)

fundamental dysfunction of multiple molecular and cellular processes in the dlPFC. This includes deficits in tuning of information processing through lateral inhibition of glutamatergic neurons, as well as suboptimal levels of dopamine signaling, leading to poor signal-to-noise ratio.

Evidence from postmortem studies in schizophrenia reveals multiple abnormalities in the connections between neurons, including excitatory glutamatergic pyramidal neurons and inhibitory GABAergic interneurons, within the dlPFC and between the dlPFC and other cortical regions, such as the parietal cortex. These abnormalities include a reduced number of dendritic spines, on which are found synaptic connections allowing neurons to communicate information back and forth (**Figure 10.16**). The dense matrix of synaptic connections between neurons, particularly in the dlPFC, is critical for tuning of information processing during executive control, as described in Chapters 8 and 9. Thus, the inability to effectively tune information processing is likely related to such structural abnormalities of prefrontal circuits in schizophrenia. Additional evidence indicates that the dysfunctional tuning associated with structural abnormalities of prefrontal circuits in schizophrenia may be exacerbated by deficits in dopaminergic modulation necessary for maintaining the signal-to-noise ratio of these same circuits.

Longitudinal neuroimaging studies further implicate abnormal development of cortical regions, particularly the dlPFC, in schizophrenia (**Figure 10.17**). Specifically, there is exaggerated loss of gray matter during the development of the PFC, which is relatively protracted in nature, leaving this brain region uniquely vulnerable to damage, as described in Chapter 8. These neurodevelopmental abnormalities are further reflected in disorganized patterns of functional connections between prefrontal and other brain regions in

dlPFC	dorsolateral prefrontal cortex
PFC	prefrontal cortex
dACC	dorsal anterior cingulate cortex

(A)

(B)

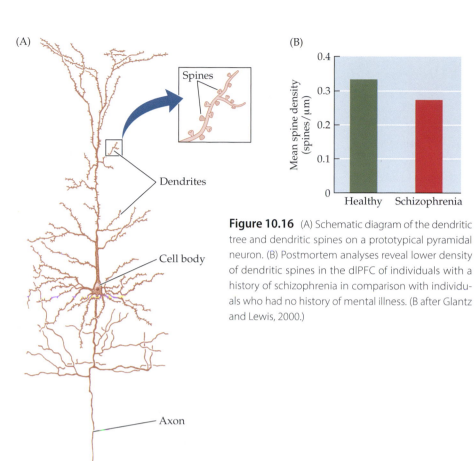

Spines

Dendrites

Cell body

Axon

Figure 10.16 (A) Schematic diagram of the dendritic tree and dendritic spines on a prototypical pyramidal neuron. (B) Postmortem analyses reveal lower density of dendritic spines in the dlPFC of individuals with a history of schizophrenia in comparison with individuals who had no history of mental illness. (B after Glantz and Lewis, 2000.)

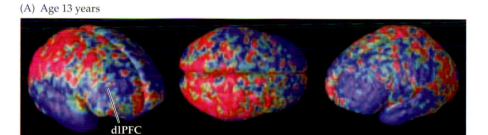

(A) Age 13 years

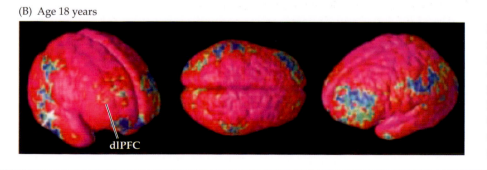

(B) Age 18 years

Figure 10.17 Although severe parietal, motor, and diffuse frontal cortex gray matter loss is evident at age 13 in individuals with schizophrenia (A), the dlPFC gray matter loss most characteristic of the disorder is not seen until age 18 (B). "Hotter" colors (pink) indicate greater gray matter loss in comparison with age-matched healthy participants. (From Thompson et al., 2001.)

RESEARCH SPOTLIGHT

There is considerable evidence that genetic differences between individuals contribute to the risk of developing psychopathology. The evidence for a genetic contribution to psychopathology can be both broad and narrow. On the broad end of the evidence spectrum, epidemiological studies clearly indicate that individuals from families with a history of psychopathology are more likely to develop disorders than those from families without such a history. This familial risk indicates that psychopathology is heritable.

While such heritability could reflect risks in the environment and experiences shared by individuals within a family, it is generally interpreted as reflecting the existence of specific genetic risk factors that are shared between relatives. This broad genetic risk is further supported by studies of twins, which find that psychopathology, particularly schizophrenia, is significantly more likely to occur in both individuals in a pair of twins if they are monozygotic (identical) rather than dizygotic (i.e., fraternal).

A search for the specific genetic factors that create the overall heritability of disorders represents the narrow end of the evidence spectrum. In candidate gene studies, investigators examine how specific differences in the DNA sequence of genes that code for molecules of known importance (e.g., dopamine receptors) predict risk for a disorder (e.g., addiction). In genome-wide association studies (GWAS), investigators look at associations between common variation in the DNA sequence across the entire genome and disorder risk in the absence of any specific targets of known importance.

Attempts to use either candidate gene studies or GWAS to identify the genetic basis of schizophrenia, which has an estimated heritability of 80%, have been the focus of intense research for more than two decades. These efforts have begun to reveal specific genetic risk factors for schizophrenia that powerfully converge to implicate dysfunctional development of prefrontal circuits. Specifically, schizophrenia has been consistently associated with common polymorphisms (i.e., genetic variation that is present in most individuals) in multiple genes encoding molecules important in the development and normal functioning of glutamatergic pyramidal neurons like those critical for information processing in the prefrontal cortex (**Figure 10.18**). Interestingly, emerging evidence suggests that antipsychotic drugs may help alleviate the positive and negative symptoms of schizophrenia by improving functioning of genetically abnormal glutamatergic neurons and, in turn, the capacity for executive control.

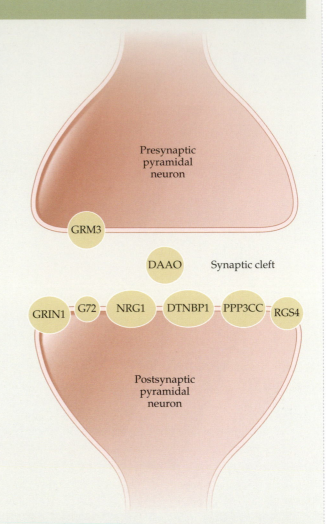

Figure 10.18 Schizophrenia susceptibility genes that can influence dlPFC function encode proteins that help regulate synaptic activity of glutamatergic pyramidal neurons. Some of these proteins are targets of current and next-generation antipsychotic drugs. GRM3 = glutamate receptor, metabotropic 3; DAAO = D-amino acid oxidase; G72 = D-amino acid oxidase activator; RGS4 = regulator of G-protein signaling 4; PPP3CC = protein phosphatase 3, catalytic subunit, gamma isozyme; DTNBP1 = dystrobrevin-binding protein 1 (dysbindin); NRG1 = neuregulin 1; GRIN1 = glutamate receptor, ionotropic, N-methyl D-aspartate 1. (After Moghaddam, 2003.)

GWAS   genome-wide association studies

schizophrenia. Importantly, loss of gray matter in cortical regions is a hallmark of normal development, reflecting experience and activity-dependent pruning of synapses, which leaves only those pathways that prove effective at processing information and generating adaptive responses while eliminating pathways that prove noisy or unnecessary. The exaggerated loss of cortical gray matter in schizophrenia, which appears to culminate in precipitous gray matter loss in the dlPFC around early adulthood, suggests over-pruning and resulting deficits in information processing.

Interestingly, early adulthood represents the peak period of risk for a psychotic break and the onset of schizophrenia. Psychotic breaks often follow periods of intense stress or mental exertion (e.g., final exams during the first semester of college), which is consistent with the prefrontal inefficiency model of schizophrenia. In this view, a circuit that was otherwise able to maintain normal behavior through relative hyperactivity finally becomes overwhelmed by the demands placed on it, leading to a breakdown of executive control and behavioral dysregulation. Unfortunately, evidence suggests that dlPFC and extended corticohippocampal circuit dysfunction in schizophrenia does not readily improve following a psychotic break. This results in the chronic inability to effectively process even routine tasks or types of information. Thus, individuals with schizophrenia become unable to keep track of even their own thoughts or maintain simple interactions with the outside world, deficits that can manifest as either positive or negative symptoms.

Summary

As perhaps best captured by the broad and pervasive symptoms of schizophrenia, dysfunction of the dlPFC hub of the corticohippocampal circuit emerges as a profound inability to process information in a logical manner. This brings chaos and disorder to the complexity of both inner experiences and interactions with the external world. While disorder of the dlPFC hub and the resulting breakdown of executive control are most prominent in thought disorders like schizophrenia and obsessive-compulsive disorder, such breakdown also manifests in other disorders. The ineffectiveness of top-down regulatory processes normally supported by the dlPFC emerges as further dysfunction of emotional responses in mood and anxiety disorders, as well as appetitive drives in substance use disorder. Specifically, deficits in the dlPFC and interconnected prefrontal regions (e.g., ventrolateral PFC, dorsal anterior cingulate cortex) further exacerbate relative hyper- or hypoactivity of the amygdala and ventral striatum hubs of the corticolimbic and corticostriatal circuits, respectively. This top-down disturbance is particularly noticeable during explicit efforts to regulate emotional responses and appetitive drives. Regardless of the specific psychopathology or constellation of symptoms, disorder of the dlPFC hub reflects abnormalities in connections between neurons, notably glutamatergic pyramidal neurons and GABAergic interneurons, that form the structural matrix of the PFC. Abnormal signaling from midbrain dopamine neurons compounds the impact of these abnormalities. Deterioration of this matrix over time, particularly in schizophrenia, results in progressive impairments in the ability to tune and maintain information processing in the service of executive control. Disorder of the hippocampal formation, in contrast, emerges as more specific deficits in long-term declarative memory. While such deficits are most obvious in amnesic syndromes (which are rare), they also represent core symptoms of more common disorders, including mild cognitive impairment. In much the same way that a symphony degrades into a cacophony when the maestro fails to conduct the orchestra, our behaviors fall into disarray when the corticohippocampal circuit fails not only in its primary functions of memory and executive control, but also in regulating both the recognition and reaction functions of the corticolimbic circuit and the motivation and action functions of the corticostriatal circuit.

dlPFC   dorsolateral prefrontal cortex
PFC   prefrontal cortex

Literature Cited & Further Reading

Ball, T. M., Ramsawhi, H. J., Campbell-Sills, L., Paulus, M. P., & Stein, M. B. (2013). Prefrontal dysfunction during emotion regulation in generalized anxiety and panic disorders. *Psychological Medicine*, 43: 1475–1486

Berlim, M. T., Van den Eynde, F., & Daskalakis, Z. J. (2013). Clinical utility of transcranial direct current stimulation (tDCS) for treating major depression: A systematic review and meta-analysis of randomized, double-blind and sham-controlled trials. *Journal of Psychiatric Research*, 47: 1–7.

Brunoni, A. R., Nunes, M. A., Pinheiro, A. P., Lotufo, P. A., & Benseñor, I. M. (2014). Bereavement and common mental disorders in middle-aged adults: Results from the Brazilian longitudinal study of adult health (ELSA-Brasil). *Journal of Affective Disorders*, 152/154: 369–374.

Bullmore, E., & Sporns, O. (2009). Complex brain networks: Graph theoretical analysis of structural and functional systems. *Nature Reviews Neuroscience*, 10: 186–198.

Callicott, J. H., Mattay, V. S., Verchinski, B. A., Marenco, S., Egan, M. F., & Weinberger, D. R. (2003). Complexity of prefrontal cortical dysfunction in schizophrenia: More than up or down. *American Journal of Psychiatry*, 160: 2209–2215.

Corkin, S. (2002). What's new with the amnesic patient H.M.? *Nature Reviews Neuroscience*, 3: 153–160.

de Toledo-Morrell, L., Dickerson, B., Sullivan, M. P.., Spanovic, C., Wilson, R., & Bennett, D. A. (2000). Hemispheric differences in hippocampal volume predict verbal and spatial memory performance in patients with Alzheimer's disease. *Hippocampus*, 10: 136–142.

DeRubeis, R. J., Siegle, G. J., & Hollon, S. D. (2008). Cognitive therapy versus medication for depression: Treatment outcomes and neural mechanisms. *Nature Reviews Neuroscience*, 9: 788–796.

Dickerson, B. C., & Sperling, R. A. (2008). Functional abnormalities of the medial temporal lobe memory system in mild cognitive impairment and Alzheimer's disease: Insights from functional MRI studies. *Neuropsychologia*, 46: 1624–1635.

Erk, S., Mikschl, A., Stier, S., Ciaramidara, A., Gapp, V., Weber, B., & Walter, H. (2010). Acute and sustained effects of cognitive emotion regulation in major depression. *Journal of Neuroscience*, 30: 15726–15734.

Glantz, L. A., & Lewis, D. A. (2000). Decreased dendritic spine density on prefrontal cortical pyramid neurons in schizophrenia. *Archives of General Psychiatry*, 57: 65–73.

Gu., B.-M., Park, J.-Y., Kang, D.-H., Lee, S. J., Yoo, S, Jo, H. J., Choi, C.-H., Lee, J.-M., & Kwon, J. S. (2008). Neural correlates of cognitive inflexibility during task-switching in obsessive-compulsive disorder. *Brain*, 131: 155–164.

Hamilton, J. P., Etkin, A., Furman, D. J., Lemus, M.G., Johnson, R. F., & Gotlib, I. H. (2012). Functional neuroimaging of major depressive disorder: A meta-analysis and new integration of baseline activation and neural response data. *American Journal of Psychiatry*, 169: 693–703.

Hart, H., Radua, J., Nakao, T., Mataix-Cols, D., & Rubia, K. (2013). Meta-analysis of functional magnetic resonance imaging studies of inhibition and attention in attention-deficit/hyperactivity disorder: Exploring task-specific, stimulant medication, and age effects. *JAMA Psychiatry*, 70: 185–198.

Hayashi, T., Ko, J. H., Strafella, A. P., & Dagher, A. (2013). Dorsolateral prefrontal and orbitofrontal cortex interactions during self-control of cigarette craving. *Proceedings of the National Academy of Sciences USA*, 110: 4422–4427.

Heller, A. S., Johnstone, T., Peterson, M. J., Kolden, G. G., Kalin, N. H., & Davidson, R. J. (2013). Increased prefrontal cortex activity during negative emotion regulation as a predictor of depression symptom severity trajectory over 6 months. *JAMA Psychiatry*, 70: 1181–1189.

Heller, A. S., Johnstone, T., Shackman, A. J., Light, S. N., Peterson, M. J., Kolden, G. G., Kalin, N. H., & Davidson, R. J. (2009). Reduced capacity to sustain positive emotion in major depression reflects diminished maintenance of fronto-striatal brain activation. *Proceedings of the National Academy of Sciences USA*, 106: 22445–22450.

Hirstein, W., & Ramachandran, V. S. (1997). Capgras syndrome: A novel probe for understanding the neural representation of the identity and familiarity of persons. *Proceedings of the Royal Society B*, 264: 437–444.

Hudson, A. J., & Grace, G. M. (2000). Misidentification syndromes related to face-specific area in the fusiform gyrus. *Journal of Neurology, Neurosurgery & Psychiatry*, 69: 645–648.

Kahn, R. S., & Keefe, R. S. (2013). Schizophrenia is a cognitive illness: Time for a change in focus. *JAMA Psychiatry*, 70: 1107–1112.

Kober, H., Mende-Siedlecki, P., Kross, E. F., Weber, J., Mischel, W., Hart, C. L., & Ochsner, K. N. (2010). Prefrontal–striatal pathway underlies cognitive regulation of craving. *Proceedings of the National Academy of Sciences USA*, 107: 14811–14816.

Lewis, D. A., & González-Burgos, G. (2008). Neuroplasticity of neocortical circuits in schizophrenia. *Neuropsychopharmacology*, 33: 141–165.

Meier, S. M., Petersen, L., Pedersen, M. G., Arendt, M. C. B., Nielsen, P. R., Mattheisen, M., Mors, O., & Mortensen, P. B. (2014). Obsessive-compulsive disorder as a risk factor for schizophrenia: A nationwide study. *JAMA Psychiatry*, doi: 10.1001/jamapsychiatry.2014.1011.

Menon, V., Anagnoson, R. T., Mathalon, D. H., Glover, G. H., & Pfefferbaum, A. (2001). Functional neuroanatomy of auditory working memory in schizophrenia: Relation to positive and negative symptoms. *NeuroImage*, 13: 433–446.

Millan, M. J., & 24 others. (2012). Cognitive dysfunction in psychiatric disorders: Characteristics, causes and the quest for improved therapy. *Nature Reviews Drug Discovery*, 11: 141–168.

Moghaddam, B. (2003). Bringing order to the glutamate chaos in schizophrenia. *Neuron*, 40: 881–884.

Perlstein, W. M., Carter, C. S., Noll, D. C., & Cohen, J. D. (2001). Relation of pre-frontal cortex dysfunction to working memory and symptoms in schizophrenia. *American Journal of Psychiatry*, 158: 1105–1113.

Pick, A. (1903) On reduplicative paramnesia. *Brain*, 26: 242–267.

Sambataro, F., Mattay, V. S., Thurin, K., Safrin, M., Rasetti, R., Blasi, G., Callicott, J. H., & Weinberger, D. R. (2013). Altered cerebral response during cognitive control: A potential indicator of genetic liability for schizophrenia. *Neuropsychopharmacology*, 38: 846–853.

Schizophrenia Working Group of the Psychiatric Genomics Consortium. (2014). Biological insights from 108 schizophrenia-associated genetic loci. *Nature* 511: 421–427.

Schuff, N. et al. (Alzheimer's Disease Neuroimaging Initiative). (2009). MRI of hippocampal volume loss in early Alzheimer's disease in relation to ApoE genotype and biomarkers. *Brain*, 132: 1067–1077.

Simon, D., Kaufmann, C., Müsch, K., Kischkel, E., & Kathmann, N. (2010). Fronto-striato-limbic hyperactivation in obsessive-compulsive disorder during individually tailored symptom provocation. *Psychophysiology* 47: 728–738.

Thompson, P. M., Vidal, C., Giedd, J. N., Gochman, P., Blumental, J., Nicolson, R., Toga, A. W., & Rapoport, J. L. (2001). Mapping adolescent brain change reveals dynamic wave of accelerated gray matter loss in very early-onset schizophrenia. *Proceedings of the National Academy of Sciences USA*, 98: 11650–11655.

Townsend, J., Bookheimer, S. Y., Foland, L. C., Sugar, C. A., & Altshuler, L. L. (2010). fMRI abnormalities in dorsolateral prefrontal cortex during a working memory task in manic, euthymic, and depressed bipolar subjects. *Psychiatric Research*, 182: 22–29.

Zeineh, M. M., Engel, S. A., Thompson, P. M., & Bookheimer, S. Y. (2003). Dynamics of the hippocampus during encoding and retrieval of face-name pairs. *Science*, 299: 577–580.

Acronyms

ACC	anterior cingulate cortex		DSM	Diagnostic and Statistical Manual of Mental Disorders
ACh	acetylcholine		ED	eating disorders
ACTH	adrenocorticotropic hormone		EEG	electroencephalography
AD	Alzheimer's disease		fMRI	functional magnetic resonance imaging
ADHD	attention deficit hyperactivity disorder		GABA	gamma aminobutyric acid
AN	anorexia nervosa		GAD	generalized anxiety disorder
ASD	autism spectrum disorders		GWAS	genome-wide association studies
ASPD	antisocial personality disorder		HF	hippocampal formation
BA	Brodmann area		HPA	hypothalamic-pituitary-adrenal axis
BD	bipolar disorders		ICMs	intercalated cell masses
BLA	basolateral complex of the amygdala		IED	intermittent explosive disorder
BMI	body mass index		LEC	lateral entorhinal cortex
BN	bulimia nervosa		LH	lateral hypothalamus
BNST	bed nucleus of the stria terminalis		LTP	long-term potentiation
BOLD	blood oxygen level-dependent		MCI	mild cognitive impairment
CA	cornu ammonis		MDD	major depressive disorder
CBT	cognitive behavioral therapy		MDE	major depressive episode
CD	conduct disorder		MEC	medial entorhinal cortex
CeA	central nucleus of the amygdala		MEG	magnetoencephalography
CS	conditioned stimulus		MID	monetary incentive delay task
CU	callous and unemotional		mPFC	medial prefrontal cortex
DA	dopamine		NAcc	nucleus accumbens
dACC	dorsal anterior cingulate cortex		NBM	nucleus basalis of Meynert
DBS	deep brain stimulation		OCD	obsessive-compulsive disorder
DG	dentate gyrus		OFC	orbitofrontal cortex
dlPFC	dorsolateral prefrontal cortex		PAG	periaqueductal gray
dmPFC	dorsomedial prefrontal cortex		PD	panic disorder
DP	dorsal pallidum		PET	positron emission tomography
DS	dorsal striatum		PFC	prefrontal cortex

PHC	parahippocampal cortex	TMS	transcranial magnetic stimulation
PO	preoptic area	US	unconditioned stimulus
PRC	perirhinal cortex	vACC	ventral anterior cingulate cortex
PTSD	posttraumatic stress disorder	vlPFC	ventrolateral prefrontal cortex
PVN	paraventricular nucleus	vmPFC	ventromedial prefrontal cortex
SAD	social anxiety disorder	VP	ventral pallidum
SN	substantia nigra	VS	ventral striatum
SSRIs	selective serotonin reuptake inhibitors	VTA	ventral tegmental area
SUD	substance use disorder (addiction)	WCST	Wisconsin Card Sorting Test

Glossary

A

adaptive response Any constellation of changes in behavior or physiology that increases an individual's survival.

agoraphobia Fear of places and situations where escape may be difficult.

Alzheimer' disease (AD) Neurological disorder characterized by initial impairments in declarative memory and progression to dementia.

anhedonia Diminished interest in and inability to experience pleasure from common activities.

anorexia nervosa (AN) Eating disorder characterized by distorted body image and excessive dieting that leads to severe weight loss, with a pathological fear of becoming fat.

anterograde amnesia The inability to create new long-term declaration memories; literally, "forward in time."

anticipatory anxiety Fear experienced only in anticipation of a threat, with no actual exposure to the threat.

antisocial personality disorder (ASPD) Characterized by disregard for the needs, safety, and well being of others, as well as an inability to follow moral, societal, or legal rules.

anxiety disorders Characterized by exaggerated fear responses to perceived threat and stress that, unlike mood disorders, are accompanied by physical as well as emotional distress.

attention Selectively concentrating on one aspect of an experience or stimulus while ignoring others to help achieve a specific goal.

attention deficit hyperactivity disorder (ADHD) Characterized by persistent inattention, impulsivity, and/or hyperactivity that exceed what is typical in children of the same age.

autism spectrum disorders (ASD) A group of disorders, including autism and Asperger's syndrome, characterized by varying degrees of intellectual dysfunction, including delayed or deficient verbal and nonverbal language skills, with persistent deficits in social and emotional behavior.

axial A horizontal plane dividing the brain into dorsal and ventral sections.

B

basal ganglia Anatomical circuit consisting of the globus pallidus together with the caudate and putamen of the dorsal striatum. Important for the proper execution and coordination of movement.

basolateral complex of the amygdala (BLA) Single term referring to the lateral, basal, and accessory basal nuclei of the amygdala. The principal input structure of the amygdala, serving to process and relay multiple inputs (e.g., sensory, contextual, regulatory) from cortical and subcortical structures on to the central nucleus of the amygdala.

bilateral symmetry Existence of the same general shape, size, and connections for structures found in both the right and left hemispheres.

bipolar disorders (BD) Characterized by typically recurring cycles of manic episodes, euthymia, and major depressive episodes.

BOLD (blood oxygen level-dependent) Signal correlated with neuronal activity and detected using fMRI.

bottom-up As used here, information processing initiated by subcortical structures, especially the amygdala and ventral striatum.

Brodmann areas (BA) Common notation for identifying cytoarchitectonically and functionally distinct subregions of the cortex, based on the work of Korbinian Brodmann.

bulimia nervosa (BN)   Eating disorder characterized by severe fear of gaining weight, but maintenance of normal weight through cycles of binge eating followed by purging, fasting, or excessive exercise.

C

callous and unemotional (CU) traits   Lack of empathy and remorse for the suffering of others.

Capgras syndrome   One form of delusional misidentification syndrome; characterized by the belief that imposters have replaced once familiar individuals.

catatonia   State of being characterized by a near-complete lack of movement and interaction with or response to others or the environment.

caudal   Refers to the back (posterior) of the brain (tailward).

central nucleus of the amygdala (CeA)   The principal output structure of the amygdala, serving to process and relay input from the BLA on to multiple downstream targets that control behavioral and physiological changes.

circuit node   Distinct brain structure responsible for a specific aspect of processing information or generating responses within a functional circuit.

classical conditioning   Passive process of learning that a previously neutral stimulus predicts a reward. Also known as Pavlovian conditioning.

conditioned stimulus (CS)   A neutral stimulus such as a tone that through fear conditioning comes to elicit a learned fear response.

conduct disorder (CD)   Characterized by delinquent and antisocial behavior during childhood and adolescence. When such behavior persists beyond age 18, it may be diagnosed as antisocial personality disorder.

conflict monitoring   Process of detecting when an outcome deviates from an expectation, which helps generate changes to plans so the desired outcome is achieved. Supported by activity in the dACC.

contralateral   Circuit node connections between the left and right hemispheres (i.e., opposite sides).

contrast image   A statistical image or map of differences in neural activity between two conditions such as an experimental task and a baseline or control state for an individual.

core symptoms   The abnormal behaviors and responses that are typically observed in a disorder.

cornu ammonis (CA)   Subregions of the hippocampus named for their curved appearance in the coronal section; literally "horns of Ammon."

coronal   A vertical plane dividing the brain into rostral and caudal sections.

cortex/cortical   Refers to gray matter (the cell bodies of neurons) on the surface of the brain.

cytoarchitectonics   Detailed cellular anatomy and arrangement of neurons; literally "cell architecture."

D

declarative memory   The conscious and often goal-directed encoding and recall of information.

delusional misidentification syndromes   A rare group of disorders characterized by delusions regarding the identity of familiar individuals.

dementia   Characterized by deterioration of cognitive and emotional functions.

depressed mood   Feeling sad, tearful, empty, or irritable; easily upset and overwhelmed by otherwise typical experiences.

difference maps   A 3-D rendering of where in the brain activity between two groups of individuals (e.g., healthy study participants compared with individuals with depression) is significantly different; derived from statistical comparisons of group maps.

dimensional symptoms   Scores derived from a variety of self-report and observational measures that reflect the severity of core symptoms in an individual.

dopamine   Neuromodulator produced in the VTA and substantia nigra of the midbrain. Important for modulating the gating function of the ventral striatum in support of motivation and action.

dorsal   Refers to the top of the brain (or the back of the body).

dorsal "where" stream   Sensory association areas encompassing the parietal lobes contributing to our perception of where objects exist in space around us.

downstream   As used here, circuit nodes that receive information from a circuit hub.

E

eating disorders (ED)   Characterized by severe disturbances in eating behavior, spanning both under- and overeating, as well as significant distress and concern about body weight or image.

endogenous opioids   Neuromodulators produced by the brain in response to reward and associated with the subjective experience of pleasure.

episodic memory   Encoding and recall of specific facts related to our unique experiences (i.e., autobiographical knowledge).

euthymia   Normal mood and affect.

executive control   The capacity to generate and orchestrate complex plans and goal-directed behaviors through attention, working memory, and response selection as well as declarative memory.

explicit recall Memory that helps guide behavior through conscious thought (e.g., declarative memory).

externalizing disorders Characterized by outwardly directed distress in the form of disruptive or destructive behaviors (e.g., violence or substance abuse).

F

fear conditioning A form of associative learning wherein a previously neutral stimulus (e.g., tone) is repeatedly paired with an aversive stimulus (e.g., electric shock) until the previously neutral stimulus alone elicits a fear response.

fear extinction A second form of associative learning, independent of fear conditioning, wherein a conditioned stimulus is repeatedly presented in a new context and in the absence of an unconditioned stimulus. Leads to the extinction of fear responses to the conditioned stimulus in the new context.

fear potentiation Increased quickness and strength of response (typically of reflexive responses like startle) when in a state of fear.

fear recall The context-dependent expression of fear conditioning or fear extinction

fMRI (functional magnetic resonance imaging) Widely used noninvasive technique for measuring neural circuit function.

G

GABA interneurons Small, inhibitory GABA neurons positioned to regulate the activity of neighboring pyramidal neurons in the cortex. (GABA is gamma-aminobutyric acid, the primary inhibitory neurotransmitter in the brain.)

generalized anxiety disorder Pervasive, "free floating" anxiety not bound to any place, thing, or situation. Highly co-morbid with and often precedes the development of major depressive disorder.

group maps A 3-D rendering of where in the brain there is activity across a group of individuals when performing the same task; created from averaging contrast images.

H

habituation The gradual decrease in amygdala activity over time when a conditioned stimulus is not followed by an unconditioned stimulus.

hedonic tone General level of pleasure an individual experiences from stimuli and activities they find rewarding. Endogenous opioids increase hedonic tone.

"high road" Term used by Joseph LeDoux for the cortical pathway from the thalamus through the sensory cortices and then to the BLA; allows sensory stimuli to be processed at higher resolution, but less rapidly than the "low road."

hub Circuit node with unique connections that allow it to coordinate the processing or flow of information throughout the rest of a functional circuit.

hypothalamic-pituitary-adrenal (HPA) axis A series of complex connections between the hypothalamus, pituitary, and adrenal glands that result in the release and regulation of cortisol in response to stress. Input from the amygdala to the paraventricular nucleus of the hypothalamus can activate this hormonal system.

I

implicit recall Memory that helps guide behavior without conscious thought (e.g., fear learning).

impulsivity The general tendency to act without full consideration of the possible consequences.

indirect fear learning Development of a conditioned fear response after only observing or hearing of the aversive consequences of others' experiences. Also known as observational fear learning.

individual differences Patterns of correlation between the magnitude of brain activity in an individual and their behaviors, including the severity of symptoms in individuals with a disorder.

instrumental (proactive) aggression The purposeful and premeditated use of violence to achieve a personal goal and (unlike reactive aggression) not in response to provocation.

intercalated cell masses (ICMs) "Islands" of inhibitory neurons that regulate communication between the amygdala's basolateral complex (BLA) and central nucleus (CeA).

intermittent explosive disorder (IED) Characterized by hypersensitivity to threat leading to episodes of grossly inappropriate (usually violent) reactive aggression.

internalizing disorders Characterized by inwardly directed distress (e.g., fear, guilt, anxiety) when confronted by threat or stressful situations.

interoception The conscious awareness of internal bodily states (e.g., gastrointestinal activity).

ipsilateral Connections between circuit nodes within the same hemisphere (i.e., same side).

L

lateral Refers to the sides.

learning trace Increased communication within specific neural pathways supporting associative learning such as fear conditioning and fear extinction.

long-term potentiation (LTP) Cellular and molecular changes resulting in strengthening of connections and communication between neurons that support learning and memory.

"low road" Term used by Joseph LeDoux for the subcortical pathway from the thalamus directly to the BLA; allows sensory stimuli to be processed rapidly, but at low resolution.

M

major depressive disorder (MDD) Commonly referred to simply as depression; characterized by typically recurring major depressive episodes (MDEs), with no occurrence of manic or hypomanic episodes.

major depressive episode (MDE) Persistent depressed mood or anhedonia, typically experienced with disturbances in appetite, sleep, or activity as well as feelings of guilt, difficulty concentrating, or suicidal ideation.

manic episodes Persistent feelings of euphoria, increased energy, diminished need for sleep, grandiosity, denial, and generally poor decision making.

medial Refers to the middle or center.

midsagittal The vertical plane that divides the brain into equal left and right sections (i.e., the left and right hemispheres).

mild cognitive impairment (MCI) Characterized by impairments in declarative memory; an early precursor in individuals with Alzheimer's disease.

mood disorders Characterized by sustained disturbance in internal emotional experiences and patterns of thinking, whether negative (depression) or positive (mania).

N

negative symptoms In schizophrenia, exemplified by the loss of emotional responsiveness and motivation, possibly to the extreme of catatonia.

neural circuit Interconnected brain structures or nodes that together function to process information to generate a discrete set of behavioral and physiological responses necessary for survival.

neuromodulators Broad class of molecules, released by a nucleus or small group of neurons, that modulate the responsiveness of other neurons. Examples include dopamine, serotonin, norepinephrine, and acetylcholine.

neuronal ensembles A complex of pyramidal neurons and interneurons in the cortex that form the foundation of information processing during executive control.

neuroticism A personality trait or disposition to experience strong negative emotions, including anxiety.

nuclei Anatomically discrete and identifiable clusters of neurons within the central nervous system.

O

obsessive-compulsive disorder (OCD) Characterized by persistent, uncontrollable intrusive thoughts or impulses (i.e., obsessions) that typically elicit a pattern of equally uncontrollable ritualized or ceremonial behaviors (i.e., compulsions).

one-trial learning A single pairing of a conditioned and an unconditioned stimulus results in a learned association (e.g., fear conditioning) that subsequently elicits a consistent fear response when encountering the conditioned stimulus alone.

operant conditioning Active process of learning that a previously neutral stimulus results in a reward only if an appropriate action is performed.

operant response Actions or behaviors performed with the goal of producing a reward.

P

panic attack Overwhelming experience of fear with severe physical symptoms that can be mistaken for a heart attack.

panic disorder (PD) Characterized by recurring, unpredictable panic attacks.

positive symptoms In schizophrenia, exemplified by powerful delusions and hallucinations that may lead to violent behavior.

posttraumatic stress disorder (PTSD) Characterized by a complex pattern of dysfunctional responses following exposure to a discrete, identifiable traumatic event or experience involving threat of death or serious bodily harm.

potentiation Increasing the responsiveness of a neuron to input (e.g., the effects of the neuromodulator acetylcholine, referred to as *cholinergic potentiation*).

primary reinforcer A stimulus that is inherently rewarding because it satisfies basic needs like hunger, thirst, and sex.

"prisoner's dilemma" Game in which participants are variously rewarded/punished for cooperation versus betrayal of another participant. When iterated (played over and over with the same participants), the game is designed to examine the factors that shape cooperation among individuals.

psychopathy Characterized by extreme callousness, selfishness, narcissism, and remorseless use of others and a persistent pattern of unstable relationships and antisocial behavior, including instrumental (proactive) aggression.

psychotic break The first, often sudden and unexpected, episode of positive symptoms in an individual with schizophrenia, often requiring emergency hospitalization.

pyramidal neurons Named for the shape of their cell bodies, these are large, glutamatergic neurons common in the brain. (Glutamate is the primary excitatory neurotransmitter in the brain.) Preeminent in the generation of sensory, motor, affective, and cognitive processes.

R

reactive aggression Anger or violence in response to perceived threat, especially from other individuals.

response selection The ability to direct and redirect our behavioral responses according to changing needs or task demands.

retrograde amnesia The inability to recall long-term declarative memories; literally, "backward in time."

rostral Refers to the front (anterior) of the brain (noseward).

S

sagittal A vertical plane dividing the brain into left and right sections.

schizophrenia Characterized by near-complete disintegration of the ability to integrate higher mental processes—including cognition, emotion, and motivation—in the service of generating adaptive behavioral responses; literally, "split mind."

secondary reinforcer A neutral stimulus (such as a sound) that over time reliably predicts a primary reinforcer through classical or operant conditioning.

semantic memory Encoding and recall of general facts (i.e., encyclopedic knowledge).

social anxiety disorder (SAD) Characterized by excessive or unreasonable fear of public scrutiny leading to persistent avoidance of social or performance situations and situationally bound panic attacks. Also known as social phobia.

specific phobia Characterized by excessive or unreasonable fear and avoidance of a specific place, thing, or situation.

state anxiety The experience of unpleasant emotional arousal such as fear in response to threat or danger.

structural dimorphism When the same structure exists in distinctively different sizes in males and females of the same species.

subcortex/subcortical Refers to the gray matter of the brain below the cortex.

substance As used in substance use disorder, refers to any rewarding stimulus (e.g., alcohol, nicotine) or activity (e.g., gambling, computer gaming) resulting in dysfunction of the corticostriatal circuit and the development of pathological motivation and action.

substance use disorder (SUD; addiction) Characterized by persistent patterns of maladaptive substance use leading to significant impairment and distress.

T

thought disorders Characterized by deficits in following or generating a logical sequence of thoughts or ideas, profound difficulty in focusing and shifting attention, and inability to adapt behavioral responses to changing demands.

top-down As used here, information processing initiated and orchestrated by cortical structures, especially the prefrontal cortex.

trait anxiety The general tendency to experience state anxiety if confronted by threat or danger.

U

unconditioned stimulus (US) An aversive stimulus such as an electric shock that is capable of directly causing bodily harm and elicits a reflexive or automatic fear response.

upstream As used here, circuit nodes that send information to a circuit hub.

V

ventral Refers to bottom of the brain (or the belly of the body).

ventral "what" stream Sensory association areas encompassing the temporal lobes contributing to our perception of what objects exists around us.

voxel A 3-D unit of brain volume (usually a cube about 2–3 mm on a side) for reporting neural activity using BOLD fMRI.

W

Williams syndrome A developmental disorder resulting from a partial deletion of chromosome 7. Associated with multiple physical and mental symptoms that include distinct patterns of disordered social and emotional behavior, notably social disinhibition and fearlessness of others.

working memory The ability to briefly maintain information in mind and subsequently manipulate that information in the service of achieving our goals.

Index

About the Book

Editor: Sydney Carroll

Project Editor: Carol Wigg

Copy Editor: Lou Doucette

Production Manager: Christopher Small

Photo Researcher: David McIntyre

Book Design: Joan Gemme

Book Layout: Jennifer Basil-Whitaker

Illustration Program: Dragonfly Media Group

Indexer: Grant Hackett

Cover and Book Manufacturer: World Print Ltd.